Lecture Notes in Pharmacy Practice

Edited by

Lilian M. Azzopardi BPharm(Hons), MPhil, PhD, MRPharmS

Associate professor

Department of Pharmacy

Faculty of Medicine and Surgery

University of Malta

Msida, Malta

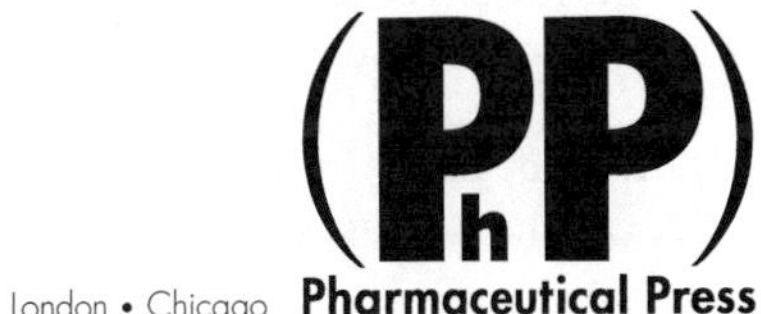

London • Chicago

Dedicated to Captain Pearce for his feline perseverance in being present during the writing of this book.

Published by the Pharmaceutical Press
An imprint of RPS Publishing

66-68 East Smithfield, London E1W 1AW, UK

First published 2009
Made ASR 2019

Typeset by New Leaf Design, Scarborough, North Yorkshire
ASR printed in Great Britain by TJ International, Padstow, Cornwall

ISBN 978 0 85369 766 4

A catalogue record for this book is available from the British Library.

Contents

Foreword

Each of us learned during our secondary school days that frogs are cold-blooded creatures. By definition, we came to know that frogs would adapt their body temperatures to their external surroundings. Through this process, the metabolic and circulatory systems of the frog could adjust the temperature of its blood and thereby survive the external environment.

In contrast to the frog, social systems and their constituents do not adapt so effectively or efficiently. This is particularly evident in healthcare systems, owing to continuous global dialogue on access to care, organisation of health delivery, financing of healthcare services and products, and assuring safety and quality. Few countries have determined perfect solutions. Some have extreme difficulty adjusting to the events of the external environment. In the developed world, it is becoming clear that current healthcare systems may not be sustainable in the future. Major human, fiscal and infrastructure resources are required in the developing and transitional countries in order to provide a basic set of essential healthcare services to their respective populations.

These phenomena are particularly applicable to pharmaceutical and biological agents and their use. Over 5000 chemical entities are currently in use around the globe. In the United States of America over 18 000 drugs and their dosage forms are approved for marketing and sales. Large protein substances have been introduced along with nanotechnological targeted delivery systems. Complex drug regimens are used daily by patients for acute and chronic conditions. And a growing number of drugs are being used for indications that have not been approved by the regulatory agencies of a number of countries.

Consequent on a dramatic increase in the number of drugs and biologicals, coupled with increased utilisation of these agents, it is not surprising that an increasing number of published reports allude to serious injury and death attributable to drug therapy gone awry. Errors of commission and omission in medication use are well documented in the professional and scientific literature. High levels of non-adherence are reported. A majority of patients do not even get their physicians' prescriptions filled. Further, a high proportion of patients do not respond to drugs the way in that they are expected to respond.

These matters have come to be debated as issues in public policy. From strengthening the regulatory oversight and approval processes to credentialing physicians in order to prescribe certain drugs, a variety of policy directions to protect patients is being taken around the world. One of these issues centres on the beginning and continuing competence of health professionals. Some countries are doing random competence assessments of pharmacists in order to determine whether licences to practise should remain valid. Other nations are requiring pharmacists to maintain dossiers for public inspection that attest to their competence. Many hospitals now require advanced credentials in order to take responsibility and accountability for expanded scopes of practice.

Like the frog in water that is becoming increasingly warmer, the profession of pharmacy must adjust and adapt to an environment that calls for improved patient care and safety in drug therapy. We must understand our limitations in competence and adjust our practice accordingly. As we expand our interest in partnering with patients and other healthcare professionals to assure appropriate outcomes associated with rational drug therapy, we need to continuously commit our learning of new developments and clinical findings and controversies in therapeutics.

That is where *Lecture Notes in Pharmacy Practice* comes in. Azzopardi and eminent faculty members and practitioners have assembled this text to aid pharmacists in their efforts to stay abreast and maintain competency. This text provides both context for its content as well as an impressively broad array of topics that represent contemporary pharmacy practice's knowledge system. It also should remind and stimulate practitioners to know what they do not know. That takes regular personal reflection and action.

This text, as the Editor notes, should be supplemented by regularly consulting the professional and scientific literature in pharmacy, the pharmaceutical sciences, medical specialty areas and other disciplines related to practice. Moreover, intense engagement with patients and other health professionals enhances good clinical judgement.

Our profession continues to evolve as a patient-centred and medication therapy-competent occupation. Our patients need us. So do our colleagues in medicine and nursing.

Henri R Manasse, Jr, PhD, ScD, FFIP
Executive vice president and
chief executive officer
American Society of Health-System Pharmacists
Bethesda, Maryland
United States of America
May 2009

Preface

Lecture Notes in Pharmacy Practice follows and complements three other books that were also edited by Professor Lilian M Azzopardi: *MCQs in Pharmacy Practice* (2003), *Further MCQs in Pharmacy Practice* (2006) and *MCQs in Clinical Pharmacy* (2007). In this fourth book Professor Azzopardi shares an insight of the developments in the field of pharmacy practice over the last few years, something that she directly experienced, has been part of and also has spearheaded from an academic as well as from a practice perspective.

This book presents pharmacy practice within the content of a social and real-life healthcare setting. It will help to prepare students for what they will experience when they start practising. And will also apply to practitioners in their day-to-day work.

'Pharmacy practice' may be misinterpreted by many as being a subject relevant only to those in the pharmacy professions. This is a great misconception as the principles for the use of medicines are relevant and applicable to any healthcare professionals, whatever their roles and responsibilities in the processes of research, manufacture, regulation, supply, prescribing, dispensing, administration and use of medicines.

The main beneficiaries of all these processes are the patients and therefore pharmacy practice must focus on patients and their needs. Patients have increased access to information on medicines and their use from various sources and through various means. The types of relationship and communication between healthcare professionals and patients have evolved, with the approach shifting from a paternalistic one to the empowerment of patients, enabling them to take a leading role in their treatment and healthcare. This evolution increases the expectations of patients and increases the need for healthcare professionals to keep abreast of ongoing developments in all areas of practice. The information presented in this book can be applied to the various cultural and professional environments in which pharmacy practice is implemented.

Through her publications Professor Azzopardi fills a lacuna in appealingly styled books in the area of pharmacy practice and the lecture notes are structured in such a way as to give a framework that helps knowledge and understanding of the basic principles in pharmacy practice. The lecture notes are useful for students and help them to get a comprehensive overview of the subject and also to revise. The lecture notes together with the MCQs provide students with a good tool to study pharmacy practice. I recommend that students start off with the lecture notes and then test their knowledge using the MCQs. The lecture notes will also appeal to practitioners, particularly those for whom pharmacy practice is a complementary subject. The lecture notes bridge classical textbooks (which most practitioners become allergic to) and specialised practice journals, which often assume a level of knowledge of the subject, and thus they are an ideal source of condensed comprehensive information on this rapidly evolving subject.

Dr Patricia Vella Bonanno
Chief executive officer
Medicines Authority
Malta
April 2009

Acknowledgements

I am deeply indebted to the many dedicated colleagues with whom I have discussed the concepts in this book and who have freely given advice, support and time. In particular I would like to thank Professor Anthony Serracino-Inglott and Dr Maurice Zarb Adami from the Department of Pharmacy for their encouragement and advice, the contributing authors for their unique contributions to the various aspects of the book, Professor Godfrey LaFerla, Dean of the Faculty of Medicine and Surgery, and Professor Juanito Camilleri, Rector of the University of Malta, for their support.

I am indebted to Henri Manasse, executive vice president and chief executive officer of the American Society of Health-System Pharmacists and Patricia Vella Bonanno, chief executive officer of the Medicines Authority of Malta for contributing to the Foreword and Preface of this publication.

I would like to especially thank my colleagues at the Faculty of Medicine and Surgery and the support staff for their assistance while I was developing this work. In the selection of material for this book I have drawn on the contributions to the curriculum by the academic staff at the department of pharmacy, namely Edwina Brejza, Marise Gauci, Mary Ann Sant Fournier, Claire Shoemake, Lilian Wismayer, as well as of a number of visiting staff at the department and members of staff from faculties at the University of Malta and from universities in other countries. In particular I would like to thank pharmacists Alison Anaskasi, Francesca Wirth and Marie Claire Zammit for their assistance in the compilation of material and colleagues from the Faculty of Medicine and Surgery who reviewed parts of the text. The preparation of this textbook draws on my experience in the teaching of pharmacy practice, which has been enjoyable due to the enthusiasm of pharmacy students whom I have had the privilege to meet during my academic career.

I would also like to acknowledge the assistance received from staff at Pharmaceutical Press, particularly Christina DeBono, Louise McIndoe and Linda Paulus, and all my staff at the Department of Pharmacy, particularly Amanda Calleja.

Finally I would like to thank my family, particularly my mum for her assistance in proofreading the text and my sister Louise, a clinical pharmacist at Mater Dei Hospital, for her comments and for reviewing parts of the text.

About the editor

Lilian M Azzopardi studied pharmacy at the University of Malta, Faculty of Medicine and Surgery. In 1994 she took up a position at the Department of Pharmacy, University of Malta as a teaching and research assistant. Professor Azzopardi completed an MPhil on the development of formulary systems for community pharmacy in 1995, and in 1999 she graduated a PhD. Her PhD thesis led to the publication of the book *Validation Instruments for Community Pharmacy: Pharmaceutical care for the third millennium* published in 2000 by Pharmaceutical Products Press, USA. She worked together with Professor Anthony Serracino Inglott who was a pioneer in the introduction of clinical pharmacy in the late 1960s. In 2003 Professor Azzopardi edited the book *MCQs in Pharmacy Practice* published by the Pharmaceutical Press, London, which was followed in 2006 by the book *Further MCQs in Pharmacy Practice* and in 2007 by the book *MCQs in Clinical Pharmacy.*

Professor Azzopardi is currently an associate professor in pharmacy practice at the Department of Pharmacy, University of Malta and is responsible for coordinating several aspects of teaching of pharmacy practice including clinical pharmacy for undergraduate and postgraduate students as well as supervising a number of pharmacy projects and dissertations in the field. She is an examiner at the University of Malta for students following the course of pharmacy and is an assessor in determining suitability to practice.

For a short period Professor Azzopardi was interim director of the European Society of Clinical Pharmacy (ESCP) and is currently coordinator of the ESCP newsletter. She served as a member of the Working Group on Quality Care Standards within the Community Pharmacy Section of the International Pharmaceutical Federation (FIP). She was a member of the Pharmacy Board, the licensing authority for pharmacy in Malta for a number of years and Registrar of the Malta College of Pharmacy Practice which is responsible for continuing education. In 1997 she received an award from the FIP Foundation for Education and Research and in 1999 the ESCP German Research and Education Foundation grant. She has practised clinical pharmacy in the hospital setting and she practises in community pharmacy.

Professor Azzopardi has published several papers on clinical pharmacy and pharmaceutical care and has actively participated at congresses organised by FIP, ESCP, RPSGB, APhA and ASHP. She has been invited to give lectures and short courses in this area in several universities. She has been a member of scientific committees for European conferences and chaired a number of oral communication sessions reporting research work in the field of pharmacy practice. She has received funding for her research projects from national and European institutions. In 2008 a European Union-funded project on automated dispensing of pharmaceuticals and pharmacist interventions was completed. In 2008 Professor Azzopardi was appointed head of the Department of Pharmacy at the University of Malta.

Contributors

Lilian M Azzopardi BPharm(Hons), MPhil, PhD, MRPharmS

Associate Professor, Department of Pharmacy, Faculty of Medicine and Surgery, University of Malta, Malta

Margarida Caramona

Professor of Pharmacology, Faculty of Pharmacy, University of Coimbra, Portugal

Benito del Castillo García

Professor and Honorary Dean, Faculty of Pharmacy, Complutense University of Madrid, Spain, Past-president of the European Association of Faculties of Pharmacy

Victor Ferrito BSc, MSc, PhD(Wales), CSci, FRSH, FIFST

Professor, Institute of Health Care, University of Malta, Malta

Steve Hudson MPharm, FRPharmS

Professor of Pharmaceutical Care, Division of Pharmaceutical Sciences, University of Strathclyde Institute of Pharmacy and Biomedical Sciences, University of Strathclyde, UK

Sam Salek PhD, RPh, MFPM(Hon)

Professor and Director, Centre for Socioeconomic Research, Welsh School of Pharmacy, Cardiff University, UK

Anthony Serracino Inglott BPharm, PharmD, MRPharmS

Professor, Department of Pharmacy, University of Malta, Malta

Vincenzo Tortorella PhD, DIC(Lond)

Distinguished Emeritus Professor, Faculty of Pharmacy, University of Bari, Italy

Maurice Zarb Adami BPharm, BPharm(Lond), PhD

Senior Lecturer, Deparment of Pharmacy, University of Malta, Malta

How to use this book

This is a text that presents salient points on the practice of pharmacy, use of medicines and therapeutics. For each chapter significant issues are highlighted in the *Practice Points* and the *Practice Summary*. The book is not meant to be a textbook of pharmacology or medicinal chemistry and though it impinges on these areas, where clinically relevant, a sound knowledge of the basics in these areas is required to grasp the points mentioned in the text.

When discussing drugs, the side-effects given reflect the most common rather than an exhaustive list. Side-effects that may be avoided or that have a significant clinical impact are mentioned. When looking at disease management, a practical approach is given as much as possible.

The book is based on real-life lectures developed over an extensive period of experience of pharmacy practice education. It should be useful as a compilation of the significant points needed to be covered in preparing for pharmacy practice assessments and in continuing professional development. The text bridges the concepts of clinical pharmacy and pharmaceutical care as encountered in both community and hospital practice.

Abbreviations

ACE	angiotensin-converting enzyme
ANOVA	analysis of variance
ANS	autonomic nervous system
API	active pharmaceutical ingredient
APTT	activated partial thromboplastin time
ARB	angiotensin II receptor antagonist
BMI	body mass index
BP	blood pressure
CEA	cost-effectiveness analysis
CHF	congestive heart failure
CHMP	Committee for Medicinal Products for Human Use
CNS	central nervous system
COPD	chronic obstructive pulmonary disease
CTD	common technical document
DVT	deep vein thrombosis
ECG	electrocardiogram
EMEA	European Medicines Agency
EPS	extrapyramidal symptoms
GABA	gamma-aminobutyric acid
GCP	good clinical practice
GDP	good distribution practice
GI	gastrointestinal
GMP	good manufacturing practice
HDL	high-density lipoprotein
IHD	ischaemic heart disease
IM	intramuscular
IV	intravenous
LDL	low-density lipoprotein
LFTs	liver function tests
LMWH	low-molecular-weight heparin
MHRA	Medicines and Healthcare products Regulatory Agency for the UK
NICE	National Institute for Health and Clinical Excellence
NREM	non-rapid eye movement
NSAID	Non-steroidal anti-inflammatory drug
PPI	proton pump inhibitor
QALY	quality-adjusted life years
QP	qualified person
REM	rapid eye movement
RLS	restless leg syndrome
RP	responsible person
SMR	standardised mortality rate
SOP	standard operating procedures
SPF	sun protection factor
SSRI	selective serotonin re-uptake inhibitor
TCA	tricyclic antidepressant
t.d.s.	three times daily
TPN	total parenteral nutrition
VTE	venous thromboembolism
WBC	white blood cell count

PART 1

Introduction to Pharmacy

1

Historical perspectives

Learning objectives:

- To highlight landmarks in the development of the pharmacy profession
- To appreciate timelines in the development of drugs and identify landmarks in drug discovery.

Tracing the origins of pharmacy

Sumerians

- The development of cuneiform writing on clay tablets during the third millennium BC included lists of drugs of animal, vegetable and mineral origin that were used in the management of diseases, and prescriptions with details of the ingredients used in their compounding.
- Many of the drugs listed were cited as having multiple uses since ailments were thought to be different manifestations of a condition.
- Use of medicines was carried out by priests (*ashipu*) and physicians (*asu*).

Egyptians

- The *Ebers Papyrus* (named after Georg Ebers, who purchased it in the nineteenth century) is a document dating back to 1550 BC, which describes prescriptions and modes of administration of drugs including gargles, inhalations, suppositories, ointments and lotions. Many of the drugs listed were included in the Sumerian documents.
- Use of medicines was carried out by priests. Imhotep who is regarded as the earliest physician, was the High Priest of Heliopolis.

India

- Ayurvedic medicine was first described around 800 BC. Documents list the use of drugs together with charms for expelling demons and make reference to the god of medicine, Dhanvantari.
- The *Charaka Samhita* includes reference to drugs of animal, plant and mineral origin used until the first century AD.

China

- In China, a comprehensive theory for diagnosis and treatment was developed.
- Manuscripts on silk and bamboo describe use of drugs of animal and plant origin.
- The text *Huangdi Neijing* listed the basic principles of pharmaceutical drug use in the third century BC.
- Shengnon Bencao Jing outlined basic theory of Chinese pharmacy.
- The Pen Ts'ao Kang Mu compilation presents details of drugs used in Chinese medicine in the late sixteenth century AD.

Greeks and Romans

- Just as the Egyptians revered Imhotep as the god–physician, the Greeks worshipped Asklepios as their god of healing.

- Later on, the use of medicines was carried out by the *rhizotomoi* (experts in medicinal plants), such as Empedocles, and the *pharmakopoloi* (preparers and sellers of drugs).

Hippocrates

- Considered to be the father of medicine.
- He is associated with a number of documents known collectively as the *Hippocratic Corpus* dating to 420–370 BC, which list 200–400 drugs of vegetable origin and describe the method of preparation of gargles, ointment and pessaries.
- His works placed emphasis on treating the patient with minimal reference to magical and religious powers.

Dioscorides

- Prepared the document *De Materia Medica* around AD 60–78. This document gives details about medicinal herbs including side-effects associated with their administration.

Galen

- A physician around AD 160.
- He compiled medical knowledge of the time drawing on the documents by Hippocrates and Dioscorides.
- He described the use of formulations made up of numerous plants which were referred to as 'galenicals'.

The Arabs

- In the Arab world, a large number of texts including documents related to medicine and works by Galen were translated into Arabic and that is how these documents have been transferred along history. Documents that were prepared included formularies, herbals and books on materia medica and toxicology.
- The use of medications consisting of complex formulations (galenic medicine) was continued.
- This required skilled preparation which was entrusted to apothecaries who opened their shops in the ninth century in Baghdad. The practice of the apothecaries was inspected by the state.
- Avicenna, a Persian philosopher, compiled the book *Canon of Medicine*, in which he merged the Greek and Arab works. The book describes the use of around 760 drugs.
- Albucasis, from the Arabic dominion in Spain, prepared documents which included a detailed description of the pharmaceutical process for the preparation of drugs in various dosage forms.

Early definition of the pharmacy profession

- After the establishment of apothecaries in Baghdad, the pharmacy profession started developing in Europe.
- Early Middle Ages: monastic medicine.
- Late Middle Ages: in the eleventh century, public pharmacies in southern Italy and southern France were established.
- Drug formulary produced by Nicolas of Salerno which described compound formulae of galenicals.
- 1231–1240: the Liber Augustalis, an edict on the profession of pharmacy, was issued by the German emperor Frederick II. The edict defined the separation of the pharmaceutical profession from the medical profession, described the official supervision of pharmaceutical practice and outlined an obligation by oath to prepare drugs reliably according to skilled art, and of a uniform, suitable quality.
- Early nineteenth century: retail pharmacies developed a separate manufacturing area, which included an area for extraction and purification, necessary for extraction of plant alkaloids such as quinine from cinchona bark used for malaria. Boehringer and Merck have their origins in community pharmacies in Stuttgart (1817) and Darmstadt (1827), Germany, respectively.
- Late nineteenth century: separation of the manufacturing business from the retail community pharmacy.

Development of medicines

- Seventeenth century: cinchona bark extract used for fever, chills – the principal active ingredient being quinine.

- Eighteenth century: foxglove plant used for the treatment of heart failure – digitalis.

Analgesics and anaesthetics

1804	Serturner isolated morphine from opium
1832	Isolation of codeine
1842	Ether used as an anaesthetic and later chloroform
1876	Stricker showed that salicylic acid had analgesic effects
1899	Development of aspirin by Bayer
1961	Development of ibuprofen
1969	Ibuprofen marketed by Boots
1983	Ibuprofen registered as an over-the-counter drug in the United Kingdom.

Antihistamines

1941	Phenbenzamine, the first histamine antagonist that was shown to be safe to use in humans
1943	Mepyramine was introduced
1946	Promethazine was synthesised
1973	Terfenadine, a non-sedating antihistamine, discovered.

Peptic ulcer healing drugs

1970	Cimetidine, a H_2-receptor antagonist, developed
1983	Ranitidine marketed
1979	Synthesis of omeprazole, a proton pump inhibitor
1989	Omeprazole marketed.

Antibacterial drugs

1891	Ehrlich coined the term 'chemotherapy'; methylene blue used for malaria
1929	Antibiotic activity of penicillin described
1935	Sulphonamides developed by Domagk
1939–41	Florey and Chain synthesised penicillin
1944–5	Streptomycin and chlortetracycline isolated
1952	Isoniazid which was followed by other antituberculous drugs
1953	Phenoxymethylpenicillin
1956	Cephalosporin structure identified
1964	Cephaloridine marketed.

Autonomic nervous system

1901	Isolation of crystalline adrenaline
1905	Theory of receptive substances postulated
1909	Acetylcholine synthesised
1926	Acetylcholine shown to be the neurotransmitter in the parasympathetic nervous system
1946	Role of noradrenaline in sympathetic nervous system identified
1947	Isoproterenol introduced as a bronchodilator
1948	Existence of alpha and beta receptors in sympathetic nervous system identified
1955	Methyldopa
1964	Propranolol
1967	Salbutamol.

Central nervous system

1912	Phenobarbitone
1937	Hydantoins
1952	Antipsychotic activity of chlorpromazine described
1957	Imipramine found to have antidepressant effects
1960	Chlordiazepoxide marketed as an anxiolytic
1990s	Development of selective serotonin re-uptake inhibitors (SSRIs) and zolpidem.

Endocrine system

1914	Crystals of thyroxine
1921–26	Isolation and crystallisation of insulin
1929	Isolation of oestrone
1934	Progesterone synthesised
1930–40	Isolation of different hormones from adrenal cortex
1959	First oral contraceptive
2006	Inhaled insulin marketed
2007	Pfizer announces that it will no longer market inhaled insulin due to marketing issues.

Anticancer agents and immunosuppressants

1946 Anticancer effect of nitrogen mustards described
1951 Mercaptopurine, an anticancer agent with an antimetabolite effect
1961 Azathioprine, an immunosuppressant
1970 Identification of paclitaxel
1992 Marketing authorisation for paclitaxel is granted
1990 Imatinib and trastuzumab developed
2000 Trastuzumab reaches registration
2002 Imatinib reaches registration
2006 Human papillomavirus vaccine hailed as the most important cervical cancer development since cervical screening.

Therapeutic proteins produced by recombinant technology

1982 Human insulin
1986 Human interferon alpha used in hepatitis B and C
1987 Human tissue plasminogen activator used in heart attacks, human growth hormone
1989 Erythropoietin used in anaemia
1991 Granulocyte–macrophage colony-stimulating factor used in neutropenia
1992–97 Human factors VIII and IX used in haemophilia
1994 Abciximab used for prevention of blood clot
1997 Rituximab approved for non-Hodgkin's lymphoma
1998 Infliximab approved for Crohn's disease and arthritis.

Adverse effects

1879–90 Sudden deaths during chloroform anaesthesia
1922 Jaundice associated with salvarsan
1937 People die after taking elixir of sulphanilamide which contained the solvent diethylene glycol
1955 Children in the USA infected with a polio vaccine due to a failure in the inactivation process
1961 Thalidomide – congenital malformations
1966 Chloramphenicol associated with blood dyscrasias
1997–99 Withdrawal of terfenadine and astemizole, the first antihistamines with a lower frequency of sedation that were marketed in the mid-1980s, due to increased risk of cardiotoxicity when taken with other drug therapy
2000 Withdrawal of cisapride which was a unique product with parasympathomimetic acivity that had a stimulating effect on serotonin receptors as well and was used in gastric conditions, due to increased toxicity in concomitant drug administration
2004 Withdrawal of rofecoxib, a COX-2 inhibitor, due to increased cardiovascular events
2006 Withdrawal of ximelagatran, the first oral anticoagulant drug to be released since warfarin, due to liver toxicity
2006 Development by Pfizer of torcetrapib, which had the main intervention of increasing high-density lipoprotein, stopped due to increased mortality
2007 Telithromycin associated with exacerbation of myasthenia gravis, occurrence of hepatoxicity, visual disturbances and loss of consciousness; revision in guidelines for its use.

Development of pharmaceutical regulation

United Kingdom

1963 As a result of the thalidomide tragedy, the Committee on Safety of Drugs was established
1968 Under the terms of the Medicines Act, the committee was renamed as Committee on Safety of Medicines (CSM). The Act

stated that medicines required a licence to reach the UK market

1989 Medicines Control Agency (MCA) created

1994 Medical Devices Agency created

2003 Medicines and Healthcare products Regulatory Agency (MHRA) established, bringing together MCA and Medical Devices Agency

2005 CSM became the Commission on Human Medicines (CHM), which provides advice to the MHRA.

European Union

1965 European directive for authorisation of medicinal products for human use presented

1975 Scientific Committee for Proprietary Medicinal Products for human use (CPMP) established

1993 Council regulation for the setting up of a European system for marketing authorisation of medicinal products and for the establishment of a European agency

1995 The European Medicines Agency (EMEA) opens in London, UK.

United States of America

1906 US Pure Food and Drugs Act which required information on contents and purity of medicines

1927 Food, Drug and Insecticide Administration takes up regulatory functions

1930 Food, Drug and Insecticide Administration renamed the Food and Drug Administration (FDA)

1938 As a result of the sulphanilamide elixir tragedy, the Food Drug and Cosmetics Act was passed which required approval by the FDA before a new drug product was marketed

1988 Food and Drug Administration Act which established the structure and responsibilities of the agency.

International

1989 At the WHO Conference of Drug Regulatory Authorities (ICDRA) plans for discussions between Europe, Japan and the USA on harmonisation started

1990 The International Conference on Harmonisation (ICH) was established. It is a forum of constructive dialogue among the three regions which aims at facilitating exchange, dissemination and communication of information.

Questions

1 List four significant developments in the history of medicines.

2 List two adverse effects that were considered tragic.

Answers

1 Four significant developments in the history of medicines:
   (a) aspirin (1899): an analgesic drug with antipyretic and anti-inflammatory properties
   (b) antibacterial activity of penicillin described in 1929
   (c) isolation and crystallisation of insulin in 1921–26
   (d) antipsychotic activitiy of chlorpromazine described in 1952.

2 Two adverse effects that were considered tragic:
   (a) people died after taking elixir of sulphanilamide that contained diethylene glycol as solvent (1937)
   (b) thalidomide led to congenital malformations when used in pregnant women (1961).

Further reading

Bryan J (2009). How the discovery of ibuprofen helped pave the way for other NSAIDs. *Pharm J* 282: 313–314.

Cowen D L and Helfand W H (1988). *Pharmacy: An illustrated history*. New York: Harry N Abrams Inc.

Fitzpatrick M (2006). The Cutter incident: How America's first polio vaccine led to a growing vaccine crisis. *J R Soc Med* 99: 156.

Mez-Mangold L (1971). *A History of Drugs*. Switzerland: F. Hoffmann-La Roche & Co.

Potzsch R (1996). *The Pharmacy: Windows on history*. Switzerland: Roche.

Rang H P, ed. (2006). *Drug Discovery and Development*. Edinburgh: Churchill Livingstone Elsevier.

Sneader W (2005). *Drug Discovery: A history*. Chichester: John Wiley & Sons.

Acknowledgements

Charles Savona-Ventura, Associate Professor, Department of Obstetrics and Gynaecology, Faculty of Medicine and Surgery, University of Malta.

2

Pharmacy practice and the healthcare system

Learning objectives:

- To identify areas within healthcare systems where pharmacists should participate
- To describe pharmacy processes within cost-effective and safe patient care systems.

Impact of pharmacy on patient care

In the United Kingdom, the *Pharmacy in a New Age* consultation launched in 1995[1] identified five main areas[2] in which pharmacy makes major contributions to health outcomes:

1. Management of prescribed medicines:
   - drug development
   - dispensing of medicine
   - counselling
2. Management of chronic conditions:
   - repeat prescribing
   - monitoring therapeutic outcomes
   - improvement in quality of life
3. Management of common ailments:
   - counselling
   - recommendation of line of action
4. Promotion and support of healthy lifestyles:
   - health education
   - health screening
5. Advice and support for other healthcare professionals:
   - provision of information on clinical and technical aspects of use of medicines
   - participation in research and development programmes to transfer science into practice.

Pharmacist interventions in the healthcare system

- *Ensuring rational use of medicines:* participation in the development of formularies, clinical guidelines and protocols, and analysis of prescribing information and drug use evaluation data.
- *Disease management:* contributing towards enhancement of compliance, adherence to evidence-based clinical guidelines and monitoring patient outcomes.
- *Management of drug therapy:* ensuring that safe and effective drug products are used and are accessible, collaboration with health professionals to ensure that prescribing is carried out for definite objectives, accessing patients' profiles and medical records, undertaking counselling about safe use of drugs, patient monitoring to identify problems and suggest actions to solve problems.

> Keep in mind the statement: 'What is not documented is not properly done.'
>
> Document all interventions.

Patient pharmaceutical needs assessment

By identifying patients who would mostly benefit from pharmacist interventions, pharmacist-dedicated services can be directed towards individual patient groups to ensure minimal drain of resources while at the same time giving patients the pharmacy service particular to their needs. Patient pharmaceutical needs assessment may be developed to identify patients who require dedicated pharmacist services. The needs assessment should take the following into consideration:

- *Access to pharmacy facilities:* Do patients who are house-bound have access to a pharmacist domiciliary service? Do patients visiting a pharmacy have access to the pharmacist? Do patients feel that they need more time with the pharmacist during outpatient visits at hospital clinics?
- *Need for compliance aids:* Do patients require memory aids or pill boxes to organise their medication?
- *Social behaviour:* Patients living on their own who may not have family or friends able to support them through their medication.
- Does the patient have special needs?

Identifying groups of patients with special needs

- Patients suffering from certain diseases, such as:
  - acute myocardial infarction
  - chronic pain
  - mental health problems
  - learning difficulties
- Age groups: extremes of age – the young and the elderly
- Drug treatment:
  - narrow therapeutic index drugs
  - expensive drugs: consider use of generic formulations – what are the pharmaceutical implications of switching to a different pharmaceutical formulation?
- Taking medicines for chronic disease:
  - repeat prescriptions
  - medication review
- Patients in particular health settings:
  - hospital, residential home, nursing home
- Patients transferring from one health setting to another.

Achieving cost-effective patient care

Within a healthcare system, pharmacists can participate in the four domains necessary for cost-effective patient care (Figure 2.1).

> When advising on the use of a drug, it is no longer enough to be assured of its efficacy. Pharmacoeconomic aspects also have to be considered. Value for money and cost-effectiveness are important considerations in selecting rational therapy. This may involve substituting a generic drug for the originator.

Quality assurance

This establishes an acceptable level of performance and incorporates mechanisms to identify when that standard of performance is not met.

Quality improvement

This comprises information-driven processes that involve the implementation of monitoring procedures to ensure that adequate standards are obtained and maintained. It has two main components: total quality management (TQM) and continuous quality improvement (CQI).

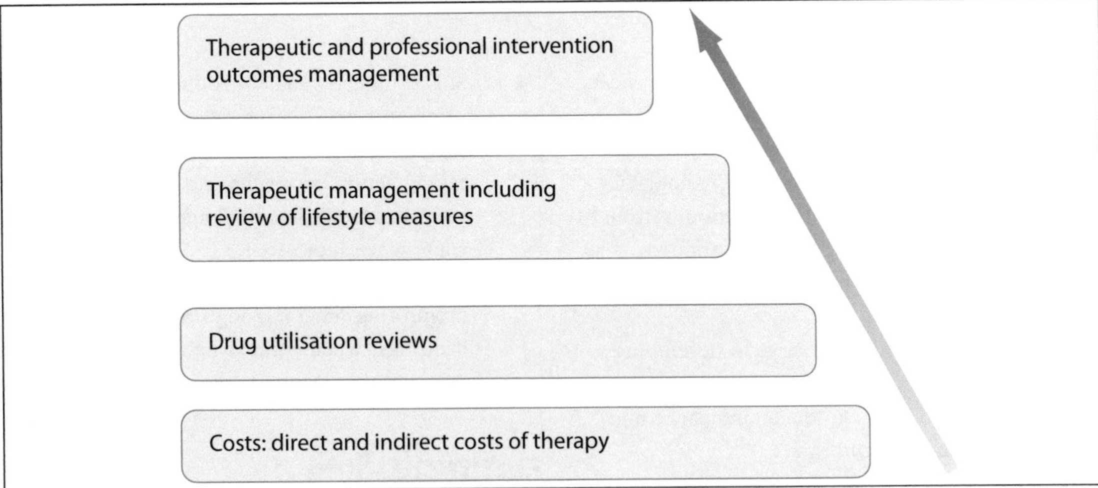

Figure 2.1 Components to achieve cost-effective drug therapy.

Total quality management (TQM)

- Defines measures of quality
- Measures current performance
- Analyses process
- Identifies improvement actions.

See Table 2.1 for a comparison of quality improvement and quality assurance.

Measuring outcomes

- Use diagnostic results
- Use medical records
- Maintain databases that provide information to allow periodical reviews
- Assess patient satisfaction.

Table 2.1 Comparing quality improvement and quality assurance

Quality improvement	Quality assurance
Prospective process	Retroactive process
Proactive	Reactive
Process based	Event based
Process approach	Inspectorate approach
Focus is to improve process	Focus is to solve problems

Assessing outcomes

- Clinical: response to treatment
- Functional: improvement in physical function
- Financial: cost-effective therapy
- Perceptual: patient's satisfaction with outcomes, care received and providers.

Difficulties in implementation of outcomes management

- Compilation of data is time-consuming
- Resistance from health professionals.

Case example for quality assessment in a hospital

- Documentation and analysis of pharmacist intervention on the ward
- Cost-effectiveness study of medications used
- Patient satisfaction questionnaire – developed to assess patient satisfaction with outcomes of therapy, care received, atmosphere on ward, communication with health professionals.

Practice summary

- Within the healthcare system, pharmacy services can contribute towards management of prescribed medicines, management of chronic conditions, management of common ailments, health promotion and health education, rational safe and effective use of medicines, and maintaining cost-effectiveness of patient care.
- Pharmacists should be proactive in developing formularies, clinical guidelines and protocols, and take an active role in the maintenance and updating of these documents.
- Pharmacists should liaise with other health professionals and with policy makers to establish therapeutic practices that include therapeutic interchange and use of generic drugs to achieve patient accessibility to drugs.
- Pharmacists should participate in exercises to monitor cost-effectiveness of patient care and in processes to ascertain quality of the professional services provided.

Question

1 List three points that could lead to improvement in the cost-effectiveness of treatment.

Answer

1 (a) Substituting a generic product for an originator product where appropriate.
(b) Preparing a drug utilisation review and taking action on results (e.g. policy to switch intravenous antibacterial agents to the oral route when indicated).
(c) Including the indirect costs of therapy (e.g. monitoring time, nursing time to change dressings) when comparing the costs of two optional therapeutic paths.

Further reading

Longley M (2006). Pharmacy in a new age: start of a new era? *Pharm J* 277: 256.

Stuart C and Ross C (2009). Why health economics is becoming ever more important in the industry? *Pharm J* 282: 255–256.

References

1 Council of the Royal Pharmaceutical Society of Great Britain. *Pharmacy in a New Age*. London: The Royal Pharmaceutical Society of Great Britain, 1995.

2 Royal Pharmaceutical Society of Great Britain. *Building the Future: A strategy for a 21st century pharmaceutical service*. London: Royal Pharmaceutical Society of Great Britain, 1997.

3

Medicine presentation and administration

Learning objectives:

- To familiarise oneself with principles of drug administration
- To list and give examples of different dosage forms
- To review main steps in development of medicines.

Background

Definition of a medicinal product

A medicinal product is any product used for the prophylaxis or management of diseases that brings about the purpose of affecting body function or is used to make a medical diagnosis.

Sources of drugs

In earlier times, plants were the primary source of substances intended for a medicinal effect. Minerals and substances of animal origin started to be used later on. Today, the largest proportion of drugs is produced by the pharmaceutical industry synthetically or semi-synthetically.

Drugs to medicines

As the purity and potency of drugs or 'active ingredients' have increased, the dose required has decreased, and many medicinal products would present great difficulties to patients to withdraw the correct amount to use at any one time. No patient would be capable of taking a dose of say 1 mg from a powdered drug supplied in bulk form. Some drugs require extraction from raw materials, while some would require preparation in sterile conditions. Therefore drugs need to be converted into medicines by the process of formulation.

Historically, pharmacists concerned themselves with extracting these active ingredients and compounding them into preparations that were convenient for patients to use. These activities of formulation, along with the discovery and testing of new active ingredients for efficacy and safety, have been taken over by the pharmaceutical industry, while community and hospital pharmacists have specialised in providing pharmaceutical care.

Administration of medicines

When introduced into the body, all drugs cause cellular changes, described as drug action, followed by physiological changes that are described as the drug effect (Figure 3.1).

The 'rights' of medicine administration

When administering medicines, it is important to ensure that the *right* medicine at the *right* dose, in the

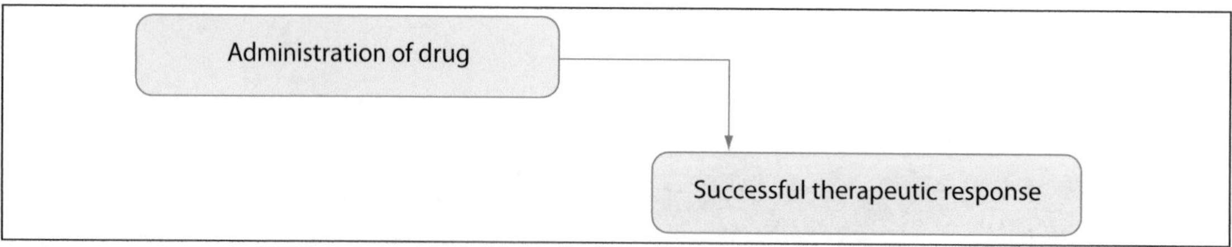

Figure 3.1 Administration of medicines.

right form is administered to the *right* patient, at the *right* time, by the *right* route, using the *right* technique, and that the *right* documentation is kept.

Pharmaceutical development

- Drugs have to undergo pre-formulation studies and formulation development to present the drug in an appropriate dosage form.
- This is a complex, time-consuming and expensive process.

Pre-formulation studies

These are carried out to investigate the physical and chemical properties of a drug including:

- solubility and dissolution rates
- chemical stability
- lipophilicity
- melting point
- particle morphology.

Formulation development

- Aims to develop formulations of the drug while overcoming shortcomings of the compound (e.g. low solubility in water for omeprazole, taste)
- Takes into account properties of drug substance and desired final dosage form.

Route of administration

Drug effects can be subdivided into:

- *systemic effect:* drug is distributed throughout the body to cause a general effect (e.g. tablets)
- *local effect:* drug is limited to the area of the body where it is administered (e.g. nose drops).

The choice of a particular route of administration of a drug may depend on many factors, including:

- desired effect (if a fast action is required, intravenous administration is preferred, e.g. in emergency situations)
- local effect desired to reduce side-effects (e.g. administration of bronchodilators and corticosteroids as inhalers in asthma)
- absorption qualities of the drug (e.g. administration of gentamicin for a systemic effect has to be done parenterally)
- the ability of the drug to withstand the conditions of the gastrointestinal tract (e.g. insulin cannot be administered orally since it is degraded in the gastrointestinal tract).

Considerations in dosage form development

- Conceal taste and odour for orally administered preparations (e.g. capsules, syrups)
- Provide protection of drug from destruction in the stomach after oral administration (e.g. enteric-coated tablets)
- Provide liquid preparations of drugs that are insoluble or unstable in a vehicle (e.g. suspensions)
- Provide rate-controlled drug action (e.g. modified-release tablets and capsules).

Routes of administration and examples of dosage forms

- Oral route:
  - solid oral dosage forms (tablets, capsules)

- liquid oral dosage forms (syrups, suspension)
- Topical route:
  - transdermal drug delivery
  - inhalation
  - nasal, ophthalmic ear drops
  - creams, ointments, lotions, powders
- Parenteral route:
  - intramuscular, subcutaneous, intravenous
  - use of pumps, implants
- Rectal route:
  - enemas, suppositories
- Vaginal route:
  - pessaries, fluid solutions, creams.

Oral route

Advantages

- Simple, convenient
- Self-administration possible.

Disadvantages

- Irregular absorption from the gastrointestinal tract (e.g. due to food)
- Drugs may be destroyed by acid or enzymes in the gastrointestinal tract
- Limitations when patient is unconscious, vomiting or in pre-/post-operative patients.

Formulations

- Tablets may be:
  - effervescent
  - enteric coated
  - modified release
- Capsules are easier to swallow but more costly to produce. They may be:
  - soft capsule: a unit that is formed from one piece and where the processes of filling and formation of the outer unit are carried out in a single operation or
  - hard capsule: consists of two separate components, namely the cap and the body.

Gelatin, which is a polymer, is used to prepare capsule shells. The source of gelatin and gelatin capsules is regulated by an EU Directive which specifies method for manufacture of gelatin so as to reduce risk of bovine spongiform encephalopathy (BSE).

Sublingual tablets

- Drug administered under the tongue (e.g. glyceryl trinitrate)
- Preferred to achieve rapid action or to bypass drug metabolism.

Buccal tablets

- Drug placed between gum and mucous membranes
- They are absorbed slowly and may be used for a local effect.

Modified-release oral preparations

- *Extended-release preparations:* preparations where the release of drug is extended to achieve sustained plasma drug concentrations, resulting in decreased requirement for frequent dosing
- *Delayed-release preparations:* preparations where the release of drug is delayed so that absorption takes place at a later stage in the gastrointestinal tract (e.g. enteric-coated preparations).

Oral liquid formulations that are sugar free are preferred to reduce risk of dental caries and when administered to diabetic patients.

Topical route

Advantages

- May be adopted to provide a localised effect
- When route used to provide systemic effect, first-pass effect is reduced.

Disadvantages

- Some dosage forms used for topical administration require particular patient advice to ensure safe and appropriate drug administration

- Local reactions may occur as side-effects
- When systemic absorption is required, lipid solubility of drugs is a required characteristic.

Transdermal drug delivery

This is a system of drug delivery where drug molecules are presented in a variety of sizes and shapes that allow for absorption through the skin and into the bloodstream at various rates.

Advantages

- Ease of application
- Effectiveness for a long period of time allowing for retention of patch for a number of hours
- Consistent blood drug level of drug is achieved.

Examples include nicotine patches and glyceryl trinitrate patches.

For discussion of ointments, creams and lotions see Chapter 47.

Metered-dose inhalers

Inhalers present the drug as an aerosol, usually as liquid, sometimes as a powder formulation, and are intended for topical application in the respiratory tract (see also Chapter 25).

- Used in the management of respiratory disease, e.g. asthma.
- Proper technique is required.
- Provide rapid onset of action and minimal side-effects due to topical action.

Examples include salbutamol, salmeterol and budesonide.

Inhalation of oxygen

Oxygen therapy is by inhalation and it is prescribed by specifying the flow rate, concentration, method of delivery and length of time of administration.

- Note that 100% oxygen may result in oxygen toxicity, presenting with symptoms such as alveolar collapse, intra-alveolar haemorrhage and disturbance of the central nervous system
- Masks are required to administer oxygen to the patient.
- Patients may require domiciliary use of oxygen and therefore access to oxygen cylinders or oxygen concentrators and patient information on the safe handling of the equipment is required.
- Pressure gauge: indicates amount available.
- Cylinder storage conditions: upright, dry well-aired room, no smoking.
- Concentrators depend on electricity supply and so back-up cylinders may need to be considered.

Ophthalmic administration

Preparation must be sterile and patient should be advised that once opened product should be discarded within 4 weeks. Good practice requires that the opening date is documented on the pack to ensure that products that have been opened more than 4 weeks previously are not used.

Patients or their carers require knowledge of the proper technique for application of the product to avoid touching the container against the eye or anything else to avoid contamination of the containers (see also Chapter 55).

- Ophthalmic preparations include:
  - eye drops
  - eye lotions
  - eye ointments.

Otic administration

- Patient must remain on his or her side for about 5 minutes to allow formulation to reach inner ear canal.
- Caution when using ear drops if patency of eardrum is not ensured (see also Chapter 58).

Nasal administration

- Nasal drops: preferred in infants due to better spread as opposed to spray.

- Nasal spray: preferred since they are less likely to be associated with postnasal drip of the drug leading to an aftertaste.

Rectal route

Advantages

- Bypasses the oral route and so is useful when when patient is nauseated or vomiting, post-operative and not able to take medicines orally.
- May be used for a local effect in the colon (e.g. in constipation).

Disadvantages

- Inconvenient and not well accepted by patients
- Erratic absorption.

Suppositories are a solid dosage form; enemas are oily or aqueous solutions. Patient should be advised to lubricate suppository tip with a water-soluble lubricant or to moisten the tip with cool water. Suppository should be inserted pointed end first until it is past the muscular sphincter of the rectum. Where patient needs to use half a suppository, the suppository should be split in half longitudinally.

Vaginal route

Advantages

- May be used to treat local infections
- Allows for local application of hormone replacement therapy.

Disadvantage

- Inconvenient and not well accepted by patients.

Examples of dosage forms available include douches, creams and pessaries.

Parenteral route

Advantages

- Allows for administration of drugs intended for a systemic effect that cannot be presented through other routes because of erratic absorption or first-pass effects
- Depending on the formulation used and the dosage form, may be used to provide a fast onset of action or a prolonged action
- Useful when patient is not cooperative.

Disadvantages

- Formulation has to be sterile
- More expensive to manufacture
- Usually requires administration by a healthcare professional
- May not be well accepted by patients.

Injections are *sterile* solutions, suspensions or emulsions presented in a suitable aqueous or non-aqueous vehicle intended for administration into the body tissues. Intravenous injections should be aqueous and should not contain particles. Whole blood and fat emulsions are exceptions.

Subcutaneous injection

- Given just below the skin and the layer of fatty tissue usually in the arm or thigh
- Not for suspensions or oily fluids
- A small volume (<2 mL) can be administered
- Example is insulin.

Intramuscular injection

- Administered into a large muscle usually in buttocks or anterior lateral thigh
- Used for aqueous and oily suspensions with the latter presenting a prolonged action
- Larger amount can be administered than subcutaneous injection (up to 5 mL)
- Absorption more rapid than subcutaneous injection but can be modified by the addition of adrenaline or hyaluronidase
- Used, for example, for immunisation.

Intravenous drug administration

- Administered usually on internal flexure of elbow, but other sites may be used.
- Aqueous solutions are administered.
- Volume varies from <1 mL to >3000 mL where the fluid is administered as an infusion.

- Used in emergency, when immediate effect is required, when drug is not available in other routes, or when large volumes of fluid are required (infusion).
- Examples include antibacterials, corticosteroids and replacement fluids (e.g. saline).

Devices required for parenteral administration

Syringes

- Sterile
- Size variability (0.5–50 mL)
- Position of hub, central for most, eccentric for intravenous
- Insulin syringes – calibrated in units (U).

Needles

- Sterile
- Gauge (G) – diameter of lumen, 16–30G; the larger the number, the smaller the diameter
- Length of needle may vary.

Implant

- Device inserted surgically under the skin for delivery of medication
- Device releases drug slowly and consistently
- Disadvantage is that termination of therapy requires surgical removal
- Example is levonorgestrel implant.

Pumps

- Medication is administered via pump to provide continuous flow into the system.
- Pump is electronically programmed to deliver a predetermined amount of drug over a predetermined amount of time. Alarms should not be overridden.
- Examples are opioid analgesia in postoperative or palliative care, insulin therapy.

Other dosage forms

- Ophthalmic administration – ocular inserts (e.g. pilocarpine)
- Oral administration – lollipops (e.g. for oral rehydration salts).

Practice summary

- When administering medicines, the choice of product and route of drug administration depends on a number of factors including patient and drug characteristics.
- Pharmaceutical development of drugs is a time-consuming process that requires a pre-formulation phase which takes into consideration drug characteristics required to establish the formulation for the different dosage forms.

Questions

1. Explain the differences between the intravenous route of drug administration and the intramuscular route of drug administration.
2. What are the advantages of transdermal drug delivery and give an example of a drug that is presented in this way?
3. Name two advantages for using the rectal route of drug administration.
4. What are the limitations to the use of eye drops?

Answers

1. The differences between the intravenous route of drug administration and the intramuscular route of drug administration are summarized in Table 3.1.
2. Advantages: easy application, effective for a long period of time, consistent blood drug level of drug. Examples: glyceryl trinitrate transdermal patches for angina.
3. Suppositories can be used in patients who are unable to ingest medications orally (e.g. confused or non-compliant patients such as infants, children, old and comatose patients). They may also be used in patients where the oral route is not available, e.g. in nausea and vomiting.

Table 3.1 Comparison of intravenous and intramuscular routes of drug administration

	Intravenous	**Intramuscular**
Site of administration	Commonly administered at the internal flexure of the elbow or the back of the hand	Administered into a large muscle, usually into buttocks or anterior lateral thigh, needle is inserted at a 90° angle
Uses	Aqueous solutions used. May be adopted in emergency situations when an immediate effect is required, when drug is not available in other routes or when large volumes of fluid are required (IV infusion).	Used for aqueous and oily suspensions in doses up to 5 mL
Volume administered	<1 mL to >3000 mL	2–5 mL
Examples	Anti-infective agents	Immunisation

4 Eye drops must be discarded 4 weeks after opening and there is risk of contamination during use. Patients should be advised not to touch the eye with the dropper during administration. Another limitation is that some patients may not be willing to use this method of drug administration due to the inconvenience.

Further reading

American Society of Health-System Pharmacists (2004). *Medication Teaching Manual*, 8th edn. Bethesda, MD: Amercian Society of Health-System Pharmacists.

Podczeck F and Jones B E (2004). *Pharmaceutical Capsules*, 2nd edn. London: Pharmaceutical Press.

Winfield A J and Richards R M E (2004). *Pharmaceutical Practice*, 3rd edn. London: Churchill Livingstone.

4

Medicine safety

Learning objectives:

- To appreciate steps undertaken in research and development of new medicines and in the development of new formulations to ensure drug safety
- To introduce concepts of safe medicine use and appreciate risks involved
- To identify pharmacists' actions in adverse drug reaction monitoring and management
- To describe medication errors and practices to minimise their occurrence.

Background

- In an attempt to improve patient safety due to different nomenclature of medicines, European law[1] requires the use of the Recommended International Non-proprietary Name (rINN), which is coordinated by the World Health Organization.
- For some medicines the British Approved Name (BAN) differed from the rINN. For example, benzhexol (former BAN) and trihexyphenidyl (rINN), frusemide (former BAN) and furosemide (rINN), dothiepin (former BAN) and dosulepin (rINN).
- Former BANs have been modified to accord with the rINN.
- Currently United States Adopted Names (USAN) are more likely to be identical to the rINN.
- A few medicines still carry synonyms that are more commonly used in some countries such as the USA. Examples include paracetamol and acetaminophen, aspirin and acetylsalicylic acid (ASA).
- Adrenaline and noradrenaline are the terms used in the European Pharmacopoeia but the names epinephrine and norepinephrine are still used in the United Kingdom.

Medical devices

A medical device is any instrument, apparatus, material, software or any other device that is used alone or in combination with accessories for the diagnosis, prophylaxis, monitoring and management of disease, injury or handicap, or for the investigation, replacement or modification of anatomy or of a physiological process or for the control of conception.[2] Examples include sutures, dressings, contact lens care products, incontinence devices (e.g. catheters, stoma care devices, such as bags).

European Directives provide for mandatory CE marking of all devices, declaring that the product satisfies the requirements essential for it to be considered safe and fit for its intended purpose. This is regarded as equivalent to a marketing authorisation.

Development of medicines

Discovery research

The basic research and discovery stages for compounds suitable for development are usually carried out by the pharmaceutical industry. Identification of a lead compound (a new chemical entity that shows potential for development into a drug) which demonstrates beneficial clinical effects with minimal side-effects leads to further development into a potential medicine. High-throughput screening may be adopted where libraries of compounds are screened to identify products that are bioactive and potent. Lead optimisation is undertaken to modify such compounds to achieve improved chemical properties.

Pre-clinical testing

Laboratory (e.g. on cells) and animal testing is undertaken to assess the safety of the new compound. The tests estimate toxicity of the product when given acutely or repeatedly, identify the organs and systems involved, and evaluate carcinogenic potential and reproductive toxicology. For animal testing, toxicological studies in two species are required and results have to be submitted to the regulatory authorities when compiling an application for registration of a new compound. Duration of pre-clinical testing is 2–4 years.

Clinical development

Clinical development is in three phases:

- *Phase I:* safety and dosage testing (tolerability, bioavailability, pharmacokinetics) in *healthy* volunteers. Results indicate dose, regimen and duration of therapy to be adopted in phase II study. Duration: 1–1.5 years.
- *Phase II:* safety and efficacy testing on *patient* volunteers. Evidence of efficacy and safety of the drug in patients is identified and optimal dose and dosing regimen are identified. Duration: 2–3 years.
- *Phase III:* safety and efficacy testing on *larger numbers of patients*. The trials aim at comparing the new treatment with placebo or comparator products in terms of safety, tolerability, efficacy, patient acceptability, compliance and pharmacoeconomic analysis. Duration: 2–5 years.

Regulatory review/approval

At this stage application is made to the regulatory authorities for marketing authorisation. Duration is 1–2.5 years.

Principles in the use of medicines

- Medicines should be used only when they are necessary.
- The benefit of administration of medicines should be considered in relation to the risk involved.

Examples of benefits vs risk of medicine use

- Antibacterials: treating infection vs occurrence of gastrointestinal side-effects
- Anticancer agents: increased life expectancy vs gastrointestinal side-effects, hair loss.

Strength of formulation

- Describes quantity of medicinal substance in the dosage form
- Some medicines available in the same dosage form but in different strengths (e.g. co-amoxiclav tablets 1 g, 625 mg or paracetamol suspension 120 mg/5 mL, 250 mg/5 mL).

Excipients

- Sugar-free oral liquid preparations: do not contain fructose, glucose or sucrose, suitable for diabetics, preferred in children for maintenance of oral health
- May include components that may be allergenic (e.g. tartrazine, arachis (peanut) oil).

Extemporaneous preparations

- This service does not cover the reconstitution of dry powders with water or other diluents.
- A product should be prepared extemporaneously when there is no product with a marketing authorisation available
- Equipment in the pharmacy must be maintained in good order
- Standard operating procedures should include acquisition of raw material, labelling, expiration date, environmental control and record keeping.

Drugs and driving

- Whenever a product that is likely to affect ability to drive is dispensed, patients should be advised
- These effects are increased by consumption of alcohol. Examples include hypnotics such as benzodiazepines (e.g. lorazepam) or antihistamines (e.g. chlorphenamine).

Safety in the home

- To keep all medicines out of reach of children (note use of child-resistant containers)
- Safe disposal of unwanted medicines
- Storage at conditions appropriate for the specific medicine: storing in the refrigerator for products required to be kept at 2–8°C (e.g. insulin and vaccines), storing in a cool place for products requiring storage temperature ranging between 8 and 15°C and storing at room temperature for products requiring storage between 15 and 25°C
- Proper labelling on container to include dosage regimen and cautionary labels (e.g. 'Warning: may cause drowsiness'). Include advisory labels (e.g. 'Shake the bottle')
- Do not change containers or remove from carton.

Cautionary labels

- Warning. May cause drowsiness. If affected do not drive or operate machinery (e.g. antihistamine-containing preparations).
- Warning. Avoid alcoholic drink (e.g. metronidazole).
- Do not take indigestion remedies at the same time of day as this medicine (e.g. enteric-coated tablets).
- Do not take indigestion remedies or medicines containing iron or zinc at the same time of day as this medicine (e.g. tetracyclines, quinolones).
- Take at regular intervals. Complete the prescribed course unless otherwise directed (e.g. antibacterial medications).
- . . . with or after food (e.g. non-steroidal anti-inflammatory drugs).
- Swallow whole, do not chew (e.g. enteric-coated and modified-release oral formulations such as bisacodyl).
- To be spread thinly (e.g. corticosteroid preparations for application on the skin).

Advisory labels

- Shake the bottle (e.g. calamine lotion).
- For external use only (e.g. for products to be applied externally).
- Discard 4 weeks after opening (e.g. eye drops).
- This medicine may colour the urine (e.g. levodopa).

Barriers to proper use of medicines

- Patient compliance and adherence with treatment
- Patient confusion
- Communication problems
- Side-effects
- Dispensing errors
- Cost of medicines
- Accessibility and availability.

Practice guidelines

Practice guidelines are adopted in clinical scenarios to provide information and reduce barriers to proper use of medicines, ensure patient safety and reduce risks. Practice guidelines are systematically developed statements designed to assist clinician and patient decisions in disease management. They may draw on evidence-based practice, which is based on research evidence, clinical expertise and patient values.

Evidence-based pharmacy

This entails conscientious, explicit and judicious use of current best evidence in decision-making in patient care. Evidence of effectiveness of therapy is based on:

- systematic literature review
- randomised controlled trials
- non-randomised experimental studies
- observational studies
- expert opinion of clinicians.

Clinical risk

Use of medicines requires a collaborative approach between different health professionals and the individual patient so as to identify rational and safe drug therapy that will achieve desired patient outcomes with minimal clinical risk. This requires:

- identification of patient needs
- patient monitoring for drug-related problems and occurrence of adverse drug reactions
- safe practice to minimise medication errors.

Examples where clinical risk led to changes in drug use include:

- rofecoxib (Vioxx), a selective COX-2 inhibitor that was approved in 1999 and withdrawn in 2004
- hormone replacement therapy, approved in 1985 for the management of menopausal symptoms. In 2003 studies indicated relationship with increased cancer risk.

Risk avoidance strategies

- Pharmacist sharing knowledge with physicians to control risk.
- Adopting an individual holistic approach to patient management and monitoring of patient characteristics which increase clinical risk with medications (e.g. patients at higher risk of presenting extrapyramidal symptoms from antipsychotic agents due to concomitant drug therapy).

Identifying patient needs

Table 4.1 summarises the factors to take into consideration in identifying patient needs.

Liver disease

- Liver disease may alter the response to drugs (e.g. due to impaired drug metabolism).
- Drug prescribing should be kept to a minimum in all patients with severe liver disease and doses need to be reviewed in patients with liver disease.

Table 4.1 Identifying patient needs

Managing therapeutic regimen	Need for treatment to be established on an individual basis (e.g. taking into account patient's lifestyle)
Diagnostic/therapeutic labelling and stigmatisation	Need for providing support and referral to patient organisations
Uncertainty	Need for information
Stress, personality, motivation	Need for psychological support

- For example, the use of paracetamol in patients with liver disease: dose-related toxicity may occur, large doses should be avoided.

Renal impairment

- The use of drugs in patients with reduced renal function can give rise to problems such as failure to excrete drug or its metabolites.
- In patients with renal impairment dose adjustment is recommended.

Drug-related problems

- Untreated indications
- Drug therapy not indicated
- Improper drug selection
- Sub-therapeutic dose
- Failure to receive drug
- Overdose or toxic dose
- Adverse drug reactions
- Drug interactions.

Adverse drug reactions

- Any drug may produce unwanted or unexpected adverse reactions.
- Detection and recording of adverse drug reactions (ADRs) are important.

Definitions

- *Side-effect:* 'Expected, well-known reaction resulting in little or no change in patient management.' The effect has a 'predictable frequency'.[3]
- *Adverse drug reactions:* 'An unexpected, unintended, undesired or excessive response' to a drug with sequelae.[3]

An ADR can lead to (sequelae of ADRs):

- drug discontinuation
- dose modification
- hospital admission
- prolonged hospitalisation
- requirement of supportive treatment
- complication of diagnosis
- negative impact on prognosis
- temporary/permanent harm, disability or death.

> Pharmacists in organised healthcare systems (hospitals, day centres, institutions, outpatient clinics and primary care practice) should develop comprehensive, ongoing programmes for monitoring and reporting adverse drug reactions.

Adverse drug reaction monitoring and reporting programmes

- ADR surveillance: monitoring occurrence.
- ADR documentation: documenting incident.
- Reporting of ADRs: reporting to national regulatory authority (e.g. MHRA in the UK). The national regulatory authority undertakes coordination and monitoring of suspected ADRs on a local and an international level.
- Pharmacists should participate in mechanisms that monitor the safety of drug use in high-risk populations (e.g. older people, children, HIV patients).
- Pharmacists should lead education of health professionals regarding potential ADRs.

Processes of an ADR monitoring programme

- Monitoring
- Detecting
- Evaluating
- Documentation
- Reporting to authorities
- Updates and discussions with healthcare team members.

Pharmacist actions in an ADR monitoring programme

- Analysis of ADR reports
- Identification of drugs and patients at high risk
- Participation in the development of policies and procedures and description of responsibilities of

healthcare professionals in the programme
- Development and maintenance of the programme in an institution
- Educating prescribers and other health professionals on the implementation and running of an ADR programme
- Dissemination of information obtained from the programme
- Reporting to authorities.

Drug interactions

- Administration of two or more drugs at the same time may lead to an exertion of their effects independently or may cause an interaction.
- The interaction may be potentiation or antagonism of one drug by the other.
- Occurrence and impact of drug interactions should be evaluated on the basis of clinical significance and potential for hazardous outcomes.
- Examples of clinically significant drug interactions:
  - aspirin/ibuprofen + warfarin = enhanced anticoagulant effect
  - aspirin/ibuprofen + phenytoin = enhanced effect of phenytoin.

Medication errors

These may occur as a result of inappropriate drug prescribing. For example, cisapride was withdrawn from the market because the drug could not be used safely due to its interaction with macrolides or due to inappropriate patient monitoring.

Types of medication errors

- Prescribing error: medication prescribed is inappropriate.
- Dispensing error: medication dispensed is inappropriate (e.g. due to incorrect interpretation of the prescription).
- Omission error: dose skipped or medication is not being administered.
- Wrong time error/improper dose error/wrong administration technique error: medication administered in an incorrect manner.
- Deteriorated drug error: medication dispensed is not of good quality.

Practices to reduce medication errors

- Avoid unnecessary use of decimal points:
  - quantities less than 1 gram should be written in milligrams
  - quantities less than 1 milligram should be written in micrograms
- Avoid use of abbreviations: micrograms and not µg, nanograms and not ng
- Names of drugs written clearly and not abbreviated.

Preventing medication errors in an institution

The following should be in place:

- policies and procedures regarding evaluation and selection of drugs
- drug use evaluation programmes
- policies for safe distribution of medicines to patients
- automated checking (e.g. barcoding).

Pharmacists and prevention of medication errors

- Participation in drug therapy monitoring
- Participation in selection of appropriate drug therapy
- Establish contact with nurses and physicians
- Maintain medication profiles
- Participation in procurement, distribution and storage of drugs in pharmacy and at ward level
- Check calculations
- Confirm confusing medication orders
- Storage guidelines: avoid having look-alike medications stored close to each

other, use of containers and labels to reduce risk of confusing medications
- Documentation systems to trace medication dispensing.

Managing medication errors

- Classification of medication error
- Determination of cause
- Documented and reported
- Corrective action identified and documented
- Supportive therapy to patient
- Quality improvement programme and dissemination of corrective action.

Classification of medication errors

The American Society of Health-System Pharmacists refers to a classification of medication errors that was initially described by Hartwig, Denger and Schneider.[4,5] This classified medication errors into six levels of severity, according to the following:

1. No clinically significant harm to the patient occurred
2. Need to increase patient monitoring but no patient harm
3. Change in vital signs but no ultimate patient harm occurred
4. Need for treatment with another drug or increased length of stay
5. Permanent patient harm occurred
6. Patient death occurred.

Poisoning

- All patients who show features of poisoning should generally be admitted to hospital.
- Poisoning may take place with immediate action poisons (e.g. alcohol (ethanol)) or delayed action poisons (e.g. paracetamol).
- It may be difficult to establish with certainty the identity of the poisoning agent and the size of dose administered, particularly in cases of premeditated poisoning.
- Supportive care is undertaken and treatment is aimed at managing symptoms (e.g. hypertension). Vital functions should be monitored.

Removal of the poison from the gastrointestinal tract

- Carried out by gastric lavage.
- Only considered if a life-threatening amount of a poison has been ingested within the preceding hour.

Prevention of absorption of poison

- Carried out by using activated charcoal.
- Charcoal binds to many poisons and reduces their absorption. It is relatively safe and the sooner it is given the more effective the procedure will be.

Use of antidotes

This is limited in that antidotes are available for only a few poisons:

- Paracetamol: acetylcysteine to protect the liver if given within 10–12 hours of ingestion of the excessive dose
- Iron: desferrioxamine which chelates iron
- Opiate poisoning presents with sedation, cough suppression and respiratory depression leading to coma. The antidote, naloxone, is an opioid receptor antagonist available as an IV injection.

Enhancing elimination of poison by alkalinisation of urine

- Aspirin is an acid.
- Poisoning with aspirin is associated with stimulation of respiratory centre (hyperpnoea) and abdominal pain, nausea, tinnitus, deafness, vertigo.
- Rehydration and alkalinisation of urine to enhance drug elimination will promote ionisation

of aspirin, thus preventing reabsorption in the kidney.

Practice summary

- The development of medicines requires a lengthy process, out of which only a few lead drugs are successfully developed into medicines.
- Regulatory aspects govern the practices involved in development of medicines.
- Use of medicines is associated with risks that include occurrence of side-effects, drug interactions, medication errors and drug misuse.
- Pharmacists may identify patient needs and characteristics that may increase clinical risk.
- Safe medicine use requires patient education about the use of medicines and requires health professionals to review patient drug therapy and ensure minimal risks for the individual patient. Risks of drug therapy have to be weighed against the benefits of therapy.
- Pharmacists are involved in developing and maintaining an adverse drug reaction monitoring and management programme.
- Pharmacists can develop guidelines and participate in strategies to minimise medication errors.
- Poisoning may occur inadvertently due to patient misunderstanding of the use of a medicine or may be deliberate. It may occur as a result of ingestion of drugs or of other substances, including household items.

Questions

1. What is meant by 'CE marking' with respect to medical devices?
2. Describe the phase I and phase II clinical testing required in the development of medicines.
3. Describe how liver disease may interfere with use of drugs.
4. Describe briefly the coordination and monitoring of adverse drug reactions (ADRs) on a local and international level.

Answers

1. The CE marking in medical devices indicates that the device satisfies the requirements essential for it to be considered safe and fit for its intended purpose. The CE marking is regarded as equivalent to a marketing authorisation. There are European Directives that provide for mandatory CE marking of all devices in EU countries.
2. Phase I is intended to assess safety and dosage in healthy individuals, while phase II is intended to assess safety and efficacy on a number of patient volunteers.
3. Liver disease may alter the response to drugs, for example due to impaired drug metabolism. Use of drugs should be kept to a minimum in all patients with severe liver disease.
4. Detection and recording of ADRs are of utmost importance. Pharmacists are urged to contribute by reporting suspected ADRs on the appropriate documents (Yellow Card prepared by the Commission on Human Medicines of the Medicines and Healthcare products Regulatory Agency in the UK) to the local medicines regulatory authority. Such an authority undertakes coordination and monitoring of suspected ADRs on a local and international level through its participation at the European Medicines Agency.

Further reading

American Society of Health-System Pharmacists (2000). ASHP statement on reporting medical errors. *Am J Health-Syst Pharm* 57: 1531–1532.

American Society of Health-System Pharmacists (2006/2007). *Best Practices for Hospital and Health-system Pharmacy*. Bethesda, MA: American Society of Health-System Pharmacists

Fidelino R J (2007). In pursuit of distinction: The method of the non-proprietary name. *J Gen Med* 5: 45–52.

Rang H P (ed.) (2006). *Drug Discovery and Development*. Edinburgh: Churchill Livingstone Elsevier.

Royal Pharmaceutical Society (2009). *Practice Guidance: Medical devices*. London: Royal Pharmaceutical Society.

Troy D B and Beringer P (2005). *Remington The Science and Practice of Pharmacy*. Philadelphia: Lippincott Williams & Wilkins.

References

1 Directive 2001/83/EC of the European Parliament and of the Council of 6 November 2001 on the Community Code relating to Medicinal Products for human use as amended by Directives 2002/98/EC, 2004/24/EC, 2004/27/EC.

2 Directive 2007/47/EEC of the European Parliament and of the Council of 5 September 2007 amending Council Directives 90/385/EEC, 93/42/EEC and 98/8/EC.

3 American Society of Health-System Pharmacists. ASHP guidelines on adverse drug reaction monitoring and reporting. *Am J Health-Syst Pharm* 1995; 52: 417–419.

4 American Society of Health-System Pharmacists. ASHP guidelines on preventing medication errors in hospitals. *Am J Hosp Pharm* 1993; 50: 305–314.

5 Hartwig S C, Denger S D and Schneider P J. A severity indexed, incident-report based medication-error reporting program. *Am J Hosp Pharm* 1991; 48: 2611–2616.

5

Community pharmacy practice

Learning objectives:

- To identify actions of community pharmacists in the provision of patient-focused services
- To describe the legal and professional issues of community pharmacy practice.

Actions of community pharmacists in society

- Procurement of medicines that are suitable for human consumption
- Storage of medicines in appropriate conditions (temperature, humidity, cleanliness, stock monitoring)
- Dispensing of medicines chosen by patient or as pharmacist-recommended products or on presentation of a prescription
- Compounding and ensuring quality of compounded products
- Patient medication review, advise patients on use of medicines and participate in adverse drug reaction reporting
- Ensuring rational and safe use of medicines by patients, developing care plans and collaborating with prescribers to establish a therapeutic plan, implement it and monitor patient outcomes
- Monitoring of self-care, responding to symptoms and identifying cases warranting referral
- Point-of-care testing
- Health promotion and promotion of healthy lifestyles (nutrition, physical activity, smoking cessation, sexual and reproductive health)
- Ensuring safe disposal of unwanted or expired medicines
- Signposting patients to other healthcare providers and support agencies
- Participating in national health service schemes to provide social pharmacy services
- Other responsibilities: nutritional supplements, special foods (e.g. gluten-free products, food for diabetic people), colostomy care and urinary incontinence devices, disability and mobility aids (e.g. wheelchairs, walking aids), oxygen supplies and ventilation equipment, veterinary medicines.

Organisation of a community pharmacy

- Personnel present: managing pharmacist, pharmacists, pharmacy technicians, pharmacy assistants, sales personnel. Staff management includes identifying training needs and providing appropriate training, management to develop a team approach, continuing professional development of professional personnel
- Premises: areas available for dispensing, storage of medicines, patient counselling, health promotion
- Equipment: dispensing equipment, diagnostic equipment for point-of-care testing (e.g. blood pressure measurement, blood testing, urinalysis)

- Documentation and information: registers to be kept at the pharmacy, IT-supported systems for documentation of pharmacist actions and for maintaining pharmacy patient profiles, drug information sources (books and electronic access).

Dispensary area

- Area should be spacious and designed in such a way as to promote communication between pharmacist and patient.
- Space should be available for patient advice and counselling in privacy.
- Consultation areas should provide for space to carry out point-of-care testing.
- Adequate facilities for dispensing must be provided – cleanable floor and surfaces, adequate fixtures and fittings, clean refrigerator with appropriate temperature monitoring and control, clean sink, logical layout of stock and a natural workflow.

Storage of medicines

- Sufficient storage space to store medicines in a dry place
- Temperature control of areas where medicines are stored
- Prescription-only medicines not accessible to the public
- Area available to store medicines that require controlled access
- Stock rotation, monitoring of expiry dates and systems to ensure that medicines are not damaged
- Pricing.

Legislation

- Pharmacists practising at the pharmacy are registered with a registering body.
- Process of community pharmacy practice is controlled by legislation.
- Legislation classifies medicines according to:
  - category of medicines that may be sold from other outlets (such as drugstores) not only pharmacies (e.g. general sales list, in countries where this is permitted)
  - category of medicines that may be sold after being recommended by pharmacists
  - category of medicines that require a prescription
  - category of medicines that are controlled (e.g. buprenorphine, diamorphine, fentanyl, methadone).
- Pharmacy services must be available for 24 hours, 7 days a week. Rosters are issued for night-time service and for service on Sundays and public holidays.

Clinical governance

- Clinical governance relates to a commitment to continuously improve the quality of professional services provided and maintain standards of practice.
- It involves development of quality standards, audit, training and development of personnel, staff management and monitoring of clinical effectiveness.
- Quality standards include the development of standard operating procedures for processes that are carried out in a community pharmacy and the implementation of audit processes (see Chapter 70).

Provision of patient-focused services from community pharmacies

- *Repeat dispensing:* pharmacists dispense medicines as a repeat prescription as directed by prescriber.
- *Supplementary pharmacist prescribing:* pharmacist prescribes medicines according to an agreed protocol with prescriber.
- *Pharmacist prescribing:* pharmacist may prescribe medicines that are designated as

pharmacist prescription drugs as long as he or she has the required competency to do so (competency is based on pharmacist skills and patient characteristics presented).

- *Electronic transmission* of prescriptions from prescriber or secondary care interface to community pharmacy.
- *Electronic patient records:* pharmacy keeps patient records which are treated as confidential and where access is limited to authorised staff. Through these records the pharmacy has a history of medicines that are taken by the patient and other relevant data. These data may be shared with prescribers and with secondary care interfaces.
- *Medicines management services:* pharmacist medication review, medicines use review, chronic medication monitoring.
- *Pharmacist consulting rooms:* where patients can discuss their health issues and drug therapy issues with pharmacists in privacy.
- *Provision of enhanced services* (e.g. preparation of extemporaneous preparations which require a dedicated area that is run according to established quality systems), dispensing of special items (e.g. gluten-free food) and provision of home deliveries.

Practice summary

- Community pharmacy practice requires management skills and involves continuing education and development of personnel.
- Setting up and maintaining a community pharmacy requires consideration of physical aspects of storage and handling of medicines as well as quality aspects.
- Documentation of processes carried out in the pharmacy is essential. Quality systems are required to ensure good standards and to promote the value of patient-focused services offered from community pharmacies.
- The development of patient-focused pharmacy services and the orientation of pharmacist actions towards individual patient care enhance the practice of pharmaceutical care in the community.
- Community pharmacy practice should be undertaken in collaboration with other health professionals and with pharmacy institutions in other settings to ensure seamless care as the patient is transferred from one setting to another.

Questions

1. What parameter should be monitored for a refrigerator that is used to store medicines in a community pharmacy? Define the range required.
2. Explain the following features of a dispensary: patient consultation area and controlled drugs cabinet.
3. Describe what is meant by an extemporaneous preparation area in a community pharmacy.

Answers

1. The temperature must be monitored. Range is 2–8°C. A large refrigerator should be temperature mapped in a loaded scenario.
2. Patient consultation area: space dedicated for patient advice and counselling in relative privacy. Consultation areas may be used to provide patient monitoring and follow-up, medication review and point-of-care testing. Controlled drugs cabinet: cabinet where medications that require limited access (e.g. methadone) are stored.
3. The extemporaneous preparation area is the part of the dispensary area dedicated to the preparation of medications (e.g. dilution of creams, mixing different creams).

Further reading

Armstrong P (2006). Standard operating procedures betray a staggering poverty of intellect. *Pharm J* 276: 262.

Avery A J and Pringle M (2005). Extended prescribing by UK nurses and pharmacists. *BMJ* 331: 1154–1155.

Blenkinsopp A, Celino G, Bond C and Inch J (2007). Medicines use reviews: the first year of a new community pharmacy service. *Pharm J* 278: 218–223.

Buisson J (2005). How to make space for a consultation room in your community pharmacy. *Pharm J* 275: 689.

Dewsbury C (2002). Guide to clinical governance: What it means for community pharmacy. *Pharm J* 268: 119.

Laaksonen R, Duggan C and Bates I (2009) Overcoming barriers to engagement in continuing professional development in community pharmacy: a longitudinal study. *Pharm J* 282: 44–48.

Royal Pharmaceutical Society of Great Britain (2009). *Medicines, Ethics and Practice: A guide for pharmacists and pharmacy technicians*. London: Pharmaceutical Press.

Waterfield J (2008). *Community Pharmacy Handbook*, London: Pharmaceutical Press.

6

Dispensing prescriptions

Learning objectives:

- To review the process of following a prescription and dispensing the medicine
- To outline pharmacist interventions in the dispensing of prescription medicines.

Receiving the prescription

The patient walks into the pharmacy and presents the prescription. At this stage, communication and interaction with the pharmacy staff take place. In the modern age of electronic documents, e-prescribing is already being practised in some countries and is expected to develop even further. In electronic prescribing, the prescription is transferred electronically and the pharmacist receives an electronic document. Once the patient presents at the pharmacy and provides the required details for retrieval of the electronic prescription, the process of communication and interaction with the patient commences.

Reading and checking of prescription

Prescription is reviewed to see which medicines are required and to note patient details. Pharmacy staff should check:

- patient's name and address
- age of patient if under 12 years
- name, dose and quantity of medicine
- date
- prescriber's name and address
- signature of prescriber
- legality and authenticity of document.

Examples of administration instructions

a.c.	before food
b.d.	to be taken twice daily
o.d.	every day
o.m.	every morning
o.n.	every night
p.c.	after food
p.r.n.	as required
q.d.s.	to be taken four times daily
stat	immediately
t.d.s.	to be taken three times daily

Collection of medicine

This step may be carried out either manually, where the pharmacy or pharmacy assistant picks up the required product from the pharmacy storage section, or mechanically, where the pharmacist requests the product through a machine interface and the product is selected from the magazine and delivered at the dispensing bench.

During this step, pharmacist intervention to decrease occurrence of dispensing errors includes:

- care in selecting appropriate medicine; there are some medicines that have very similar names (e.g. amlodipine and amiloride, Lescol and Losec)
- care in selecting the appropriate strength; there are medicines that are available in different strengths (e.g. amoxicillin 250 and 500 mg capsules, atenolol 25, 50 and 100 mg tablets)
- care in selecting the appropriate dosage form; there are medicines that are available in different dosage forms (e.g. diclofenac gel, tablets, modified-release tablets, suppositories).

Label production

The label should be clear and legible to ensure that the patient takes the medicine as prescribed. The information presented has to be understood by the patient.

Details to be included on label:

- patient's name
- date of dispensing
- name of pharmacy
- name of medicine
- strength
- dosage form
- quantity dispensed
- dose with clear instructions
- cautionary labels.

To avoid confusion, where several containers of the same medicine have to be dispensed, it should be indicated on the label that there is more than one container of the same medicine (e.g. 1 of 4, 2 of 4).

For cautionary and advisory labels see Chapter 4.

Containers

If, during the dispensing process, there is a requirement to repack the medicines, the appropriate container should be chosen for the medication. This includes taking into consideration stability of the product and interaction of the product with the material used for the container. Usually repacking takes place in a controlled area under a quality assurance system and pre-packs are produced to be available for the pharmacist during the dispensing.

In the UK, original pack dispensing is required, whereby the pharmacist can dispense branded or generic products as packaged in the original form as produced by the manufacturer.

Rechecking

Recheck that the prescription and the medicine prepared are consistent and that the right medicine in the right dosage form and strength has been identified, that the right label is attached and that the right patient instructions are provided.

Handing over the medicine

The pharmacist hands over the medicine and explains to the patient when and how to take the medication. Refer to Chapters 8 and 9 for discussion on communication, patient counselling and compliance.

Practice summary

- The pharmacist should ensure that the dispensing process implemented in the pharmacy implies the correct attitude and transfer of knowledge from reading the prescription to the handing over of the medicine to the patient.
- The dispensing process includes communication and interaction between the patient and the pharmacist. The way that this interaction takes place may influence the efficacy of the dispensing process.
- The dispensing process employed could be outlined in good dispensing procedures to ensure standardisation of the dispensing process within a pharmacy.
- Pharmacist intervention should ensure that the process eliminates dispensing errors. Factors that

decrease dispensing errors include: dispensary layout and workflow, systems of drug storage, lighting, limitation of noise and use of electronic equipment (e.g. scanners).

- Pharmacist intervention should ensure that the patient understands the use of the medicine, its correct application and information about any side-effects expected and action that might need to be taken in the case of missed doses.
- When the customer is not the patient but a proxy, emphasis should be placed on the need for correct onward transmission of the information to the patient or carer.

Questions

1. For each of the following abbreviations, which may be used on prescriptions, give a brief explanation and an example of a product for which this abbreviation is used, stating generic name and dosage form(s): p.c., p.r.n.
2. For each of the following cautionary and advisory labels, give one example of a drug where the label should be used:
   (a) May cause drowsiness
   (b) Do not take milk, indigestion remedies and medicines containing iron or zinc at the same time of day as this medicine
   (c) Take at regular intervals. Complete the prescribed course unless otherwise directed.
3. Give two examples of products that should be taken after food. Give reasons for your choice.

Answers

1. p.c. – after food, ibuprofen (tablets, suspension). p.r.n. – when required, paracetamol (tablets, soluble tablets, suspension, suppositories).
2. (a) May cause drowsiness – hydroxyzine.
   (b) Do not take milk, indigestion remedies and medicines containing iron or zinc at the same time of day as this medicine – ciprofloxacin.
   (c) Take at regular intervals. Complete the prescribed course unless otherwise directed – co-amoxiclav.
3. (a) Diclofenac potassium tablets – should be taken after food to minimise gastrointestinal irritation. (b) Itraconazole capsules – should be taken after food to ensure optimal absorption.

Further reading

Azzopardi L M (2000). *Validation Instruments for Community Pharmacy: Pharmaceutical care for the third millennium*. Binghamton, NY: Pharmaceutical Products Press.

Royal Pharmaceutical Society of Great Britain (2007). Developing and implementing standard operating procedures for dispensing. Guidance documents. http://www.rpsgb.org/pdfs/sops.pdf.

Waterfield J (2008). *Community Pharmacy Handbook*, London: Pharmaceutical Press.

7

Health promotion

Learning objectives:

- To identify the intervention of the pharmacist in health promotion
- To develop skills required to participate in health promotion.

Background

- Health promotion: a process enabling people to increase control over and to improve their health.
- Health education: giving information and working towards improving individual attitude and behaviour changes to sustain healthy living.

In health promotion, pharmacists provide information and skills to individuals so that they can prevent specific diseases and participate in services for early detection and treatment of disease. The process involves a behavioural change approach such as in advising individuals on the importance of preventing and managing obesity.

Health promotion activities from community pharmacies include the organisation of theme-oriented weeks where patrons are advised on the theme, and written and other visual aids are available in the pharmacy for further information and for shop window dressing.

Themes of health promotion in community pharmacies

- Smoking cessation programmes
- Diet, exercise and body weight
- Cardiovascular disease risk factors and prevention
- Sun exposure
- Travel medicine
- Patient concordance with treatment
- Immunisation programmes
- Sexual health
- Screening tests
- Alcohol and drug abuse.

Sustainable development and public health are closely related. Through health promotion activities pharmacists can contribute towards the reduction of carbon footprints and to practices that tackle climate change. This can be achieved by:

- acting as role model and educators
- serving as a resource (e.g. collecting used batteries)
- promoting proper use and disposal of medicines
- distributing literature on ways to save the environment.

Information transmitted

The information presented should be educational but at the same time acceptable to busy patrons. An entertaining presentation helps to make the information attractive and prompts the individual to take notice of the message being transmitted (Figure 7.1).

The impact of the information transmitted depends on the methods used to convey the information. The information presented has to be understandable by the individual. Pharmacists are in a position of interpreting scientific information so as to convey the message to the individuals in an understandable manner (Figure 7.2).

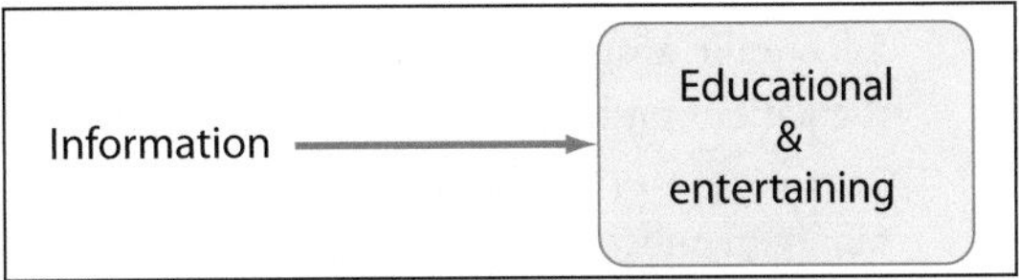

Figure 7.1 Information that is conveyed in health promotion programmes.

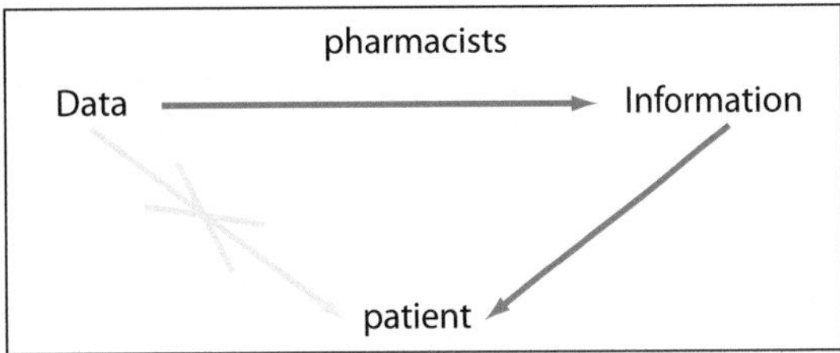

Figure 7.2 Pharmacists act as conveyers of patient-understandable information.

Factors influencing health-promotion activities in community pharmacies

Positive factors

- Environment within the pharmacy conducive to health promotion
- Accessibility of the pharmacy
- Communication skills of community pharmacist
- Strong pharmacist–patient relationship.

Negative factors

- Lack of resource materials
- Lack of space
- Lack of confidentiality
- Improper time management of the pharmacy personnel.

Planning a health promotion campaign

- Identify area(s) to be addressed
- Establish targets to be achieved
- Identify resources that can be used and are already available
- Develop a practical and realistic implementation programme
- Establish evaluation methods
- Set an action plan.

Practice summary

- Pharmacists are accessible health professionals who can play a very proactive role in promoting health.
- Pharmacists should actively promote healthy lifestyles including discouraging smoking, pointing out the importance of exercise and highlighting the benefits of a healthy diet.
- Pharmacists in any practice setting should encourage positive behavioural changes.

Question

1 List five points helpful in counselling patients on smoking cessation.

Answer

1 (a) Act as a role model by not smoking and not allowing smoking on the premises (e.g. putting up no smoking signs).
(b) Provide patient with information on the risks associated with smoking (e.g. use patient leaflets about smoking).

(c) Encourage abstinence by directly advising the patient on how to quit and highlighting benefits of stopping smoking (e.g. effects on family members particularly patients with cardiovascular disease and children).
(d) Refer patient to smoking cessation support groups (e.g. programmes organised by the local health promotion centre).
(e) Follow up on the use of smoking cessation products and maintenance strategies (e.g. schedule a follow-up visit).

Further reading

Anderson C, Blenkinsopp A and Armstrong M (2009). The contribution of community pharmacy to improving the public's health: Summary report of the literature review 1990–2007. London: Pharmacy-HealthLink.

McClelland C and Rees L (2000). A foundation for health promotion in pharmacy practice. In: Gard P (ed.) *A Behavioural Approach to Pharmacy Practice*. London: Blackwell Science.

Root G (2008). Help the public and the planet by engaging in sustainable development. *Pharm J* 281: 596–597.

8

Communication skills and patient counselling

Learning objectives:

- To identify good communication skills
- To appreciate pharmacist intervention in patient counselling on health-related issues and the use of medicines
- To identify factors that should be considered when developing individual patient counselling.

Background

For effective pharmacist actions in the promotion of health, responding to symptoms and management of disease states, it is necessary to use communication skills that convey the correct information to the patient and encourage discussion of health-related problems.

Patient counselling is undertaken by pharmacists:

- during dispensing
- in disease management
- in providing advice on self-care: advice on product selection and use, non-drug self-care, referral and health assessment.

Pharmacist actions and communication with patients

- Ensuring safe and correct use of medicines
- Responding to symptoms
- Discussing patient health-related and social problems that impact on health status
- Empowering individuals to be active in health promotion and preservation.

Communication process

- Understanding perception of individual
- Rapport building
- Non-verbal communication and body language
- Questioning and listening
- Responding and explaining.

Understanding perception of individual

- Through the communication process, anticipate different perceptions according to the individual's needs (e.g. social problem associated with occurrence of acne may impact differently on individuals).

Rapport building skills

- Convey friendliness and warmth
- Express genuine interest and concern

- Refer to previous encounters when relevant
- Provide reassurance
- Preserve confidentiality.

Non-verbal communication and body language

- Close conversational distance
- Direct eye contact
- Direct body and facial orientation
- Open, forward leaning posture
- Smiling and using pleasant facial expressions
- Voice intonation denoting interest and appropriate speech speed.

Questioning and listening skills

- Use effective questions by adopting open questions to obtain information that is necessary.
- Ask only one question at a time.
- Structure the flow of questions to follow a logical pattern.
- Use probing questions to follow up patient's response. Patients may not be aware that certain information must be known by the pharmacist to suggest appropriate line of action.
- Encourage patient participation by pausing both after asking a question and after the initial response.
- Practise active listening.

Responding and explaining skills

- Place the most important points at the beginning of the communication session.
- Emphasise key issues.
- Give specific, concrete instructions.
- Limit the information to the essentials to prevent cognitive overload.
- Simplify complicated messages.

Barriers to communication

- Environmental factors such as lack of privacy, lack of space in the pharmacy
- Time available for pharmacist to dedicate to the patient for listening
- Patient characteristics such as speech defect, inability to communicate.

Dont's in communicating with patients

- Don't ask 'why' questions
- Don't use 'should' and 'ought'
- Don't blame the patient
- Don't automatically compare the patient's experience with your own
- Don't invalidate the patient's feelings.

Pharmacist skills needed

In addition to a sound knowledge of drugs and the ability to adopt a comparative approach between possibilities of treatment, the pharmacist also needs the ability to:

- explain information clearly and in terms that are understandable to patients of different backgrounds
- pose the right questions to patients without putting them off
- listen to the patient.

- Well-informed patients are more likely to use their medications correctly.
- The intervention of the pharmacist in the provision of advice on medicines improves medicine safety.

Counselling in the community pharmacy setting

- This should be an integral part during dispensing of medicines.
- Pharmacists should be visible and accessible for patients to request advice.

Counselling in the hospital setting

- On admission
- During hospitalisation: needs assessment

- On discharge
- At outpatient clinics
- In rehabilitation settings.

Objectives of patient counselling by pharmacists

- To ensure that patients are adequately informed about their medication
- To predict any problems which might cause loss of efficacy of the drug or be detrimental to health of patient
- To identify any drug-related or health-related problems.

Counselling process during dispensing of medicines

- How and when to take or use a medicine
- How much to take or use
- How long to continue treatment
- What to do if a dose is missed
- How to recognise side-effects and minimise their occurrence
- Lifestyle and dietary changes
- Drug–drug and drug–nutrient interactions.

Pharmacist counselling process

- Recognising the need for counselling: extent of counselling required varies from one individual to another.
- Assessing and prioritising the needs: what points need to be emphasised?
- Checking assessment methods: to identify outcomes and follow-up counselling process.
- Environment in pharmacy: must be conducive to privacy and to induce patients to ask for professional advice from the pharmacist.
- Professional appearance of pharmacist: to project a professional appearance that enables individuals, including those who feel that they have a very sensitive issue to discuss, to address the pharmacist with confidence.

Recognising the need for counselling

- *Is it a repeat medication?* Patients who have already taken the medication also require counselling to ensure proper use of medicines. If the patient is taking medication for the first time more information is required.
- *Polytherapy:* patients who are taking more than one medicine need more support to manage the drug-handling process.
- *Complex instructions:* with medicines that have a complex drug regimen or require an unusual drug-taking pattern (e.g. bisphosphonates) the pharmacist needs to provide counselling and must ensure that the patient has understood the drug regimen.
- *Narrow therapeutic index drugs:* the risk associated with these medications (e.g. warfarin) is higher if patient is not aware of how to take medication, which side-effects should be reported and the necessity of relevant routine checks.
- *Patient characteristics:* the pharmacist needs to adapt the counselling session according to patient characteristics and to individualise the session (e.g. elderly, frail, psychiatric conditions).

Assessing and prioritising needs

Patient needs vary according to a number of factors. The counselling process has to be developed according to each individual patient's needs. Patient priorities in life (e.g. lifestyle) should be taken into consideration during the counselling session if maximum patient benefit is expected. Information about patients that will help to prioritise the needs includes:

- educational background
- available support
- sight or hearing problems
- pregnancy and breast-feeding.

Follow-up counselling sessions

During follow-up counselling sessions, which may take place during dispensing of a repeat medication, identification of the following factors should be considered:

- patient problems with medication (side-effects, complex drug regimen, drug therapy interfering with lifestyle)
- deterioration in health status requiring pharmacotherapy review
- medication errors
- medication mismanagement.

Written information

- Patient-specific written information
- Patient information leaflets
- Warning cards (e.g. used for lithium, anticoagulant therapy, steroids, benzodiazepines)
- Leaflets on drug administration (e.g. pessaries, inhalers, nebulisers).

Practice summary

When communicating with patients, establishing a good rapport with the patient, active listening, relevant questioning and appropriate body language enhance the process. Pharmacist counselling programmes can be developed focusing on themes such as:

- Lifestyle measures:
  - counselling on exercise and diet
  - monitoring of body weight, lipid profile, glucose levels and blood pressure
- Smoking cessation:
  - counselling on nicotine replacement therapy (transdermal nicotine patch, chewing gum, inhalator) and smoking cessation psychological behaviour
- Diabetes:
  - giving information on condition, advising on proper techniques for insulin storage and administration
  - identifying and providing guidance on actions to monitor and compensate for aberrations in glucose levels, dietary and exercise management, and foot care
- Asthma:
  - providing information on condition, medicines and pharmaceutical dosage forms
  - identifying and providing guidance on actions to compensate for aberrations in peak flow meter readings and exercise management
- Hypertension:
  - providing counselling on significance of monitoring blood pressure
  - carrying out drug therapy review
  - advising patients on lifestyle measures
- Anticoagulant therapy:
  - giving information on identification of symptoms indicating haemorrhage
  - providing education on anticoagulant–food interactions and drug–drug interactions
  - explaining significance of monitoring of prothrombin time
- Hormone replacement therapy:
  - providing counselling on impacts of drug therapy, lifestyle measures and requirement for continuous monitoring.

Question

1 List factors that could hinder communication with patients in a community pharmacy.

Answer

1 (a) Environment such as lack of space
(b) Time
(c) Patient factors: not responsive to pharmacist advice
(d) Administrative factors: access to pharmacist.

Further reading

Beardsley R S, Kimberlin C L and Tindall W N (2007). *Communication Skills in Pharmacy Practice*, 5th edn. Philadelphia: Lippincott, Williams & Wilkins.

Hargie O D W, Morrow N C and Woodman C (2000). Pharmacists evaluation of key communication skills in practice. *Patient Educ Couns* 39: 61–70.

Kreit K (2008). Enhancing and using negotiation skills. *Dermatol Nurs* 20: 140.

Maguire T (2002). Barriers to communication – how things go wrong. *Pharm J* 268: 246.

Schnipper J L, Kirwin J L, Cotugno M C, Wahlstrom S A, Brown B A, Tarvin E *et al.* (2006). Role of pharmacist counseling in preventing adverse drug events after hospitalization. *Arch Intern Med* 166: 565–571.

Waterfield J, Aspinall V and Hall S (2009). The use of digital video media in the teaching of communication skills. *Pharm J* 282: 135.

9

Compliance, adherence and concordance

Learning objectives:

- To appreciate factors that increase risk of a patient's inability to follow drug therapy and recommendations made by health professionals
- To develop skills necessary for pharmacists' actions in promoting adherence.

Compliance

This is a term that has been established to describe a patient's degree of conformity with the advice and recommendations given by health professionals. The term *non-compliance* was used to describe significant failure to conform with the advice and recommendations to an extent that it interferes with achieving the patient outcomes planned. Since this term has a negative nuance for the patient and overrides the concept that the patient may have a problem with the medication or recommendations, the term non-compliance is not very much supported today.

The concept of compliance seems to denote a relationship in which the patient has a passive role and is expected to follow the doctor's orders. Since the term does not emphasise patient participation, there has been a shift towards the use of 'adherence' as a term instead.

Adherence

As opposed to the concept of compliance, adherence seems to denote a relationship in which the patient has an active role and is expected to contribute to the establishment of the treatment to be followed. In the concept of adherence the patient is free to decide whether or not to adhere to recommendations by health professionals and failure to do so should not be a reason to blame the patient. Health professionals have a responsibility to facilitate adherence.

Concordance

This term is used to denote the degree to which the patient and the health practitioner agree about the nature of the illness and the need for management, and the relative risks and benefits of the proposed line of treatment. In the concept of concordance, the patient's views are taken into account during the prescribing phase in order to increase the likelihood of better compliance.

Categories of non-adherence

- Primary non-adherence: patient does not have access to medicine
- Secondary non-adherence: patient has access to medicine but does not take it due to:

- accidental non-adherence: forgets to take medication or is unable to take medication due to lifestyle
- triggered non-adherence: cannot take medication due to drug-related problem
- intentional non-adherence: decides not to take medication.

Classification of non-adherence

- The ideal situation – adherence achieved
- Few errors (0–15%) – partial adherence
- Major default (>15%) – partial/non-adherence.

It is still hard to quantify the consequences of poor adherence to medication. There is no consensus as to the quantification of partial adherence (number of missed doses).

Measurement of non-adherence

- *Direct methods:* observation of ingestion of the drug or by detecting its presence in body fluids
- *Indirect methods:* assume ingestion based on proxy evidence such as patient's self-reporting, number of dosages remaining, number of dosages removed from a container through data recorded in medication compliance aids. These include:
  - tablet counts: counting number of units left in container
  - patient diary cards: reporting by patient
  - electronic monitors: incorporation of electronic devices into the medicine container recording time and date of usage
  - clinicians' estimates and therapeutic outcomes
  - patient self-reporting on health status and how the condition has improved.

Causes of non-adherence

- *Therapy-related factors:* type of dosage form (e.g. large solid oral dosage forms, inability to use metered dose inhalers), problems with handling container (e.g. opening of child-resistant containers, blister packs), polypharmacy (e.g. patient has to handle a number of different drugs), dosage frequency (e.g. multiple daily dosing), occurrence of side-effects
- *Condition-related factors:* non-adherence particularly noted in conditions where patient is not seeing benefit from drug therapy (e.g. hypertension), in conditions that are associated with a social stigma (e.g. psychiatric disorders, HIV), where patients may not be ready to accept medications for the condition (denial of illness or of need for medications)
- *Patient-related factors:* patient's knowledge, beliefs about and attitudes towards medicine and disease state
- *Health-system factors:* relationships with the healthcare team, ability to get prescription and medicines, inadequate patient education
- *Social and economic factors:* social factors such as lack of patient support and income, problems with living conditions and problems at home, level of education and literacy.

One helpful final question that may be asked to confirm likelihood of adherence would be: How have we agreed that you are going to take the medicines?

Strategies to improve patient adherence

- Labelling: large (font size), clean (printed), simple, specific
- Packaging: while taking into account stability of the product, ensure patient accessibility and acceptance of product appearance
- Compliance aids: use of devices that can be used to remind patient to take medication, dispensing medication in blister pack according to dosage regimen, preparing medicine reminder charts, administration devices (e.g. eye-drop applicators)
- Review patient prescriptions and medications: to reduce dosing frequency and multiple drug therapy where relevant
- Improve patient–pharmacist–doctor rapport
- Ensure effective patient information

- Maintain patient contact and regular pharmacist follow-ups
- In January 2009 in the UK, the National Institute for Health and Clinical Excellence prepared a guideline on medicines adherence.[1]

Practice summary

- It can be difficult for patients to take medicines and follow recommendations by health professionals due to a number of factors.
- Factors that interfere with adherence should be evaluated for each individual patient so as to minimise occurrence of non-adherence.
- Pharmacist skills required to improve adherence include communication techniques with the patient and the prescriber, availability and accessibility.
- Pharmacist actions to improve adherence include the initiation and facilitation of discussion with patient on drug therapy, eliciting the patient's view and experience of treatment, undertaking regular review of all medications taken, providing information that meets patient's needs, liaising with other health professionals to ensure continuity of care, acting as the navigator in the healthcare system and collaborating with prescribers to identify and/or improve treatment protocols.

Question

1 List three interventions that help to promote adherence to therapy.

Answer

1 (a) Initiate discussion with patient on drug therapy
(b) Carry out regular medicines use reviews (MURs)
(c) Provide information on medicines and conditions managed

Further reading

Bellingham C (2008). Pharmacies work to improve access. *Pharm J* 280: 684.

Gray N and Celino G (2008). Why adherence is a sensitive issue. *Pharm J* 281: 169–172.

Reference

1 Malson G. Helping patients take their medicines as prescribed. *Clin Pharm* 2009; 1: 64.

10

Mathematical principles of drug therapy

Learning objectives:

- To familiarise oneself with metric units
- To calculate concentrations in amount strength, ratio strength, parts per million, percentage concentration
- To be able to work out dilutions
- To understand density, displacement volumes and displacement values
- To include the meaning of molecular weights as involved through calculations
- To calculate the amount of ingredients and doses, including consideration of body weight and body surface area
- To determine rate of flow of intravenous solutions
- To develop mathematical skills required in the handling of drug therapy.

Metric units

The metric system (or the SI) is the system most commonly used for expression of quantities in pharmacy. The metric system is a decimal system of weights and measures.

1 Complete the following:
   (a) 15 g = 0.015 kg = 15 000 mg
   (b) 0.004 L = 4 mL = 4000 microlitres

The apothecaries' system is the historic system of weights and measures used in pharmacy. Today, on a metrically written prescription, the dram symbol ʒ is used with reference to a dose; it means a teaspoonful, which is today considered to be equivalent to 5 mL.

Concentration

- Concentration may be expressed as quantity per volume, percentage concentrations, ratios and parts.
- Concentration is expressed in percentage as % weight/volume (w/v), % weight/weight (w/w) and % volume/volume (v/v).
- Quantity per volume gives the amount or weight of drug (moles or grams) in a volume of solution.
- Ratio concentration is the number of parts of a solvent in which one part of the drug is dissolved or dispersed.

Amount strength

2 Calculate the weight per millilitre for:
   (a) 27 g in 40 mL. *The weight per millilitre is 0.675 g/mL (27/40)*

(b) 0.625 kg in 500 mL. *Since 0.625 kg is equivalent to 625 g, the weight per millilitre is 1.25 g/mL (625/500).*

3 Ten millilitres of distilled witch hazel are made up to 70 mL of solution. Express the concentration of the final solution as an amount strength. *In 1 mL there is 0.143 mL of distilled witch hazel (1/70 × 10).*

Ratio strength

4 Fluocortolone is available as 0.25% w/w cream. Express this as a ratio strength. *The ratio strength of this preparation is 1 in 400 (1/0.25 × 100).*

5 Mometasone is available as 0.1% w/w cream. Express this as a ratio strength. *The ratio strength of the cream is 1:1000 (100/0.1).*

Parts per million

6 The carbon monoxide content in medical oxygen should not exceed 5 ppm. Express this as a percentage strength (v/v). *The carbon monoxide content should not exceed 5 mL in 1000 000 mL of oxygen, therefore the percentage strength is 0.0005% v/v (5 × 100/1000 000).*

Percentage concentration

7 A patient dissolves two 500 mg paracetamol tablets in 250 mL of water. What is the percentage strength of the solution? *Two 500 mg tablets are equal to 1 g. The percentage strength is 0.4% w/v (100/250).*

8 Ofloxacin is available at a concentration of 1.5 mg/0.5 mL. Express this in % w/v. *Since 1.5 mg is equivalent to 0.0015 g, ofloxacin is available at a concentration of 0.3% w/v (0.0015 × 100/0.5).*

9 Xalacom eye drops contain 50 micrograms latanoprost and 5 mg timolol per mL. Calculate the percentage strength for latanoprost. *Fifty micrograms are equivalent to 0.00005 g and the percentage strength for latanoprost is 0.005% w/v.*

> One millimole solution of sodium chloride contains 1 mmol (equivalent to 0.058 g) of the compound dissolved in 1 litre of solution.

Dilutions

- Dilution means to diminish the strength often by adding a diluent.
- In a dilution, the weight of the active ingredient will stay the same throughout: $c_1 \times v_1 = c_2 \times v_2$.
- The strength of a pharmaceutical preparation is based on the quantity of the primary ingredient relative to the quantity of the whole preparation. A dilution of the preparation means a preparation of a lesser strength is prepared.
- Concentration is the opposite of dilution, namely, to render a preparation to a greater strength (e.g. by evaporation).

10 If 100 g of aqueous cream are added to 30 g of cream containing azelaic acid 15% what is the strength of the resulting cream expressed as a percentage? *30 g of cream contains 4.5 g of azelaic acid (30/100 × 15). The new preparation contains 4.5 g in 130 g of cream (100 + 30), therefore the percentage strength w/w is 3.46% (3.5%).*

11 A prescription is presented for Betnovate ointment 2 parts with 3 parts aqueous cream. Express the amount of aqueous cream required if you start with 30 g Betnovate ointment. *Forty-five grams of aqueous cream need to be mixed with 30 g of Betnovate ointment (3 × 30/2).*

12 What volume of chlorhexidine gluconate solution 0.2% w/v is required to prepare 250 mL of a 0.1% w/v solution? *A 250 mL volume of a 0.1% w/v solution contains 0.25 g of chlorhexidine gluconate (0.1 × 250/100). This is present in 125 mL of the 0.2% solution (100 × 0.25/0.2).*

A stock solution is a relatively concentrated solution of a substance used as the source of that substance to prepare a solution of lesser concentration. The strength of stock solution is expressed in percentage strength or in ratio strength.

Density, displacement volumes and displacement values

- The density of a liquid is the weight per unit volume expressed as grams per millilitre.
- Displacement volume is the quantity of solvent that will be displaced by a specified quantity of a solid during dissolution.
- Displacement value is used in calculations when solids are incorporated into another solid.
- Displacement values are commonly used in preparing extemporaneous preparations such as suppositories. In the preparation of suppositories, displacement values are used to calculate the amount of suppository base required when an amount of a drug has to be incorporated in the base.

13 Calculate in kilograms the weight of 5 L of glycerol. The density of glycerol is 1.25 g/mL. *Since 1 mL weighs 1.25 g, 5000 mL weigh 6250 g, equivalent to 6.25 kg.*

The density of a substance is required to convert a volume of a product to its weight or vice versa.

14 Calculate the volume of diluent required to be added to 250 mg of drug when a concentration of 400 mg/mL is required given that the displacement value of the drug is 0.5 mL/350 mg. *Since a concentration of 400 mg per 1 mL is required, 250 mg should be present in 0.625 mL (250/400). With a displacement volume of 0.5 mL/350 mg, 250 mg occupies 0.357 mL (0.5 × 250/350). Therefore 0.268 mL of diluent should be added to 250 mg of drug (0.625–0.357).*

The displacement value is used to calculate the volume that will be occupied by a known amount of solid.

Calculations involving molecular weights

- A number of calculations in pharmacy involve the need to know the molecular weight or the molecular structure of the drug. Molecular weights are given in a number of reference books (e.g. *Martindale: The Complete Drug Reference*), pharmacopoeias or may be calculated from the atomic weights if the chemical formula is known.
- All the atoms in a molecule must be included in the calculation of molecular weight.
- Associated water molecules (e.g. water of crystallisation) must also be included in the calculation of molecular weight.
- It is sometimes important when calculating a specific dosage to express it in terms of the base or in terms of the salt. This is especially relevant when the indicated dosage was calculated from clinical studies based on only one part of the molecule since only that part is pharmacologically active.

Molecular weight of a drug is the sum of all the atomic weights of the individual atoms in the molecule given in grams.

15 Calculate the milligrams of ferrous chloride ($FeCl_2$) that will contain the same amount of iron ion as 150 mg of ferrous sulphate (relative molecule mass (rmm) chlorine = 35.452, iron = 55.845, oxygen = 15.999, sulphur =

32.066). *One mole of ferrous sulphate weighs 151.907 g (55.845 + 32.066 + 4(15.999)). In 150 mg of ferrous sulphate there is 55.144 mg of iron (55.845 × 150/151.907). One mole of ferrous chloride weighs 126.75 g (55.845 + 2(35.452)) and 55.144 mg of iron are present in 125.15 mg of ferrous chloride (126.75 × 55.144/55.845).*

16 A patient is receiving 2 L of potassium chloride 0.3% w/v and glucose 5% w/v intravenous infusion. For each litre, 40 mmol of potassium are delivered. How many grams of potassium is the patient receiving every day? (rmm of potassium = 39). *For every 2 L of potassium chloride, the patient is receiving 80 mmol of potassium (40 × 2). One millimole of potassium weighs 39 mg and 80 mmol of potassium weigh 3120 mg (39 × 80), equivalent to 3.12 g.*

It is often helpful when required to calculate the molecular weight from a structural formula first to form the empirical formula. Figure 10.1 shows the calculation of the molecular weight of aspirin, for example.

Calculating the amount of ingredients

- Tables and capsules are used to prepare liquid dosage forms for children and adults who are unable to swallow solid dosage forms (see Chapters 49 and 50).

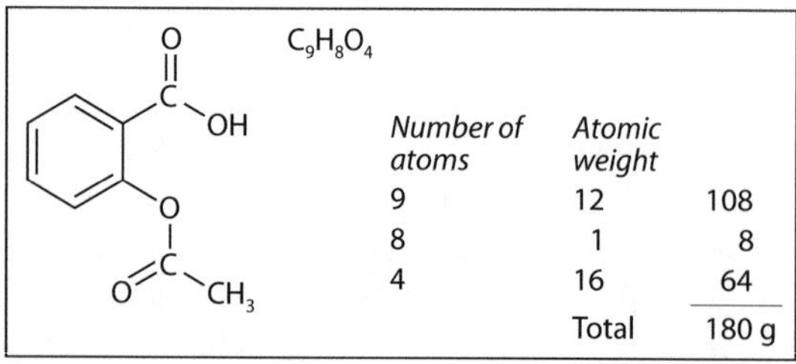

	Number of atoms	Atomic weight	
	9	12	108
	8	1	8
	4	16	64
		Total	180 g

Figure 10.1 Calculating the molecular weight of aspirin from its structural formula.

- Extemporaneous preparations should be prepared only when commercial preparations with a marketing authorisation are not available.
- Uncoated tablets are preferred over coated tablets to use for extemporaneous preparations.
- Controlled-release dosage forms are to be avoided in the preparation of extemporaneous preparations.
- The use of fewer tablets or capsules is preferred over the use of a larger number (e.g. use two 100 mg atenolol tablets if one requires 200 mg of atenolol for a preparation rather than eight 25 mg atenolol tablets).

17 How many 25 mg amitriptyline tablets are required to prepare 80 mL of a paediatric preparation containing 10 mg amitriptyline per millilitre? *The paediatric preparation contains 800 mg of amitriptyline (10 × 80). Thirty-two tablets are required to prepare the solution (800/25).*

18 Cetirizine is available as an oral solution containing 5 mg/5 mL presented in 200 mL containers. How many grams of cetirizine are present in one container? *One container contains 200 mg (5 × 200/5), equivalent to 0.2 g.*

19 Calcipotriol cream contains 50 micrograms/g. What is the amount of cream that contains 30 mg of calcipotriol? *Fifty micrograms is equivalent to 0.05 mg. Thirty milligrams are present in 600 g of cream (30/0.05).*

20 Gaviscon Advance contains 500 mg sodium alginate and 100 mg potassium bicarbonate per 5 mL. What is the quantity of sodium alginate in kilograms that is required to prepare 50 containers of 500 mL? *The total amount to prepare is 25 000 mL (50 × 500). The total amount of sodium alginate is 2500 000 mg (500 × 25 000/5), equivalent to 2.5 kg.*

21 Calculate the amount of white soft paraffin that is required to be added to 100 g of

Betnovate ointment to prepare an ointment according to the following formula:

- white soft paraffin 30%
- Betnovate ointment 40%
- salicylic acid 30%

According to the formula, 75 g of white soft paraffin should be added to 100 g of Betnovate ointment (30 × 100/40).

22 A sugar-free suspending agent is prepared according to the following formula:

- methylcellulose 1 g
- saccharin sodium 0.3 g
- benzoic acid 0.2 g
- water q.s. 100 mL

What are the quantities required of each ingredient when 30 mL of the suspending agent solution is required? *The quantities required for each ingredient are 0.3 g of methylcellulose (30/100), 0.09 g of saccharin sodium (0.3 × 30/100) and 0.06 g of benzoic acid (0.2 × 30/100).*

23 Ten millilitres of an ophthalmic preparation contain 0.2% w/v ciprofloxacin and 1% w/v hydrocortisone. What weight in grams of ciprofloxacin is required to increase the concentration of ciprofloxacin to 0.3% w/v? *In order to obtain a concentration of 0.3% w/v, 0.03 g of ciprofloxacin are required in 10 mL of solution (0.3 × 10/100). The 0.2% w/v solution contains 0.02 g in 10 mL (0.2 × 10/100). The amount of ciprofloxacin required to increase the concentration is 0.01 g (0.03–0.02).*

24 Tetramil eye drops contain 0.3% pheniramine and 0.05% tetrazoline. Calculate the amounts of active ingredients in 10 mL. *Tetramil eye drops contain 0.3 g of pheniramine in 100 mL and 0.05 g of tetrazoline in 100 mL. In 10 mL, 0.03 g of pheniramine and 0.005 g of tetrazoline are present.*

25 Elidel cream consists of 1% w/w pimecrolimus and is available in 15 g tubes. How many milligrams of pimecrolimus are required to manufacture 30 tubes? *For a 1% w/w cream, 1 g of pimecrolimus is present in 100 g of cream. Thirty tubes contain 450 g of cream (15 × 30), and 4.5 g of pimecrolimus are required for 30 tubes (450/100). This is equivalent to 4500 mg.*

Calculation of doses

- Calculation of dosage may be carried out according to body weight or body surface area.
- A dosage is often calculated to obtain a certain drug concentration and to maintain this concentration a dosage regimen is often established.
- Drug concentrations achieved depend on the maintenance dose, the dosage interval and the elimination half-life (see Chapter 13).
- In order to calculate the correct dose for certain drugs specific data on the drug or the patient such as body weight, body surface area, pharmacokinetic parameters or clinical laboratory values (such as liver and renal function tests) may be required.

26 A patient receives 20 micrograms of ethinylestradiol daily for 28 days. How much ethinylestradiol in milligrams does the patient receive in 28 days? *The patient receives 560 micrograms in 28 days (20 × 28). This is equivalent to 0.56 mg.*

27 A salbutamol inhaler presents 100 micrograms/metered inhalation and each inhaler presents 200 doses. How many milligrams of salbutamol are there in each inhaler? *Each salbutamol inhaler contains 20 mg (100 × 200/1000).*

28 How many millilitres of 100 units/mL soluble insulin should be administered to achieve a dose of 40 units? *One hundred units are available in 1 mL. Forty units are available in 0.4 mL (40/100).*

29 Nicotine patches are available as packs of seven where each nicotine patch of 22 cm^2 delivers 21 mg over 24 hours. How much nicotine in grams is delivered in 6 weeks? *The amount of nicotine delivered in 6 weeks is 882 mg (21 × 7 × 6), equivalent to 0.882 g.*

30 A patient is prescribed 2.5 mL co-trimoxazole suspension every 12 hours. Co-trimoxazole is available as a suspension where 5 mL contain 40 mg trimethoprim and 200 mg sulphamethoxazole. How many milligrams of each ingredient is the patient receiving per dose? *The patient is receiving 2.5 mL per dose and this* *contains 20 mg trimethoprim (40 × 2.5/5) and 100 mg sulphamethoxazole (200 × 2.5/5).*

31 A patient is prescribed 75 micrograms per day of levothyroxine. Levothyroxine is available as 50 microgram tablets and each pack contains 28 tablets. How many packets should be dispensed for a 2-month supply? *The patient takes 1.5 tablets daily, which is equivalent to 90 tablets in 2 months (1.5 × 60). Therefore four packs should be dispensed.*

32 A patient receives one tablet Fosavance a week which contains 70 micrograms of colecalciferol and 70 mg of alendronic acid. How much colecalciferol in milligrams does the patient receive in 4 weeks? *Seventy micrograms is equivalent to 0.07 mg and the patient receives 0.28 mg in 4 weeks (0.07 × 4).*

33 How many millilitres are required per dose if a patient is prescribed gentamicin by intravenous injection at a daily dose of 210 mg in three divided doses? Gentamicin injection is available as 40 mg/mL in 2 mL vials. *Each individual dose should contain 70 mg (210/3) and 70 mg is available in 1.75 mL (70/40).*

34 Doxorubicin is available as 25 mL vials at a concentration of 2 mg/mL. The dose required is 200 mg. How many vials are required? *Each vial contains 50 mg of doxorubicin (25 × 2), and 200 mg is present in four vials (200/50).*

Body weight

35 An obese child weighing 70 kg is prescribed amprenavir at a dose of 20 mg/kg every 12 hours at a maximum daily dose of 2.4 g. How many milligrams of amprenavir per day should the patient receive? *The child should receive 2800 mg daily but this exceeds the maximum daily dose so the child should receive 2400 mg daily, which is the maximum daily dose.*

36 Vancomycin should be administered to children at a dose of 5 mg/kg every 6 hours. What is the daily dose administered to a child weighing 4.2 kg? *The daily dose that should be administered is 21 mg every 6 hours (5 × 4.2) and 84 mg in 24 hours (21 × 4).*

37 Filgrastim is available as 300 micrograms/mL injection. A patient with a body weight of 95 kg is prescribed 5 micrograms/kg daily. How many millilitres are required to present the daily dose? *The patient should receive 475 micrograms of filgrastim (95 × 5), which is present in 1.58 mL (475/300).*

Body surface area

38 How many millilitres of paclitaxel are required to prepare a dose of 100 mg/m^2 for a patient whose estimated body surface area is 1.68 m^2 ? Paclitaxel is available as 6 mg/mL. *The patient should receive 168 mg (100 × 1.68). This is available in 28 mL of solution (168/6).*

- The dosage interval may depend on whether the dosage form is a controlled release or a normal release. Controlled-release preparations often achieve a better compliance but take longer to be eliminated from the body, which is especially relevant if an adverse reaction such as allergic reaction occurs (see Chapter 9).
- Calculating the dose using the body surface area is preferred for patients receiving cancer chemotherapy and for paediatric patients.

Rate of flow of intravenous solutions

- For intravenous solutions, the dosage administered is often calculated through the rate of flow of the solution.
- The rate of flow is usually determined by the use of an administration pump or through measuring number of drops per minute.
- The volume of intravenous solution that delivers a particular amount of drug over a specific time period may be calculated.
- Sometimes the administered solution is required to be isotonic. (Calculations of isotonicity are described in textbooks of pharmaceutics and pharmaceutical calculations.)

39 If 60 mg disodium pamidronate are diluted to 250 mL in sodium chloride solution, how many millilitres are required per minute to deliver 60 mg at a rate of not more than 1 mg/min over not more than 100 minutes? *One milligram of disodium pamidronate is present in 4.17 mL (250/60). To administer the solution at a rate not exceeding 1 mg/min, not more than 4.17 mL/min should be delivered. By delivering 4 mL/min, the solution would be administered in 62 minutes, resulting in an administration time of less than 100 minutes.*

40 A patient is receiving 25 micrograms of a drug per hour. The syringe driver has a volume of 2.5 mL and a length of 25 mm. It is set to deliver 2 mm/h. What is the concentration of the infusion solution in micrograms per millilitre? *Twenty-five micrograms of drug is available in 2 mm and 312 micrograms are therefore available in 25 mm (25 × 25/2). Since 312 micrograms are present in 2.5 mL, the patient is receiving 125 micrograms/mL.*

41 Pantoprazole injections are available as powder for reconstitution in 40 mg strength. The dose for infusion is 40 mg. Each vial is diluted with 100 mL sodium chloride 0.9%. If the time for infusion is 1 hour, how much is the rate of delivery in mg/min? *Since 40 mg is delivered over 60 minutes, the delivery rate is 0.67 mg/min (40/60).*

42 Isosorbide mononitrate is available as 0.05% w/v injections. How many millilitres of isosorbide mononitrate injection should be drawn into a syringe to deliver 5 mg? *For a 0.05% w/v solution, 50 mg (0.05g) of isosorbide mononitrate are present in 100 mL and 5 mg are present in 10 mL (100 × 5/50).*

43 A 300-mL infusion containing 100 mg dacarbazine is to be administered over 150 minutes. A giving set which delivers 20 drops/mL is used. What is the infusion rate in drops/minute that should be used? *The patient should receive 2 mL every minute (300/150). This is equivalent to 40 drops (20 × 2). Therefore the infusion rate should be 40 drops/minute.*

44 The infusion rate for intravenous insulin is 0.1 unit/kg per h until glucose level drops to 250 mg/dL. The insulin is prepared in 100 mL 0.9% saline at a concentration of 0.05 unit/mL. What is the infusion rate in millilitres per hour for a patient with a body weight of 85 kg? *The patient should receive 8.5 units/hour (0.1 × 85). Since the insulin solution is prepared at a concentration of 0.05 units/mL, 8.5 units are delivered with 170 mL (8.5/0.05). The infusion rate should be set at 170 mL/h.*

45 Disodium pamidronate 60 mg is diluted to 250 mL in sodium chloride solution. Calculate the number of millilitres required per minute to deliver 60 mg at a rate of not more than 1 mg/min over 90 minutes. *The disodium pamidronate should be delivered at a rate of 2.78 mL/min (250/90). This will deliver 0.67 mg/min, which is less than 1 mg/min (60 × 2.78/250).*

When injecting a small amount of drug directly into the vein it is often indicated to be administered over a period of time. This is best achieved through dilution in a suitable solution such as physiological saline (0.9% w/v sodium chloride in water).

Further reading

Ansel H C and Prince S J (2004). *Pharmaceutical Calculations: The pharmacist's handbook*. Philadelphia: Lippincott Williams & Wilkins.

Ansel H C and Stoklosa M J (2001). *Pharmaceutical Calculations*, 11th edn. Philadelphia: Lippincott Williams & Wilkins.

Coben D and Atere-Roberts E (2005). *Calculations for Nursing and Healthcare*, 2nd edn. New York: Palgrave Macmillan.

Bonner M C, Wright D J and George B (2000). *Practical Pharmaceutical Calculations*. London: LibraPharm Ltd.

Rees J A and Smith I (2006). *Pharmaceutical Calculations Workbook*. London: Pharmaceutical Press.

Rees J A, Smith I and Smith B (2005). *Introduction to Pharmaceutical Calculations*. London: Pharmaceutical Press.

11

Point-of-care testing

Learning objectives:

- To become familiar with possibilities for point-of-care testing in a community pharmacy or hospital outpatient setting
- To identify background necessary to develop point-of-care testing services
- To give examples of tests that could be carried out within a point-of-care service.

Background

Point-of-care testing (POCT) is defined as any analytical test performed for a patient by a healthcare professional outside a conventional laboratory setting. It involves the use of kits to diagnose or monitor a wide variety of conditions including pregnancy, abnormal levels of cholesterol, glucose and prostate-specific antigen, blood pressure, coagulation, occurrence of *Chlamydia* and detection of faecal blood. Equipment such as weighing scales is available in pharmacies for weight management of clients. For examples, see Table 11.1.

Table 11.1 Examples of point-of-care testing

Blood analysis	Cholesterol, coagulation, glucose
Urinalysis	Pregnancy tests, glucose, red blood cells, leukocytes, nitrites, occurrence of menopause and ovulation prediction
Faeces	Occult blood
Microbiological analysis	*Helicobacter pylori*, streptococci

The provision of point-of-care testing in pharmacies:

- presents potential economic benefits
- identifies signs of ill-health
- assists the monitoring of treatment
- increases pharmacist participation in rapid response, chronic disease management and patient follow-up.

- *Non-invasive test:* a test that does not entail penetration of the skin or the body with a needle or other device (e.g. blood pressure monitoring, urinalysis, monitoring of exhaled air).
- *Invasive test:* a test that requires penetration of the skin or body to obtain blood (e.g. blood glucose and cholesterol testing).

Invasive tests require more preparation, such as segregation, storage and disposal of clinical waste, and dealing with spillage and accidental needle-stick injuries.

Sensitivity, specificity, accuracy and precision

To ensure that a point-of-care service is of a high quality, the sensitivity, specificity, accuracy and precision of the tests must be known:

- *Sensitivity:* ability of the test to identify true positives. In a quantitative test, sensitivity also refers to the range over which the quantitative result is accurate.
- *Specificity:* ability of the test to identify true negatives. In a quantitative test, specificity refers to the degree to which results are not affected by other factors (e.g. other substances in the sample).
- *Accuracy:* extent to which the mean measurement reflects the true value.
- *Precision:* reproducibility of the results.

These characteristics are achieved by:

- inherent quality of device
- appropriate location where test is carried out
- careful maintenance of equipment
- good handling of consumables
- competent operators.

Point-of-care testing

- May be carried out at a community pharmacy or a hospital outpatients setting
- Is required to confirm suspected diagnosis (e.g. urinary infection), to detect disease recurrence, to monitor patient outcomes
- May be adopted as screening tests as part of a health promotion activity (e.g. serum cholesterol, blood glucose levels, blood pressure)
- Characteristics that are required for the test to be practical include: fairly simple to carry out, highly sensitive, easy to interpret results, not expensive
- Quality assurance of the testing carried out and the professional service provided should be in place to ensure reliability and robustness of service provided
- Record keeping should include date of testing, strip-reagent used, batch number, result, operator and patient identity.

Limitations of point-of-care testing

- Costs
- Area where to provide service
- Time
- Responsibility for payment
- Safety.

Advantages

- Rapidly available test results
- Enhances patient care in primary care settings
- Supports pharmacists' actions in identifying required line of action (starting appropriate treatment, referring patient)
- Reduces chances of analytical error due to inappropriate storage of sample, inappropriate labelling, mishandling of results.

Disadvantages

- Waste material disposal
- Quality assurance and quality control of test performance and devices used
- Documentation required
- Misuse or misinterpretation of results.

Make contact with an accredited local laboratory to get advice on:

- purchase of the right equipment
- CE marking requirement (see Chapter 4)
- continuing education and training
- interpretation of results and results review
- quality control and assurance including external assessment
- health and safety issues
- preparation of standard operating procedures (see Chapter 70)
- maintenance assistance

Home testing

In home testing patients are encouraged to participate in disease management. Examples of home testing include blood glucose, blood pressure, pregnancy and body weight monitoring. Pharmacist interventions in home testing include:

- patient education on use of test
- choice of test and maintenance of device where applicable
- support in interpretation of results.

Up-to-date knowledge of tests and interpretation of results is required from pharmacists providing the service. Provision of the service should adopt a holistic approach whereby individual patient management is implemented. Risk factors should be identified and the patient should be advised on behavioural changes to follow a healthy lifestyle (e.g. exercise, diet, smoking cessation).

Monitoring of body weight

The monitoring of body weight in babies is used as an indicator of development. In adults, monitoring of body weight is used to evaluate occurrence of obesity and overweight. The body mass index (BMI) is calculated after measuring the weight and height of an individual. See Table 11.2 for classification of body weight for adults.

Table 11.2 Classification of body weight for adults

	BMI (kg/m^2)
Underweight	<18.5
Average	18.5–24.9
Overweight	25–29.9
Obese	>30

Blood pressure measurement

The auscultatory method is the mainstay of blood pressure measurement, involving the Korotkoff technique – measuring the appearance of clapping sounds (phase I) as the systolic and the disappearance of the sounds completely as the diastolic (phase V) pressure. See also Chapter 20.

The patient should be seated and relaxed for about 10 minutes before the blood pressure is measured. When a high blood pressure reading is obtained, the pharmacist should recommend that the patient should have his or her reading checked on two further occasions.

Blood pressure-measuring equipment

- Mercury sphygmomanometer: not used in some places due to environmental impact
- Aneroid sphygmomanometer
- Semi-automatic apparatus
- Automatic apparatus including electronic devices.

- Mercury sphygmomanometers are the gold standard for clinical measurement and are used to test other sphygmomanometers.
- Aneroid sphygmomanometers require calibration at regular intervals.
- Finger manometers are considered as inaccurate.
- Wrist manometers require further evidence and are therefore not recommended, although they may be useful for obese patients. They should be held at the level of the heart.

Cuff size

Error in blood pressure measurement is large when the cuff is too small relative to the patient's arm circumference. The length of the cuff also plays a

Table 11.3 Cuff size guidelines

Arm circumference (cm)	Cuff size (cm)	Designation
22–26	12 × 22	Small adult
27–34	16 × 30	Adult
35–44	16 × 36	Large adult
45–52	16 × 42	Adult thigh

part in the accuracy of blood pressure measurement. See Table 11.3 for cuff size guidelines.

Testing of body fluids

- The specimen collection and the test itself must not be undertaken within the dispensary area.
- Apply simple protective measures designed to avoid contamination of the person or clothing and use good basic hygienic practices.
- Control surface contamination by blood and body fluids by disinfection.
- Dispose of waste safely.
- When using lancing devices for blood sampling avoid cross-contamination.

Diabetes monitoring

Blood glucose testing

- Diagnosis and monitoring of diabetes mellitus
- Indication of high levels of blood glucose:
  - random blood glucose more than 11.2 mmol/L
  - fasting plasma glucose more than 7.8 mmol/L
- Equipment: blood glucose meter, test strips.

Blood glucose meters

Blood glucose meters use the principle that the sample reacts with glucose oxidase, generating electrons and producing a current proportional to the glucose content, which is measured electronically.

Instructions for a point-of-care blood glucose testing

- Meter should be calibrated often (e.g. for every new batch of test strips).
- Test strips used should correspond to a specific meter.
- Test strip is inserted into the meter.
- Clean puncture site with mild soap and water.
- Rinse and dry thoroughly.
- Puncture the skin and obtain sample of capillary blood.
- Deliver a full blood drop on the test area or touch the tip of the test strip with the drop of blood depending on the type of meter being used.
- Result appears on the display screen.

Alternative site testing

- Blood samples for glucose may be taken from alternative sites other than the fingertips.
- Variations may occur when sample is taken from other sites (e.g. forearm, palm, abdomen or thigh).
- The variation is more significant for alternative sites when the measurement is taken when levels are changing rapidly (e.g. post-prandially, after insulin administration and with exercise).

- When alcohol is used to clean puncture site, dry thoroughly before puncturing.
- Do not use alternative sites to fingertip pricking if:
  - testing time is less than 2 hours after a meal, after taking medication or performing exercise
  - area of puncturing is not free from hair or visible veins
  - participation in risky activities (e.g. car driving and operating machinery) is envisaged
  - hypoglycaemia symptoms are not recognised easily (hypoglycaemia unawareness).

Glycated haemoglobin

- Used to monitor management of diabetes
- Indicates long-term blood glucose control

- The same meter may often be used to carry out tests for creatinine and albumin levels. These are indicators of kidney disease
- See also Chapter 38.

Lipid profile

Blood testing is carried out to analyse cholesterol and triglyceride levels. This has been adopted as a screening test, to monitor patients who have hyperlipidaemia and to assess cardiovascular risk.

Cholesterol is produced endogenously in the liver and is also taken up from foods of animal origin. It is used in the synthesis of steroid hormones, vitamins and bile acids.

Cholesterol monitoring devices

A common reaction used to measure the amount of cholesterol is the Trinder reaction, in which the cholesterol ester is hydrolysed by cholesterol esterase to form cholesterol which is subsequently oxidised to produce hydrogen peroxide by cholesterol oxidase. Hydrogen peroxide reacts with a substrate (an indicator) in the presence of cholesterol peroxidase to give a coloured dye.

- When a fasting sample is required, it is best to take the sample in the morning (e.g. for a full lipid profile).
- Two or more cholesterol measurements are required to diagnose high blood cholesterol due to factors (e.g. day-to-day and time) that may influence readings.
- Assess therapeutic efficacy of treatment for hyperlipidaemia after 4 weeks of initiation of therapy.
- See also Chapter 23.

International normalised ratio

- Blood testing is carried out as a point-of-care test to measure prothrombin time.
- The international normalised ratio (INR) range for the patient is usually established in a secondary care environment. Anticoagulant therapy requires regular INR measurement. This can be done in community pharmacies and in outpatient settings.
- Pharmacists can monitor patients who are taking anticoagulants to monitor therapy and to monitor patient outcomes when treatment is adjusted or new drugs included.

- In the interpretation and actions following an INR test from a point-of-care test the use of computer decision support software (CDSS) may be used. CDSS standardises dosage adjustments carried out following INR testing. Pharmacists still need to take into consideration individual patient features (e.g. change in diet due to travel, introduction of a new drug therapy, alcohol consumption, missed doses, bruising or bleeding, patient general well-being) when following the CDSS-recommended dose adjustments.
- Dose of warfarin should be indicated to patients both in milligrams and by colour of tablets.

Referral back to secondary care

- Suspected sensitivity or intolerance to medications
- Alcohol dependence causing difficulties in stabilising dosage regimen
- Liver dysfunction
- Pregnancy or breast-feeding
- See also Chapter 24.

Helicobacter pylori identification

- *Helicobacter pylori* is associated with the occurrence of peptic ulcer disease and is tested for in patients with gastric pain. See also Chapter 16.

- *H. pylori* testing is considered cost-effective in the initial management of patients with dyspepsia in primary care, especially after failure of initial acid suppression.
- It can be carried out as a follow-up test to confirm eradication of *H. pylori* after eradication therapy.
- Testing may be carried out by serology, urea breath test and faecal antigen test.

Serology test

- This is the most widely used *H. pylori* test.
- Sensitivity 90% and specificity 88%. Large number of false positives and false negatives possible.
- It is an invasive technique: requires a finger prick.
- Test is based on diffusion of antibodies from a drop of serum or whole blood obtained by finger puncture through a membrane and an immunogen reaction.
- Since antibodies remain after a few months of eradication, the serology test is not indicated to be used to test treatment outcomes after eradication of therapy.

Urea breath test

- Orange juice may be administered before test to delay gastric emptying.
- Samples are taken 20 minutes after administration of urea.
- Simple kits available to collect sample (exhaled air) are easy to use.

Faecal antigen testing

- This is a non-invasive test based on monoclonal antibody testing.
- It is the least frequently used test but developments are expected to take place to establish it for point-of-care testing.

> - A number of positive serology tests could be false positives.
> - Positive serology tests can be confirmed with a laboratory breath or stool test.
> - A negative serology test can be relied on.
> - Serology may not clearly distinguish active infection from occurrence of antibodies due to previous infection.

Urine specimen sampling

- First morning urine
- Carry out test within 4 hours of specimen collection to avoid:
  - a bacterial reduction of glucose and the formation or reduction of nitrite,
  - an increase in pH due to ammonia produced as a result of bacterial reduction of urea
  - decomposition of leukocytes and erythrocytes
- Containers should be clean and free from detergent traces.

Pregnancy testing

- Various commercial kits available
- Morning urine sample is recommended
- Specimen is tested for urinary gonadotrophin
- Notwithstanding the result of the test, the patient should be strongly advised to consult her general practitioner
- Patients planning a pregnancy should be advised to take folic acid supplementation daily before conception and on initiation of pregnancy. See Chapter 51.

Urinalysis

- May be adopted in the monitoring of therapy (e.g. for urinary tract infection) and as a screening in preventive medicine.

Complete urinalysis

- Leukocytes
- Nitrite
- pH
- Protein

- Glucose
- Ketone bodies
- Urobilinogen
- Bilirubin
- Blood: erythrocytes, haemoglobin.

Carrying out a urinalysis test

1 Dip the test strip briefly in the urine.
2 Wipe test strip along rim of vessel to remove excess urine.
3 After 30–60 seconds compare reaction colour with chart.

Indicators of kidney disorders and lower urinary tract infection

- Leukocyturia
- Proteinuria
- Nitrite
- Alkalinity.

Glycosuria

Glycosuria is the occurrence of glucose in urine. It is no longer considered a reliable diagnostic test for diabetes since there is great inter-individual variation in the renal threshold above which glucose appears in urine.

Urobilinogen

- Formed from bilirubin and is usually completely reabsorbed
- Presence in urine indicates damage in enterohepatic circulation
- Conditions that may present with urobilinogen in urine include hepatitis, hepatic congestion and myocardial infarction.

Bilirubin

- Occurs in urine when there is jaundice which reflects liver disorders or an underlying condition that is precipitating jaundice.

Haematuria

- Presence of erythrocytes in urine
- Indicates renal or urogenital disease (e.g. infection).

Haemoglobinuria

- Presence of free haemoglobin in urine
- Occurs in anaemia, myocardial infarction, burns.

Practice summary

- Point-of-care testing is a convenient way to identify and monitor disease states.
- Test sensitivity, specificity and practical implications should be considered when assessing service development.
- A high-quality point-of-care testing service requires close cooperation with other healthcare providers.
- The interpretation of results and patient counselling are essential to complement the service.

Questions

1 What devices are necessary to diagnose the following conditions: hypertension, pyrexia, haematuria?
2 How is blood pressure measurement undertaken?
3 List four conditions for which it is recommended that a patient undergoes blood cholesterol testing.
4 List ten principles that need to be checked before providing a diagnostic service.

Answers

1

(a) Hypertension – sphygmomanometer or digital blood pressure meter
(b) Pyrexia – mercury-in-glass or digital thermometer
(c) Haematuria – urine test strips for urinalysis.

2 The patient should be seated and relaxed for about 10 minutes before the blood pressure is measured. When a high blood pressure reading is obtained the pharmacist should recommend that the patient should have the reading checked on two further occasions. Blood pressure can be measured using a mercury sphygmomanometer, a semi-automatic apparatus or an automatic apparatus.

3 Family history or personal history of heart disease, hypertension, diabetes, overweight.

4 Training of staff, proper environment, quality control and assurance of the service, contact with accredited laboratory, insurance, health and safety rules especially regarding handling of body fluids and sharps, guidelines on requirement for patient consent, record keeping, method of interpretation of results, quality and maintenance of equipment.

Further reading

Braden B, Teuber G, Dietrich C F, Caspary W F and Lembeke B (2000). Comparison of new faecal antigen test with C-urea breath test for detecting *Helicobacter pylori* infection and monitoring eradication treatment: prospective clinical evaluation. *BMJ* 320: 148.

Delaney B C, Qume M, Moayyedi P, Logan R F, Ford A C, Elliott C, *et al.* (2008). *Helicobacter pylori* test and treat versus proton pump inhibitor in initial management of dyspepsia in primary care: multicentre randomized controlled trial. *BMJ* 236: 651–654.

Elwyn G, Taubert M, Davies S, Brown G, Allison M and Phillips C (2007). Which test is best for *Helicobacter pylori?* A cost-effectiveness model using decision analysis. *Br J Gen Pract* 57: 401–403.

Hobbs F D R, Fitzmaurice D A, Murray E T, Holder R, Rose P E and Roper J (1999). Is the international normalised ratio (INR) reliable? A trial of comparative measurements in hospital laboratory and primary care settings. *J Clin Pathol* 52: 494–497.

International Pharmaceutical Federation (2004). FIP statement of policy: Point of care testing in pharmacies. http://www.fip.nl/www/uploads/database_file.php?id=161&table_id= (accessed June 2009).

Megraud F and Lehours P (2007). *Helicobacter pylori* detection and antimicrobial susceptibility testing. *Clin Microbiol Rev* 20: 280–322.

Pickering T, Hall J E, Appel L J, Falkner B E, Graves J, Hill M N *et al.* (2005). Recommendations for blood pressure measurement in humans and experimental animals (Part 1). *Hypertension* 45: 142–161.

Royal Pharmaceutical Society of Great Britain (2009). Practice guidance: Diagnostic testing and screening services. http://www.pharmacyplb.com/servicespracticeguidance.aspx (accessed June 2009).

Rust G, Gailor M, Daniels E, McMillan-Persaud B, Strothers H and Mayberry R (2008). Point of care testing to improve glycemic control. *Int J Health Care Qual Assur* 2: 325–335.

Urban R, Hirst L and Hildebrandt M (2009). Pharmacists with a special interest in anticoagulation raise standards. *Clin Pharm* 1: 145.

PART 2

Clinical Pharmacy and Pharmacotherapeutics

12

Pharmaceutical care plans

Learning objectives:

- To appreciate the practice of pharmaceutical care in the primary and secondary care settings
- To identify steps required in the development and handling of pharmaceutical care plans.

Background

- Clinical pharmacy (CP) is the discipline concerned with the use of medicines in patients. It requires the application of pharmaceutical science in order to solve drug therapy problems in individual patients.
- Pharmaceutical care (PC) is the integration of clinical pharmacy knowledge, skills and attitudes into a system of multidisciplinary care which aims to provide quality assurance of medicines in use (Figure 12.1).

Pharmaceutical care process:

Quality assurance of pharmacotherapy

Pharmacotherapy in the real world setting: factors to be considered

- Comorbidity
- Polypharmacy
- Incomplete information about the patient's background and drug history

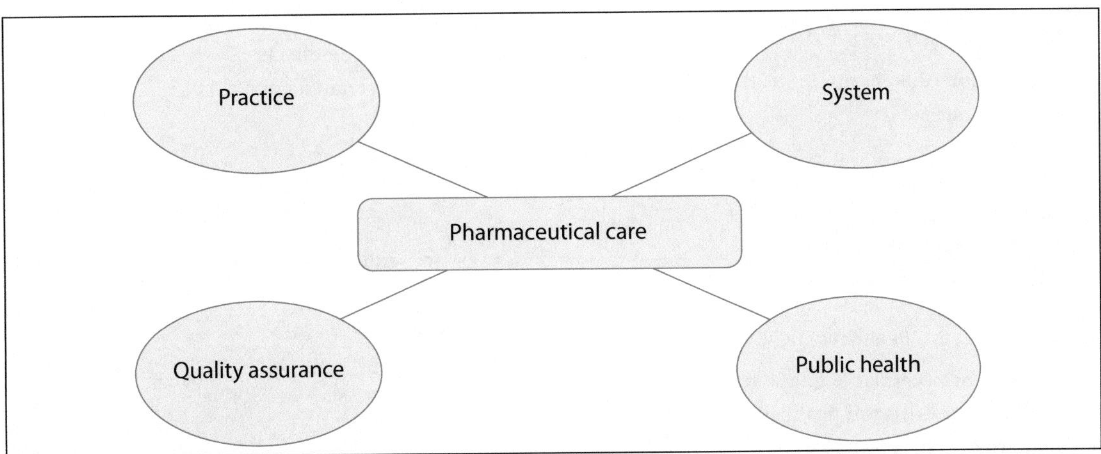

Figure 12.1 The concept of pharmaceutical care.

- Clinical uncertainty
- Patients' responses may be unpredictable
- Evidence base for use of a medicine or a combination may be lacking
- Pharmaceutical care is a monitoring and enquiry strategy to *validate* the treatment plan.

The practice

Achieving rational drug therapy

- Accurate diagnosis
- Knowledge of the pathophysiology of disease
- Knowledge of basic pharmacology and pharmacokinetics
- Ability to transfer knowledge into effective bedside action
- Reasonable expectations of these relationships so as to anticipate the effect of drugs
- Plan of therapy.

Medication-related problems

- Untreated indication
- Improper drug selection
- Subtherapeutic dosage
- Failure to receive medication
- Overdosage
- Adverse drug reactions
- Drug interactions.

The system

Preparing a pharmaceutical care plan

The preparation of a pharmaceutical care plan can be divided into four stages:

1 Define the patient's healthcare needs
2 Specify pharmacotherapeutic goals
3 Identify therapy recommendations
4 Develop patient monitoring.

Define the patient's healthcare needs

- All actual or potential (e.g. due to co-morbidities) healthcare problems
- To alleviate actual problems
- To avoid potential problems.

> **Case study – diabetes**
>
> Ms XZ, a 55-year-old patient living on her own, has hyperglycaemia. She has been diagnosed with type 2 diabetes for 2 years and is receiving treatment. She is receiving human insulin treatment but the patient states that she does not take the medicine regularly because sometimes it makes her dizzy.
>
> Needs:
> - control blood glucose levels
> - avoid any adverse effects from medication
> - prevent complications from disease.

> **Case study – cancer**
>
> Mr BW is a 60-year-old patient with prostate cancer. He is complaining of severe pain that is interfering with his daily activities. He takes paracetamol with codeine, when needed, for pain and has received treatment for prostate cancer.
>
> Needs:
> - control pain
> - control potential side-effects
> - treat cancer.

Specify pharmacotherapeutic goals

- Management of condition
- Prevention of side-effects
- Prevention of related conditions.

> **Case study – diabetes**
>
> Goals:
> - optimise blood glucose control
> - prevent hypoglycaemia due to medications
> - prevent onset of disease sequalae (e.g. retinopathy, skin infections).

Case study – cancer

Goals:
- optimise pain control
- prevent side-effects of pain medication
- treat cancer.

Identify therapy recommendations

- Drug selection
- Dose and dosing frequency
- Route of administration
- Length of therapy.

Case study – diabetes

Drug selection:
- oral antidiabetic agents: sulphonylureas (e.g. gliclazide) or biguanides (e.g. metformin)
- insulin – short acting (e.g. insulin aspart) or intermediate acting (e.g. insulin zinc suspension)

Dose and dosing frequency:
- insulin mixture or biphasic preparation (e.g. biphasic insulin aspart – 30% insulin aspart, 70% insulin aspart protamine)
- number of doses per day vs meal times

Route of administration:
- syringe vs injection device (pen).

Once the patient's healthcare needs are defined and the pharmacotherapeutic goals established (pharmaceutical care issues), healthcare providers need to collaborate and go through a decision-making process to identify a therapeutic regimen which may include non-pharmacological approaches. This therapeutic plan has to be verified and confirmed by different members of the healthcare professions (Figure 12.2).

Patient monitoring

- Quantitative and qualitative parameters (i.e clinical assessment)
- Define pharmacotherapeutic end-points
- Determine monitoring frequency.

See Figure 12.3 for monitoring treatment delivery.

Case study – diabetes

Patient monitoring:
- glucose control (blood glucose, HbA1c)
- assessment of quality of life
- assessment of onset of side-effects due to medications (e.g. nausea, hypoglycaemic attacks).

Case study – cancer

Patient monitoring:
- use of pain scales to assess pain perception
- assessment of quality of life
- assessment of onset of side-effects due to medications (e.g. nausea, constipation).

Example of pharmacist care plan in community pharmacy setting

- Patients with diabetes participate in monthly consultations with community pharmacists.

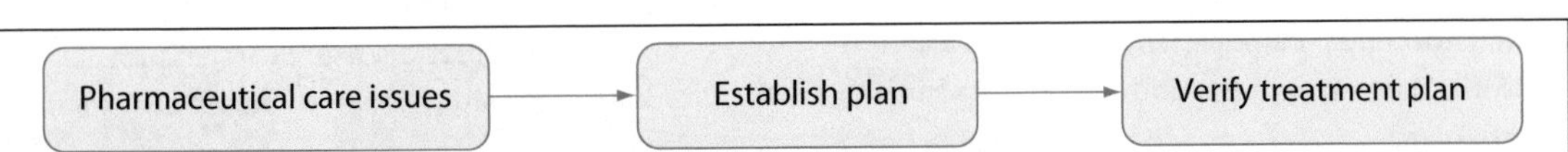

Figure 12.2 Verification of treatment plan.

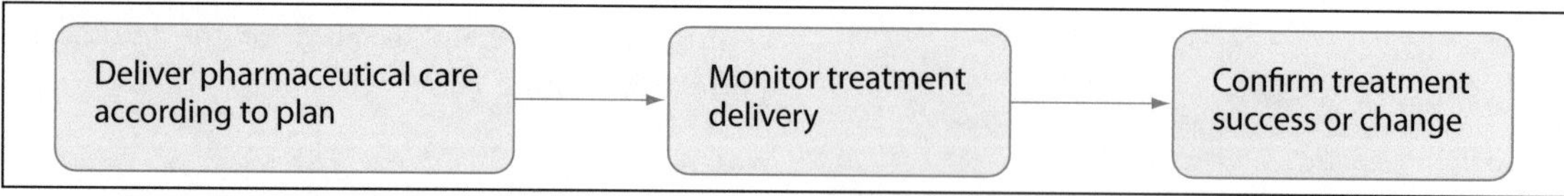

Figure 12.3 Monitoring treatment delivery.

- Pharmacist contributes to education of the patient, clinical assessment and recommending referrals as necessary.

Education

- Glucose and lipid management
- Training on self-monitoring blood glucose and interpretation of results
- Medication management.

Clinical assessment

- Feet, skin, blood pressure, body weight.

Follow-up and referral

- Referral as needed

Outcome measures

- HbA1c
- Home blood glucose measurements
- Health-related quality-of-life measurement
- Evaluation of patient satisfaction with pharmacy services.

Practice summary

- Pharmaceutical care requires integration of clinical pharmacy knowledge which has a pharmaceutical science baseline within a multidisciplinary approach.
- Pharmaceutical care is practised in both primary and secondary care settings.
- Documentation is required in the practice of pharmaceutical care: patient profile, medication profile, laboratory tests and the pharmaceutical care plan.
- Checks and changes to the pharmaceutical care plan are required to ensure quality assurance of the care provided.
- Checks require patient monitoring using clinical cues such as patient interviews, laboratory markers, quantitative tools to establish disease progression, and occurrence of signs and symptoms.
- Changes take place when there is modification of the original pharmaceutical care plan during plan verification, treatment monitoring and patient outcomes evaluation.

Question

1 Outline the features to be considered in a pharmaceutical care plan for a patient with chronic hypertension.

Answer

1 (a) Determine the objectives of care in hypertension.
(b) Establish the importance of non-pharmacological measures (e.g. diet and exercise).
(c) Use evidence-based guidelines to devise a treatment plan.
(d) Identify the optimal treatment options for the particular patient, taking into consideration co-morbidities and individual patient risks.
(e) Promote adherence to therapy and lifestyle modifications.
(f) Identify signs of comorbidities (e.g. ischaemic heart disease, heart failure, kidney disease, diabetes, impairment of vision).

(g) Monitor blood pressure regularly and encourage patient to take up self-monitoring.
(h) Monitor clinical parameters (e.g. blood glucose levels, lipid profile, creatinine clearance).
(i) Monitor for the occurrence of drug-related problems (e.g. side-effects, patient safety).
(j) Verify compliance, assess outcomes and confirm treatment or suggest changes.
(k) Refer patient back to prescriber or secondary care interface as necessary.

See also Chapter 20.

Further reading

Sexton J, Nickless G and Green C (2006). *Pharmaceutical Care Made Easy*. London: Pharmaceutical Press.

13

Medicine action

Learning objectives:

- To understand how drugs work at the molecular level
- To identify mechanisms underlying inter-individual responses.

Pharmacodynamics

- Pharmacodynamics is the study of how drugs act.
- Medicines act by:
  - targeting macromolecules usually proteins: receptors (e.g. adrenaline, histamine, sympathomimetics) or enzymes (e.g. ACE inhibitors such as enalapril)
  - interfering with membrane ionic channels, such as the movement of sodium, calcium and potassium (e.g. calcium channel antagonists such as amlodipine)
  - cytotoxic actions, such as damage to DNA and other macromolecules (e.g. antibacterial and anticancer drugs).

Medicines are used to:

- cure disease (e.g. antibacterial drugs)
- alleviate symptoms (e.g. analgesics)
- replace deficiencies (e.g. insulin)
- prevent disease (e.g. vaccines).

Drug action: receptors

- *Receptors:* specific molecules usually protein to which endogenous substances (e.g. neurotransmitters or hormones) or drugs bind.
- *Agonists:* elicit a physiological or biochemical response that is similar to the response achieved when the neurotransmitter attaches to the receptor. The chemical structure of an agonist is often similar to that of the neurotransmitter.
- *Antagonists:* bind to receptors but do not elicit a physiological response and prevent the neurotransmitter from attaching to the receptor. The chemical structure of an antagonist is similar to that of the neurotransmitter so that it allows the drug to attach to the receptor but the fit with the receptor is very sluggish due to a bulky structure.

Receptors involved in the action of commonly used drugs

Drugs act as agonists or antagonists on the various receptors; some have an equal effect on all types of the receptors while others have a more predominant action on one type of receptor rather than on others.

Adrenoceptors

These are subdivided into alpha and beta receptors.

Alpha receptors

- $Alpha_1$ receptors: phenylephrine, an agonist producing vasoconstriction, and prazosin, an antagonist producing vasodilatation
- $Alpha_2$ receptors: moxonidine, an agonist producing hypotension.

Ephedrine is an agonist that acts on both $alpha_1$ and $alpha_2$ receptors.

Beta receptors

- $Beta_1$ receptors: dopamine, an agonist that increases heart rate; atenolol, an antagonist that decreases heart rate
- $Beta_2$ receptors: salbutamol, an agonist causing bronchodilatation and uterine relaxation.

Propranolol is an antagonist acting on both $beta_1$ and $beta_2$ receptors causing a decrease in heart rate and blood pressure and bronchoconstriction. See also Chapter 20.

Cholinergic receptors

These are subdivided into muscarinic and nicotinic receptors:

- Muscarinic receptors: bethanechol, an agonist acting on gut and urinary motility; atropine, an antagonist that increases heart rate and causes mydriasis
- Nicotinic receptors: suxamethonium which effects the contraction of striated muscle.

Histamine receptors

These are subdivided into H_1 and H_2 receptors:

- H_1 receptors: chlorphenamine, an antagonist that is an antihistamine
- H_2 receptors: ranitidine, an antagonist that decreases gastric acid secretion.

5-Hydroxytryptamine (5HT) receptors

This is also known as serotonin and is divided into subgroups (e.g. $5HT_{1A–D}$, $5HT_3$, $5HT_4$).

- $5HT_{1A}$ receptors: buspirone, an agonist with anti-anxiety and antidepressant properties
- $5HT_{1D}$ receptors: sumatriptan, an agonist causing vasoconstriction
- $5HT_3$ receptors: ondansetron, an antagonist with antiemetic effect
- $5HT_4$ receptors: cisapride, an agonist with effects on the gastrointestinal tract which was withdrawn (see also Chapter 1)
- Re-uptake inhibitors: may act by inhibiting the re-uptake of transmitters (e.g. fluoxetine), which selectively inhibits the re-uptake of serotonin (SSRI).

Dopamine receptors

- Bromocriptine, an agonist that is an anti-parkinsonian drug
- Domperidone, an antagonist that is an antiemetic.

Opioid receptors

These are subdivided into mu, kappa and delta receptors. Examples include:

- morphine and fentanyl, agonists acting on mu, kappa and delta receptors with analgesic and narcotic properties
- naloxone, an antagonist acting on mu, kappa and delta receptors which reverses opioid-induced respiratory depression
- nalorphine, an antagonist at the mu and kappa receptors
- buprenorphine, a partial agonist at the mu receptors and an antagonist at the kappa receptors; it is an adjunct in the management of opioid dependence.

Some drugs act as antagonists for different lengths of time. Those acting for a short time are termed *competitive* (reversible). Those acting for a longer time are termed *non-competitive* (irreversible). In practice this means that the action of a competitive antagonist can be stopped by an agonist. For example, the action of the beta-antagonist atenolol, can be stopped by the beta-agonist isoprenaline.

Drug action: enzymes

These are mostly protein molecules and may be either activated or inhibited. The action of some drugs is explained by their inhibition of enzymes – for example, aspirin inhibits cyclo-oxygenase, carbidopa inhibits decarboxylase, allopurinol inhibits xanthine oxidase, phenelzine inhibits monoamine oxidase.

The side-effects of vigabatrin, an antiepileptic that acts as an irreversible inhibitor of the enzyme gamma-aminobutyric acid aminotransferase, may last for some time after the drug has been stopped.

Drug action: cytotoxic

- Cytotoxic actions often result in death of cells (e.g. bacteria, cancer cells).
- Cell death occurs through toxic action on receptors or enzymes.
- Alkylation caused by drugs could damage DNA and other cell structures.
- Antibacterial action could be either bactericidal or bacteriostatic (see Chapter 34).

Potency and efficacy

- Potency for a drug is the biological activity per unit weight.
- Potencies are compared on the basis of doses that produce the same effect.
- Efficacy is the intrinsic activity of the drug, the magnitude of response.
- Efficacy is related to the tendency of the drug to combine with the receptor (affinity) and the number of receptors occupied.

The potency of a drug is relatively unimportant. Pharmacists often confuse potency and efficacy. High potency is often overrated as an advantage in pharmacotherapeutics. The fact that a drug is more potent than another is often irrelevant in clinical pharmacy practice. It may influence pharmacoeconomic considerations in establishing the cost of manufacture and of the finished product. A drug with greater efficacy may accomplish results that are unattainable with one that is less efficacious (e.g. furosemide is more effective than chlorthiazide).

Pharmacogenetics and inter-individual variation in drug responses

Drug responses differ in different individuals as a result of variation:

- in concentration of endogenous agonists (e.g. catecholamines)
- in receptors (e.g. downregulation or upregulation, abnormalities in structure)
- in metabolism (e.g. drug metabolism, tissue metabolism disorders such as glucose-6-phosphate dehydrogenase (G6PD) deficiency)
- due to anatomical disorders (e.g. fatal reactions by digitalis in hypertrophic subaortic stenosis).

Pharmacogenetics

Inter-individual differences may be due to genetic factors. For example, people who are slow acetylators of isoniazid are more prone to develop peripheral neuropathy, while rapid acetylators respond less favourably to isoniazid as a treatment for tuberculosis.

The acetylator phenotype may be determined by administering sulfamethazine. Slow or rapid acetylators are classified according to the concentration ratio of acetylsulfamethazine to sulfamethazine in plasma determined at specific times.

Patient characteristics

- Identical doses of drugs can produce large differences in pharmacological response.
- Body weight, body mass index, age, gender, concomitant diseases and physical activity influence drug action.
- For discussion of body weight and body mass index (difference in children, elderly and adults) see Chapters 49 and 50.
- Other factors include:
  - diseases (e.g. penicillin distribution in meningitis)
  - physical activity (lower clearance of digoxin during immobilisation).

It is not always clinically relevant to make dosage adjustments in adults according to the individual patient's body weight unless there is a difference of more than 50% from the average weight, taken to be 70 kg. In practice, dosage adjustments for body weight are made for children, unusually small or obese adults, and for specific therapy such as anaesthesia and cancer chemotherapy.

Therapeutic equivalence and index

- *Therapeutic equivalence:* two similar drugs that have comparable efficacy and safety are said to have therapeutic equivalence.
- *Therapeutic index:* the ratio of toxic dose to effective dose of a drug. With drugs that have a narrow therapeutic index (e.g. warfarin) the effective dose is very close to the toxic dose.

Amoxicillin is an example of a drug that has a broad therapeutic index.

Pharmacoepidemiology, biostatistics and pharmacoeconomics

The relevance and quantification of drug action may be enhanced through pharmacoepidemiological, biostatistics and pharmacoeconomic reviews by estimating the probability of beneficial effects, adverse reactions and drug use in populations.

- *Pharmacoepidemiology:* study of effect of drugs on populations.
- *Biostatistics:* study of the significance of the results to identify drug action; it aids in understanding risks of medicine use and reduces errors in clinical practice (e.g. t-values, chi-squared values, standard errors, probability (P values), variation).
- *Pharmacoeconomics:* study of drug treatment in terms of cost and effectiveness.

Evaluation

- Descriptive: describe disease, exposure (epidemiology); calculate rates (e.g. incidence, prevalence, drug utilisation (biostatistics)).
- Analytical: observational (case–control, cohort studies) (e.g. randomised clinical trials, statistical hypothesis testing studies (differences between exposed group and control group)).

Pharmacovigilance

- Continuous monitoring for the occurrence of unwanted effects and other safety-related aspects of drug action.
- Considers drugs that are already on the market.
- See also Chapter 69.

Risk–benefit ratio of drugs

Drug action presents a risk to patients due to the possibility of occurrence of unwanted effects.

Pharmacotherapy should identify the benefits against the risks for individual patients. Risks and benefits vary between drugs and from patient to patient.

Beneficial effects of a drug

- Reduced morbidity
- Effectiveness
- Ease of administration
- Selective toxicity
- Improved quality of life.

Disadvantages of a drug

- Adverse effects
- Cost
- Inconvenience.

Practice summary

It is useful to be able to deduce the action of a drug and its expected side-effects from the pharmacological classification of the drug. In the autonomic nervous system, drugs can be classified as *fast* or *slow* acting.

Fast-acting drugs

- Adrenergic agonists (sympathomimetics): fright, fight and flight reaction (e.g. adrenaline (epinephrine)). Action: increase blood pressure, heart rate, nervousness and glycosuria; reduce bronchospasm.
- Cholinergic blockers (parasympatholytics, anticholinergics, antagonist effect): drying, dilatation and decreased motility (e.g. atropine; antiemetic, antinausea, antispasmodic). Action: increase heart rate, dilate pupils, dry mouth, urinary retention, constipation, confusion.
- Monoamine oxidase inhibitors (MAOIs): vasopressor action (hypertensive crisis) (e.g. phenelzine, isocarboxazid; antidepressants). Action: decrease depression, increase accumulation of amine neurotransmitters (e.g. clinically significant interaction with concomitant administration of sympathomimetics found in cough and cold preparations and with tyramine found in food).

Slow-acting drugs

- Cholinergic agonists (parasympathomimetics): resting mode and gastrointestinal motility (e.g. betanechol, pilocarpine). Action: decrease respiration, intraocular pressure, heart rate; constrict pupil, increase secretions, peristalsis, bladder contractions, muscle strength, nausea, vomiting, diarrhoea, sweating.
- Beta-adrenergic blockers (sympatholytics): decrease blood pressure and pulse rate (e.g. propranolol). Action: decrease blood pressure, pulse, blood glucose; increase fatigue, depression, bronchoconstriction.
- Cholinesterase (acetylcholinesterase, AChE) inhibitors: enhance neuromuscular transmission in muscle, cognitive enhancement (e.g. edrophonium, neostigmine, malathion (insecticide)). Action: decrease heart rate, blood pressure, intraocular pressure, pupil size; increase acetylcholine neurotransmitters, cognition, bronchoconstriction, bronchial secretions, sweating, salivation, diarrhoea, lacrimation, micturition.

Question

1 What are the clinical implications for a drug with a narrow therapeutic index?

Answer

1 Drugs with a narrow therapeutic index (i.e. drugs with a little difference between toxic and therapeutic doses) such as warfarin, lithium and digoxin require extensive therapeutic drug monitoring (TDM) both to achieve therapeutic levels and to minimise toxicity. Drugs with a broad therapeutic index such as amoxicillin are safer as very high doses are required to result in toxicity. Therapeutic index = toxic dose/effective dose.

Further reading

Durham T A and Turner J R (2008). *Introduction to Statistics in Pharmaceutical Clinical Trials*. London: Pharmaceutical Press.

Elliott R and Payne K (2005). *Essentials of Economic Evaluation in Healthcare*. London: Pharmaceutical Press.

Jekel J F, Katz D L and Elmore J G (2001). *Epidemiology, Biostatistics and Preventive Medicine*, 2nd edn. Philadelphia: Saunders.

14

Clinical pharmacokinetics

Learning objectives:

- To understand the principles of pharmacokinetics
- To familiarise oneself with the clinical relevance of pharmacokinetic parameters
- To describe inter-relationships of drug dose, drug concentrations, response and toxic effects.

Pharmacokinetics

- Pharmacokinetics is the study of drug movement in the body over time.
- Processes (LADME):
  - liberation
  - absorption
  - distribution
  - metabolism
  - excretion.

See Figure 14.1 for movement of orally administered drugs in the body.

Factors affecting rate and degree of absorption (oral route of administration)

The rate and degree of absorption of a drug may be affected by various factors including the chemical and physical properties of the drug, the surface area of the absorbing surface, intestinal motility, blood flow and pharmaceutical factors.

Chemical and physical properties of drug

- Most drugs are weak acids or weak bases.
- Degree of ionisation is determined by the surrounding pH and their pK_a.
- Weak bases are better absorbed from the small intestine.
- Weak acids are better absorbed from the stomach.

Surface area

- The surface area of the small intestine from where a number of drugs are absorbed may be reduced by surgery and inflammatory bowel disease.

Intestinal motility and presence of food

- A short transit time and a rapid gastric emptying can decrease rate of absorption of drugs.

Blood flow

- The extent of blood perfusion affects the rate of distribution of drugs.

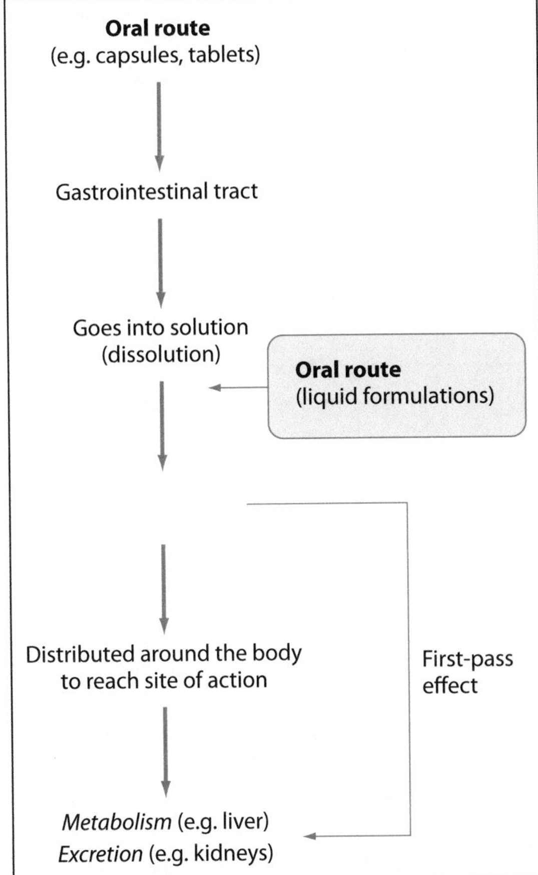

Figure 14.1 Movement of orally administered drugs in the body.

Pharmaceutical factors

- Dosage form: drug absorption increases in the following order: tablets, capsules, suspensions, solutions.
- Slow-release preparations: designed for controlled dissolution and consequently prolonged absorption.

Bioavailability

- Bioavailibility is the extent of absorption of a drug following its administration by routes other than by intravenous administration.
- When a drug is given intravenously, 100% of the dose enters the circulation.
- Factors that account for a low bioavailability include:
  - absorption (e.g. low lipid and water solubility), lack of mechanism facilitating passage through membrane (active transport), drug interaction (e.g. antacids can reduce the absorption of drugs such as quinolone antibacterials by binding with them in the gut)
  - first-pass effect: drug is metabolised in the liver before reaching systemic circulation (e.g. when glyceryl trinitrate is administered orally).

Distribution – plasma protein binding

- In plasma, most drugs are partly in solution and partly bound to plasma proteins.
- Only the unbound fraction is able to transfer across membranes and produce an effect.
- Acidic drugs mainly bind to albumin.
- Basic drugs mainly bind to α_1-acid glycoprotein.
- Warfarin is extensively protein bound.

Distribution – tissue distribution

Tissue distribution depends on:

- organ blood flow
- drug lipophilicity – increased lipophilicity increases ability of the drug to cross membranes, such as the blood–brain barrier (e.g. anaesthetics)
- drug hydrophilicity (e.g. gentamicin crosses membranes poorly).

Volume of distribution (V_d)

Volume of distribution is the apparent volume into which a drug distributes, based on the amount of drug in the body and the measured concentration in the plasma and serum. For example, volumes of distribution (L/kg): chloroquine 200, digoxin 7, propranolol 4, phenytoin 0.65, gentamicin 0.25, aspirin 0.14, warfarin 0.10.

- For drugs that have a low lipid solubility, low tissue binding or high plasma protein binding, the volume of distribution is low.
- For drugs that have a high lipid solubility, high tissue binding and low plasma protein binding, the volume of distribution is high.

> Knowledge of volume of distribution may be used to determine the size of the loading dose for a quick response when drug response takes days to develop with a regular dose (e.g. digoxin). Care has to be taken that the loading dose does not produce adverse effects.

Metabolism

- Metabolism of a drug may lead to:
  - active metabolite(s)
  - inactive metabolite(s)
  - active substance(s) from an inactive form (pro-drug).
- Metabolism involves processes of oxidation, reduction and hydrolysis.
- It is based on enzymes such as cytochrome P450 enzymes and any drug that interferes with these enzymes has a high potential for drug–drug interactions.

Variation in metabolism

Inter-individual variation in metabolism may occur as a result of various factors:

- genetic (slow metabolisers)
- disease induced (e.g. liver disease)
- induction of cytochrome P450 enzymes (e.g. carbamazepine, phenytoin)
- inhibition of cytochrome P450 enzymes (e.g. erythromycin, ciprofloxacin).

> Patient monitoring is required in individuals who are prone to a variation in metabolism of a drug due to disease states or concomitant drug therapy. Patient monitoring includes detection of occurrence of side-effects, monitoring of liver function and identifying clinically significant potential drug interactions.

Excretion

- Some drugs are mainly excreted without metabolism from the kidney (e.g. atenolol).
- Excretion from the kidney depends on glomerular filtration rate and tubular secretion.
- In renal disease, lower dosage is required so as to avoid reaching toxic drug blood levels due to a low excretion rate.
- Other routes of excretion include: bile, saliva, sweat, tears and lungs.

> Patient monitoring is required in patients who could be prone to changes in excretion rate due to disease states or concomitant drug therapy. Renal function is assessed through evaluating creatinine clearance.

Elimination parameters

Half-life

Half-life is the time taken for drug concentration to fall to half its original value. Unit: hours. Examples: chlorpropamide 24–72, glipizide 6–12, nitrazepam >20, diazepam 20–50, lorazepam 10–20, triazolam 1.5–5, amlodipine >40, nifedipine 4–6, irbesartan 15–17, valsartan 5–9.

Clearance

Clearance is the measurement of drug elimination from the body. Unit: volume/time (L/h).

- Knowledge of half-life or clearance provides a quantitative measurement of persistence of drug in the body.
- For drugs eliminated by first-order kinetics it takes four half-lives after intravenous administration for the amount of drug in the body to be reduced to one-tenth of the original amount.
- Half-life may sometimes be used to estimate duration of effect and dosing frequency.
- A drug with a shorter duration of action is often preferred in the elderly and in patients with renal or hepatic impairment to reduce risks of drug therapy (e.g. glipizide rather than chlorpropamide to reduce risk of hypoglycaemia, lorazepam rather than diazepam to reduce risk of morning-after hangover effects).

Practice summary

- When administering a drug the interaction of the drug with the biological system depends on the physical and chemical properties of the drug, the pharmacokinetic profile and the pharmacodynamic effect.
- Bioavailability of a drug differs between one route of administration and another, and may differ from one preparation to another preparation of the same dosage form due to the formulation (excipients used, method of production) of the dosage form.
- When identifying drug therapy for a patient, consideration of the pharmacokinetic profile of the drugs and patient characteristics is required to obtain optimum therapeutic effect and decrease risks from drug therapy.
- Biopharmaceutics describe the relationship of the drug product's physical and chemical properties to its bioavailability, LADME activity, and pharmacodynamic and toxic effects.
- Bioequivalence describes two related drugs showing comparable bioavailability.

Questions

1. Differentiate between the terms pharmacokinetics and pharmacodynamics.
2. Which route of administration is associated with the highest bioavailability rate and why?

Answers

1. Pharmacokinetics is the study of drug movement in the body over time while pharmacodynamics is the study of how drugs act.
2. Intravenous (IV) route – when a drug is given intravenously 100% of the dose enters the general circulation.

Further reading

Allen L V, Popovich N G and Ansel H C (2005). *Ansel's Pharmaceutical Dosage Forms and Drug Delivery Systems*, 8th edn. Baltimore: Lippincott Williams & Wilkins.

Dhillon S and Kostrzewski A (2006). *Clinical Pharmacokinetics*. London: Pharmaceutical Press.

15

Constipation and diarrhoea

Learning objectives:

- To understand diarrhoea and constipation
- To appreciate factors that may contribute to constipation and diarrhoea
- To develop skills required to identify signs that warrant referral
- To review management of simple constipation and diarrhoea.

Definitions

- *Constipation:* a change from the normal body habits, where normal body habits vary from one individual to another, ranging from several stools a day to the passage of one stool every 2–3 days.
- *Diarrhoea:* an increased frequency of bowel movements and the production of soft or watery stools resulting in fluid and electrolyte loss.

Constipation and diarrhoea can be a symptom of an underlying condition and require investigation if occurrence persists. A good history of normal body habits, change in habits, introduction of new drugs and underlying conditions is required.

Constipation

Incidence of constipation

- About 10–20% of individuals believe that they suffer from constipation because their normal bowel habits are not occurring on a daily basis.
- Patient groups at risk of constipation include:
  - elderly patients: due to sedentary lifestyle and poor mobility which diminishes colonic activity, due to multiple disease states and polypharmacy, and due to decreased food and fluid intake
  - pregnant women: due to fetal pressure and increased progesterone levels, which cause a decrease in peristaltic movements
  - bed-ridden patients: due to decreased mobility.

Aetiology of constipation

- Inadequate intake of dietary fibre
- Dehydration
- Lack of exercise and poor mobility
- Failure to recognise or answer normal call to stool
- Medical causes
- Drugs.

Drugs causing constipation

- Antacids
- Antidiarrhoeal agents
- Anticholinergic drugs

- Antihistamines
- Anti-parkinsonian drugs
- Phenothiazines
- Tricyclic antidepressants
- Diuretics
- Iron.

Medical causes of constipation

- Gastrointesinal disease (e.g. haemorrhoids)
- Neurological disorders (e.g. Parkinson's disease)
- Psychiatric disorders (e.g. stress, depression)
- Metabolic disorders (e.g. diabetes, hypothyroidism).

Symptoms of constipation

- Inability to pass stools at regular intervals
- Production of abnormally hard stools
- Straining at stool, abdominal pain and discomfort
- Sensation of incomplete evacuation
- Mild abdominal distension, headache, slight anorexia.

Rome criteria for diagnosis of constipation[1]

- Straining >25% of the time
- Hard stools >25% of the time
- Sensation of incomplete evacuation >25% of the time
- Manual manoeuvres required >25% of the time
- Fewer than three bowel openings per week.

Constipation – predominant inflammatory bowel disease

- Inflammatory bowel disease is characterised by day-to-day variability in gastrointestinal motility.
- In the constipation-predominant variant, frequent passage of hard stools occurs.
- Urgency, diarrhoea, abdominal pain and bloating are all common.

Investigation required

Investigation is required if:

- there is recent onset of symptoms
- change in bowel habits is detected.

Treatment: general measures

- High-fibre diet
- High fluid intake
- Regular exercise.

Laxatives

These may cause retention of fluid in colonic contents. They act directly or indirectly on the colonic mucosa to decrease net absorption of water and electrolytes or increase intestinal motility, causing less absorption of salts and water due to reduced transit time. There are four main types:

- bulk-forming laxatives: e.g. ispaghula husk (powder)
- osmotic laxatives: e.g. lactulose (liquid)
- stimulant laxatives: e.g. senna (tablets), bisacodyl (tablets, suppositories), sodium picosulphate (liquid), glycerol (suppositories)
- saline laxatives: e.g. magnesium salts (powder).

Bulk-forming laxatives

These are polysaccharide and cellulose derivatives that are not digested. They exert an effect within 12–72 hours of administration and are useful in hard stools.

- Example: ispaghula husk
- Action:
  - bind water and ions in the colonic lumen
  - support growth of colonic bacteria thereby increasing bulk, fibre digested by bacteria to metabolites which have a laxative effect
- Side-effects: flatulence and borborygmi
- Counselling: to take an adequate supply of fluid otherwise they may further precipitate constipation
- Contraindications: intestinal obstruction, faecal impaction, colonic atony, difficulty in swallowing.

Note: methylcellulose may interfere with absorption of drugs such as digoxin.

Stimulant laxatives

These stimulate intestinal motility, probably through an effect on the myenteric nerve plexus, decrease absorption of electrolytes and water, and increase synthesis of prostaglandins which reduce transit time.

They have a rapid onset of action which makes them suitable for the management of a chronic attack. An effect is expected within 6–12 hours after oral administration and within 15–30 minutes when administered rectally.

- Examples:
  - senna: anthraquinone group, which may cause discoloration of the urine, dose: adults: 15–30 mg, 2–4 tablets at night
  - bisacodyl: diphenylmethane derivative available as enteric-coated tablets which should be swallowed whole not crushed, to reduce occurrence of abdominal cramps, or as suppositories. The oral formulation should not be taken within 1 hour of ingesting antacids or milk. Dose: adults: 5–10 mg at night
- Side-effects: may colour urine, dehydration, gastric irritation
- Counselling: not for chronic use since prolonged use may cause diarrhoea and cathartic colon
- Contraindication: intestinal obstruction.

Glycerol suppositories and enemas

Glycerol (glycerin) is a rectal stimulant that is effective where intestinal obstruction or impaction is suspected. It is safe to use in paediatrics (see Chapter 50).

- Suppositories: child 1.5 g, adult 3 g
- Enemas: child 2–5 mL, adult 5–15 mL.

Osmotic laxatives

- Example: lactulose
- Poorly absorbed, acts in the distal ileum and colon where it is metabolised by the bacteria to fructose and galactose which increase osmotic strength
- Increases amount of water in the intestines by osmosis. This increased volume results in distension of the lumen which promotes peristalsis
- Reduces proliferation of ammonia-producing organisms and for this reason it is useful in hepatic encephalopathy
- Takes 48 hours to act
- Side-effects: flatulence, cramps, abdominal discomfort, loss of fluid, hypernatraemia
- Contraindications: galactosaemia, intestinal obstruction
- Dose: adult 15 mL twice daily orally.

Saline laxatives

- Examples: magnesium hydroxide, magnesium sulphate, Epsom salts
- Increase amount of water in the intestine
- Cause a very rapid action, used where complete evacuation is required (e.g. prior to diagnostic or surgical procedure)
- May lead to electrolyte imbalance, fluid retention.

Note: use of enemas, bowel cleansing solutions, before interventions that require bowel cleansing (e.g. endoscopy).

- Contraindications: gastrointestinal obstruction, acute gastrointestinal conditions, perforated bowel, congestive heart failure
- Side-effects: systemic absorption, significant dehydration.

See Table 15.1 for classification of laxatives and Figure 15.1 for management of constipation.

Conditions that may present with constipation that requires further investigation include:

- possible intestinal obstruction
- appendicitis
- intestinal perforation
- faecal impaction
- abdominal pain of unknown origin
- nausea and vomiting.

Table 15.1 Classification of laxatives

Softening of faeces	
Onset:	1–3 days
Bulk-forming laxatives	Ispaghula husk Bran Methylcellulose
Side-effects:	Bloated feeling, blockage and impaction
Counselling:	Maintain adequate fluid intake
Osmotic laxative	Lactulose
Side-effects:	Flatulence, belching
Soft/semi-fluid stools	
Onset:	6–8 hours
Stimulant laxatives	Bisacodyl Senna
Side-effects:	Belching, cramping
Counselling:	Avoid prolonged use
Watery evacuation	
Onset:	1–3 hours
Saline laxatives	Magnesium sulphate Magnesium hydroxide
Side-effects:	Sodium and water retention
Counselling:	Maintain adequate fluid intake

Diarrhoea

Diarrhoea may be acute or chronic. There are three main types:

- *Osmotic diarrhoea:* non-absorbable solute retains water in the intestine lumen. Examples include osmotic substances such as sorbitol (found in sugar-free sweets) and drugs such as magnesium-containing antacids.
- *Secretory diarrhoea:* damage to intestinal wall leading to increased secretion in contrast to absorption of electrolytes (e.g. infectious diarrhoea).
- *Motility diarrhoea:* decreased contact time of faeces in intestine resulting in fluidy faeces (e.g. inflammatory gastrointestinal disease, drugs).

Common causes of diarrhoea

- Gastroenteritis
- Irritable bowel syndrome
- Crohn's disease
- Ulcerative colitis
- Neoplasms
- Metabolic disorders (e.g. hyperthyroidism, diabetes).

Drugs that may cause diarrhoea

- Antibacterial drugs
- Antacids
- NSAIDs
- Iron preparations
- Diuretics.

Symptoms of diarrhoea

- Sudden onset
- Mild abdominal cramping pain
- Flatulence
- General weakness
- Nausea and vomiting may also be present,

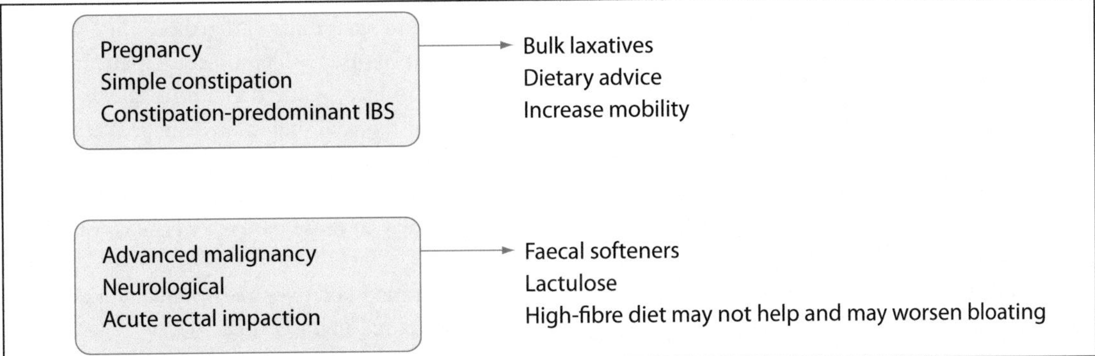

Figure 15.1 Management of constipation. IBS, irritable bowel syndrome.

particularly in infective diarrhoea.

Lifestyle measures

- To use oral rehydration salts to rehydrate and replace lost electrolytes
- To avoid dairy products.

Oral rehydration salts

Oral rehydration salts (ORSs) provide fluid and electrolyte replacement. They are presented in the form of powder for reconstitution, consisting of sodium, potassium and glucose. The intestinal absorption of sodium and water is enhanced by glucose.

Patients should be advised to reconstitute ORSs with potable water and any unused reconstituted solution should be discarded within 1 hour after preparation unless stored in a refrigerator where it can be kept for up to 24 hours. Factors that affect patient acceptance are palatability and flavouring.

> Rehydration, orally or intravenously, is extremely important to prevent circulatory collapse in severe diarrhoea.

Antimotility drugs

These relieve symptoms by reducing peristalsis through stimulation of the mu opioid receptors on the intestinal wall. They are not recommended for use in children.

- Examples: codeine, loperamide
- Side-effects: abdominal cramps, constipation
- Chronic use may cause paralytic ileus and toxic megacolon
- Dose for loperamide: adults 4 mg followed by 2 mg after each unformed stool.

> Opioid antidiarrhoeal drugs should be avoided in children. The use of oral rehydration salts in patients using antidiarrhoeal agents should be emphasised.

Practice summary

- Many drugs may cause constipation or diarrhoea.
- When constipation or diarrhoea occur, confirm that symptom is not secondary to another condition.
- Lifestyle changes in constipation and adequate rehydration in diarrhoea are mainstay of treatment.
- Bulk-forming laxatives, osmotic laxatives, stimulant laxatives and saline laxatives differ in the mode of action, time for onset of action and side-effects to be expected.

Questions

1. Discuss the management of constipation-predominant inflammatory bowel syndrome.
2. Compare a bulk-forming laxative with a stimulant laxative considering mode of action, onset of action, dosage regimen and side-effects.

Answers

1. Inflammatory bowel syndrome is a chronic condition that may present with a higher frequency of occurrence of constipation as opposed to symptoms of diarrhoea. In constipation-predominant disease, patients are advised to increase fluid and fibre intake, avoid intake of fats and undertake regular exercise. In addition, regular use of a bulk-forming laxative such as ispaghula husk may be considered, particularly in those patients whose diet lacks fibre.
2. Bulk-forming laxatives and stimulant laxatives are compared in Table 15.2.

Table 15.2 Comparison of bulk-forming laxatives and stimulant laxatives

	Bulk-forming laxative	**Stimulant laxative**
Active ingredient	Ispaghula husk	Bisacodyl
Dosage forms	Sachets (granules)	Tablets, suppositories
Adult dosage regimen	1 sachet dissolved in water morning and evening (twice daily)	1–2 tablets at bedtime (once daily) or 1 suppository at bedtime
Mode of action	Increase faecal mass in small and large intestines. Useful in hard stools	Stimulate enteric nervous system to promote intestinal motility in the small and large intestine
Onset of action	May take several days for full effectiveness: 12–24 hours and up to 72 hours, are indicated for chronic constipation	Act within 6–12 hours (tablets) or within 15–30 minutes (suppositories), therefore much faster onset of action when compared with bulk-forming laxatives and are indicated for acute constipation
Side-effects	Bloated feeling, blockage and impaction – very important to maintain adequate fluid intake	Belching, cramping, and prolonged use may cause diarrhoea; avoid in intestinal obstruction

Further reading

Elringham M and Yiannakou Y (2003). Constipation: current approaches to treatment. *Prescriber* 19 April: 69–76.

McNair A and Henderson R (2003). Diarrhoea management. *Prescriber* 19 September: 39–42.

Reference

1 Cash B D and Chey W D. The role of serotonergic agents in the treatment of patients with primary chronic constipation. *Aliment Pharmacol Ther* 2005; 22: 1047–1060.

16

Gastro-oesophageal reflux disease and peptic ulcer disease

Learning objectives:

- To understand acid secretion in the stomach
- To appreciate presentation of upper gastrointestinal disorders
- To recognise the role of *Helicobacter pylori* in gastrointestinal ulceration
- To identify properties of antacids and ulcer-healing drugs
- To develop skills to manage patients presenting with upper gastrointestinal disorders.

Background

In the parietal cells acid secretion is activated by stimulation of gastrin receptors, histamine type 2 receptors and muscarinic type 3 receptors. After stimulation, there is a common pathway through the H^+/K^+-dependent ATPase proton pump which releases H^+ into the stomach lumen. Secretion is decreased by the stimulation of prostaglandin E_2 (PGE_2) receptors. Synthesis of the prostaglandin PGE_2 is mediated via pathways involving cyclo-oxygenase type 1 (COX-1).

Gastro-oesophageal reflux disease

- Reflux into the oesophagus of the gastric or intestinal contents occurs which causes oesophagitis due to acidic contents coming into contact with the oesophagus.
- Patient complains of heartburn (see Chapter 60).
- Risk factors: pregnancy, obesity, foods with high fat content, spices, citrus fruit, coffee.
- Occurrence increases at night when patient is in supine position.

Extra-oesophageal complications of gastro-oesophageal reflux disease

- Laryngopharyngeal disorders
- Dental erosion
- Sinus problems
- Reflux-induced asthma.

Lifestyle measures

- Achieve ideal body weight.
- Decrease cigarette smoking.
- Avoid foods that irritate gastric mucosa (spicy foods, citrus, tomato extracts), lower oesophageal sphincter pressure (chocolate, alcohol, peppermint, fatty food) or stimulate secretion (cola, beer).
- Elevate head of bed.

Dyspepsia

This is described as persistent or recurrent abdominal discomfort in the upper abdomen. Of patients presenting with dyspepsia:

- 50% have an underlying cause
- 20% have abnormalities
- 30% have no underlying cause or physical abnormality.

Management guidelines for dyspepsia

- Symptom evaluation and history:
  - alarming symptoms or age >50 years: endoscopy
  - no alarming symptoms, age <50 years
  - symptoms <4 weeks: treat and monitor.
- Test for *Helicobacter pylori*:
  - positive result: eradication therapy
  - negative result: empirical therapy: H_2-receptor antagonists, or proton pump inhibitors.

See also Chapter 11.

Alarm symptoms in the presentation of gastrointestinal disorders

- Anaemia
- Dysphagia
- Epigastric mass
- Gastrointestinal bleeding
- Jaundice
- Odynophagia
- Persistent vomiting
- Previous history of peptic ulceration
- Use of NSAIDs
- Weight loss.

Peptic ulcer

This is the occurrence of discontinuity in the entire thickness of the gastric or duodenal mucosa that persists and results from acid and pepsin in the gastric juice.

Epidemiology

Diseases associated with peptic ulcer include:

- chronic pulmonary disease
- cirrhosis of liver
- chronic renal failure
- pancreatic insufficiency.

Potential risk factors are:

- cigarette smoking
- psychological stress
- genetic factors
- diet
- *H. pylori* infection.

Pathogenesis

- *H. pylori* infection: 95% of duodenal ulcers and 80–85% of gastric ulcers are due to the occurrence of this microorganism in the gastrointestinal tract.
- Use of NSAIDs may cause:
  - superficial erosions and haemorrhages
  - silent ulcers
  - ulcers causing clinical symptoms and complications.

Enteric-coated preparations of NSAIDs prevent physical damage during drug dissolution but do not reduce ulcer risk since damage is due to systemic action by reducing mucosal prostaglandin production.

Clinical manifestations

- Upper abdominal pain
- Anorexia
- Weight loss
- Nausea and vomiting
- Heartburn and eructation
- Haemorrhage, chronic iron deficiency anaemia, perforation.

Investigations

- Endoscopy: very sensitive and reliable test, invasive and some patients refuse to undergo this investigation
- Radiology: using double-contrast barium radiography
- *H. pylori* detection: using serological tests to detect antibodies.

Goals of therapy in uncomplicated peptic ulcer disease

- To provide relief from pain and other ulcer symptoms
- To promote healing
- To prevent complications of peptic ulcer disease
- To maintain adequate nutrition
- To prevent recurrence.

The European *Helicobacter pylori* Study Group (1997) recommendations

When patients are diagnosed with *H. pylori* infection, the triple therapy eradication technique should be adopted.

One week of triple therapy using a proton pump inhibitor,[1] e.g. omeprazole 20 mg twice daily plus:

- amoxicillin 1 g twice daily and clarithromycin 500 mg twice daily
- amoxicillin 500 mg three times daily plus metronidazole 400 mg three times daily
- metronidazole 400 mg twice daily plus clarithromycin 250 mg twice daily.

Drugs used for prophylaxis of NSAID-induced ulceration

In patients at risk of developing an ulcer such as elderly patients, patients who are taking drugs that may increase risk (e.g. SSRIs) or patients with a past history of gastrointestinal haemorrhage, prophylaxis may be considered using:

- misoprostol 200 micrograms twice to four times daily
- ranitidine 150 mg twice daily
- omeprazole 20 mg every day.

Drugs used in the treatment of peptic ulcer

- Antacids: to counteract symptoms
- Drugs that inhibit acid secretion:
  - H_2-receptor antagonists
  - proton pump inhibitors
  - prostaglandin analogues
- Drugs that do not inhibit acid secretion, but have a cytoprotective effect:
  - chelated bismuth salts
  - sucralfate.

Antacids

- These products are weak alkalis that bring about neutralisation of the acidic pH in the stomach.
- They provide symptomatic relief in dyspepsia, peptic ulceration and gastro-oesophageal reflux.
- Antacids may be used when symptoms occur and provide relief generally within 5–15 minutes of administration.
- They should be administered between meals and at bedtime (relief duration ranges from 1 hour to 3 hours).

Systemic antacids : sodium bicarbonate

- After oral administration it is absorbed and may cause alkalosis.
- It is usually present in compound indigestion remedies.
- It should be used with care in patients on salt-restricted intake (e.g. patients with hypertension).
- To be used for short-term periods.

Systemic antacids : calcium-containing salts

- These can induce rebound acid secretion and so should not be used for prolonged periods.
- Prolonged high doses may cause hypercalcaemia and alkalosis.

Non-systemic antacids

These are antacids that are not absorbed. They include aluminium salts, magnesium salts and aluminium–magnesium compound preprations (mixture).

Side-effects

- Aluminium: constipation, phosphate depletion
- Magnesium: diarrhoea, hypermagnesaemia

- Calcium carbonate: acid rebound, hypercalcaemia, renal calculi
- Sodium bicarbonate: hypernatraemia, bicarbonate alkalosis.

Factors to consider when choosing an antacid

- Mechanism of action: systemic or non-systemic
- Dosage form: liquid preparations more effective than solid formulations
- Administration and dosage regimen
- Side-effects
- Taste: flavour of liquid formulation or chewable tablets
- Packaging: convenience to carry around
- Price.

Other active ingredients in combination with antacids

- Antiflatulents: simeticone (used also in infant colic – see Chapter 50), activated charcoal
- Alginates: protectants against gastro-oesophageal reflux (e.g. aliginic acid).

> Antacids may be used in addition to H_2-receptor antagonists or proton pump inhibitors to manage occurrence of symptoms.

H_2-receptor antagonists

These products are structural analogues of histamine. They act as antagonists to the histamine type 2 receptors which are predominantly found in the gastric parietal cells. Examples include cimetidine, ranitidine, famotidine and nizatidine. All have similar effectiveness and all have rapid absorption after oral administration. Cimetidine and ranitidine (Figure 16.1) are primarily metabolised in the liver while famotidine and nizatidine are primarily excreted from the kidneys.

- Cimetidine has an imidazole ring as found in histamine.
- Ranitidine, famotidine and nizatidine have other heteroaromatic rings instead of the imidazole ring.

Side-effects

- Common: dizziness, fatigue, rash
- Rare: headache, liver dysfunction, blood disorders, bradycardia, confusion, gynaecomastia (cimetidine).

Drugs interacting with cimetidine

Cimetidine binds to the cytochrome P450 enzymes and it may cause clinically significant drug interactions particularly for drugs with a narrow therapeutic index. Examples include:

- benzodiazepines
- beta blockers
- calcium channel blockers
- imipramine
- phenytoin
- theophylline
- warfarin.

Proton pump inhibitors

Proton pump inhibitors act by irreversibly binding to K^+/H^+ ATPase. They have a prolonged duration of action. Examples include omeprazole, esomperazole, lansoprazole, pantoprazole and rabeprazole. They are used in gastro-oesophageal reflux disease, *H. pylori* triple therapy eradication programme and acid-NSAID peptic ulcer disease.

They are rapidly absorbed after oral administration and are eliminated by hepatic metabolism. Side-effects include diarrhoea, nausea and vomiting, and headache. Dosage frequency: once daily.

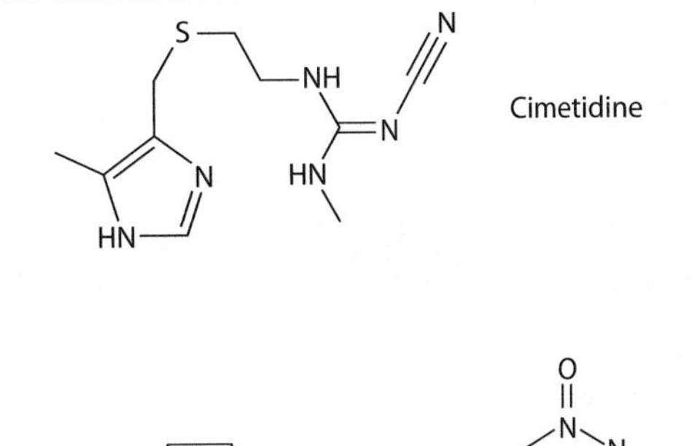

Figure 16.1 Chemical structures of cimetidine and ranitidine.

Interactions for proton pump inhibitors

Proton pump inhibitors bind to P450 enzymes. Clinically significant drug interactions may occur with the following:

- Antiepileptics – omeprazole and esomeprazole: effects of phenytoin may be enhanced
- Warfarin: possibly enhanced anticoagulant effect.

H_2-receptor antagonists and proton pump inhibitors are compared in Table 16.1.

- Stability of proton pump inhibitors: the active ingredient is unstable
- Patients unable to take a solid dosage form: proton pump inhibitors only available as solid dosage forms for oral administration
- In triple therapy for patients sensitive to penicillin: use a regimen that contains metronidazole, macrolide and a proton pump inhibitor.

Prostaglandin analogues

Synthetic prostaglandin analogues, such as misoprostol, exhibit antisecretory and protective properties. They promote healing of ulcers and are used to prevent NSAID-associated ulcers.

- Side-effects: crampy abdominal pain, diarrhoea
- Contraindication: pregnancy since it may cause miscarriage.

Nocturnal gastric acid suppression

Bedtime ranitidine is more effective than bedtime omeprazole on residual nocturnal acid secretion. This is clinically significant for patients taking a proton pump inhibitor twice daily who remain symptomatic during the night.

Acute upper gastrointestinal bleeding

- Around 50% of cases of acute upper gastrointestinal bleeding are due to peptic ulceration.
- Stabilisation of blood pressure is required and endoscopy should be planned.
- In vitro studies suggest that platelet aggregation and blood coagulation are impaired when the pH of gastric fluids is below 6.8.
- Therefore haemostasis may be promoted by suppressing acid secretion using proton pump inhibitors.
- Use of intravenous injection or tablets of omeprazole reduces risk of continued bleeding or re-bleeding.

Case presentation

Patient presents at the community pharmacy with upper abdominal discomfort, retrosternal pain, heartburn, with or without nausea and vomiting.

Table 16.1 Comparison of H_2-receptor antagonists and proton pump inhibitors (PPIs)

Drugs	Cautions	Common side-effects
H_2-receptor antagonists	Hepatic and renal impairment, pregnancy, breast-feeding	Gastrointestinal disturbances, headache, dizziness, rash, tiredeness
PPIs	Hepatic impairment, pregnancy, breast-feeding	Gastrointestinal disturbances, headache

Case management

- Check: any weight loss, blackened stools
- Treatment: consider use of antacids for symptom management
- Recommend use of H_2-receptor antagonist
- Refer if alarming symptoms or if unresponsive to treatment
- Lifestyle advice: to decrease weight, smoking and alcohol consumption, heavy meals and consumption of fried and spicy food

Practice summary

- Drugs used in hyperacidity include antacids that are used to control the symptoms, H_2-receptor antagonists and proton pump inhibitors which aim to reduce acid secretion and the triple therapy used to eradicate *H. pylori* that is associated with occurrence of gastric ulcers.
- Advise patients on use of ulcer-healing agents prescribed, dose, duration of treatment and response to therapy; advise on triple therapy where appropriate.
- Monitor frequency of medicine requests to identify worsening of the symptoms.
- Advise patient on use of adjunct therapy: antacids.
- Gastrointestinal investigations are based on *H. pylori* tests and endoscopy.
- Abnormal biochemical and haematological test results may occur in perforation or bleeding ulceration.
- Assess concurrent drug therapy and other diseases.

Questions

1 Give an example of an antiflatulent and state reasons for its use.

2 Comment on the following statement: Particular care is required in using proton pump inhibitors in those presenting with 'alarm features'.

Answers

1 Simeticone added to an antacid as an antifoaming agent is used to relieve flatulence. It is also licensed for infant colic.

2 Proton pump inhibitors may mask symptoms that indicate occurrence of conditions that require referral and further investigation such as carcinoma. The occurrence of gastro-oesophageal reflux disease and gastric pain in patients who are older than 55 years or patients who present with alarm features such as weight loss, anaemia (or signs of anaemia) and vomiting require referral to check for other underlying conditions.

Further reading

Dominici P, Bellentani S, Di Biase A R, Saccoccio G, Le Rose A, Masutti F *et al.* (1999). Familial clustering of *Helicobacter pylori* infection: population based study. *BMJ* 319: 537–541.

Griffin S M and Raimes S A (1998). Proton pump inhibitors may mask early gastric cancer. *BMJ* 317: 1606–1607.

Hatlebakk J G, Hyggen A, Madsen P H, Walle P O, Schulz T, Mowinckel P *et al.* (1999). Heartburn treatment in primary care: randomised, double blind study for 8 weeks. *BMJ* 319: 550–553.

Jafri N S, Hornung C A and Howden C W (2008). Meta-analysis: Sequential therapy appears superior to standard therapy for *H. pylori* infection in patients naive to treatment. *Ann Intern Med* 148: 923–931.

Peghini P L, Katz P O and Castell D O (1998). Ranitidine controls nocturnal gastric acid breakthrough on omeprazole: a controlled study in normal subjects. *Gastroenterology* 115: 1335–1339.

Stewart D (1999). Upper gastrointestinal disease management. *Primary Care Pharm* 1: 24–27.

Reference

1 Martin J, ed. *British National Formulary,* 57th edn. London: Pharmaceutical Press, 2009, pp. 43–44.

17

Inflammatory bowel disease and other chronic bowel disorders

Learning objectives:

- To identify characteristics of inflammatory bowel disease and other chronic bowel disorders
- To develop skills required for drug therapy monitoring and evaluation.

Background

Inflammatory bowel disease represents disorders occurring in the gastrointestinal tract which are chronic and relapsing. Routine treatment involves mainly steroids and aminosalicylates.

- Crohn's disease: may affect any part of the gastrointestinal tract, from the lips to the anal margin but ileocolic disease is the most common. In contrast to ulcerative colitis, inflammation extends through the bowel wall. Drugs that exert a topical effect are less effective in Crohn's disease than in ulcerative colitis.
- Ulcerative colitis: affects colon and rectal mucosa and the terminology used to describe the area affected is:
  - rectal mucosa – proctitis
  - rectum and sigmoid colon – proctosigmoiditis
  - other parts of the colon – colitis.

Crohn's disease

Aetiology

- Genetic factors
- Diet high in refined carbohydrates
- Infective agents possibly related to infections by anaerobic Gram-negative bacteria.

Clinical manifestations

- Ill-health, lassitude, fever
- Abdominal pain, nausea, diarrhoea, anorexia, abdominal tenderness
- Weight loss
- Intestinal obstruction
- Rectal bleeding, iron-deficiency anaemia
- Extra-intestinal illnesses
- Oedema
- Osteoporosis
- Finger clubbing
- Erythema nodosum
- Peripheral arthritis
- Liver disease
- Deficiency of calcium, magnesium, vitamins C, K, B_{12}, folate, iron.

Ulcerative colitis

Aetiology

- Genetic factors
- Environmental factors: infective agents, diet and psychosocial stress.

Clinical manifestations

- Diarrhoea
- Abdominal pain
- Rectal bleeding.

Investigations for inflammatory bowel disease

- Radiological: double-contrast barium enemas
- Pathological: biopsies taken during endoscopy
- Clinical assessment: clinical index – assessment of occurrence of symptoms; lab parameters (which indicate an inflammatory condition, though not specific to inflammatory bowel disease): C-reactive protein, erythrocyte sedimentation rate, platelet count.

Complications of inflammatory bowel disease

- Toxic dilatation and perforation
- Stricture formation
- Fistulae and fissures
- Carcinoma.

Drugs that may precipitate relapse

- NSAIDs
- Antibiotics
- Oral contraceptives
- Antidiarrhoeal drugs.

Description of a severe attack of ulcerative colitis

- Bloody diarrhoea: >6/day
- Fever: >37.5°C
- Tachycardia: >90 beats/min
- ESR: >30 mm/h
- Anaemia: Hb <10 g/dL
- Serum albumin: <30 g/L.

Treatment of inflammatory bowel disease

- Treatment is aimed at treating acute attacks, maintaining remission and assessing the risk of colonic carcinoma.
- Surgical intervention is resorted to in treatment failure.

Management

- Smoking cessation
- Diet
- Aminosalicylates*
- Corticosteroids
- Methotrexate*
- Azathioprine*
- Ciclosporin*
- Infliximab*
- Adalimumab*
- Metronidazole.

*Also used to maintain remission.

Surgery

Surgery is considered when there is (are):

- failure of medical therapy or uncontrollable drug-related complications
- complications: impaired quality of life, perforation, acute dilatation
- failure to grow in children.

Nutrition

Foods that may cause bolus obstruction if there is an intestinal stricture should be avoided. Patients are advised to avoid intake of:

- segments of oranges and any other citrus fruit
- sweetcorn, peas
- coleslaw, uncooked vegetables, salads
- nuts
- popcorn.

Corticosteroids

Corticosteroids are the mainstay of treatment especially during the acute attack. Their use is limited by the occurrence of side-effects. Prednisolone oral therapy is usually the preferred treatment. It is usually given for 4–8 weeks after which gradual dose reduction should be started. However, some patients require longer treatment with prednisolone to counteract the inflammatory disease. During a severe acute attack, hydrocortisone or methylprednisolone as a parenteral administration is usually used.

The corticosteroids used are compared in Table 17.1.

Corticosteroids

The use of enteric-coated preparations of oral steroids reduces the risk of gastrointestinal damage. The use of these preparations in patients who have already undergone intestinal surgery, leading to a smaller surface area for absorption, may result in poor absorption of the drug.

Aminosalicylates

- Efficacy in Crohn's disease is less well established.
- Example: sulfasalazine, which is composed of sulphapyridine that acts as a carrier (sulphonamide) and 5-aminosalicylic acid; the newer aminosalicylates (e.g. balsalazide, mesalazine, olsalazine) do not contain the sulphonamide carrier and are therefore free of the side-effects associated with this component.
- Dosage forms with the newer aminosalicylates have been developed to increase local delivery of the aminosalicylate to the lower intestine and decrease systemic absorption so as to minimise side-effects. However, this localised effect decreases efficacy in Crohn's disease.
- Side-effects: diarrhoea, nausea, vomiting, abdominal pain, headaches, dizziness, and idiosyncratic reactions, namely occurrence of skin rash, hepatic and pulmonary dysfunction, aplastic anaemia.

Aminosalicylates

- Monitor for maintenance of remission
- Risk of blood dyscrasias (agranulocytosis, aplastic anaemia, leukopenia, neutropenia, thrombocytopenia): patient advised to report any unexplained bleeding, sore throat or fever, and carry out FBC (full blood count) routinely
- Avoid in salicylate hypersensitivity
- Concomitant therapy: avoid lactulose or drugs which alkalinise the gastrointestinal tract since this interferes with the formation of 5-aminosalicylic acid
- Use with care in renal disease.

Immunosuppressants

- Examples: azathioprine, 6-mercaptopurine, ciclosporin, methotrexate.
- Used in patients with severe disease who have not responded to aminosalicylates and corticosteroids or for patients who cannot be weaned off corticosteroids to maintain remission.

Table 17.1 Comparison of corticosteroids used

Drug	Clinical effectiveness	Dosage forms
Hydrocortisone	u.c. +++, c.d.	Foam, IV, suppositories
Prednisolone	u.c. +++, c.d.	Oral, enema, suppositories
Budesonide[a]	u.c. +++, c.d. ++	Oral

u.c., ulcerative colitis; c.d., Crohn's disease.

[a]Associated with a lower occurrence of side-effects but may be less effective than oral prednisolone.

- Azathioprine, 6-mercaptopurine and methotrexate have a long onset of effect while ciclosporin has a more rapid onset of action.

Infliximab

- Used for the management of severe active Crohn's disease and moderate-to-severe ulcerative colitis that has not responded to corticosteroids and immunosuppressants
- Cytokine modulator – monoclonal antibody that inhibits proinflammatory cytokine
- Administered by intravenous infusion and a rapid onset is expected.

Adalimumab

- Used in severe active Crohn's disease in patients who have not responded to corticosteroids and immunosuppressants
- Administered by subcutaneous injection.

Antibiotics used in the treatment of Crohn's disease

When there is an infective component during an acute attack, metronidazole is considered. Metronidazole is also associated with immunosuppressive properties. Ciprofloxacin is considered an alternative to metronidazole.

Treatment of acute severe colitis

- First line: intravenous hydrocortisone 100 mg 6 hourly
- Second line: intravenous ciclosporin
- Check electrolyte and fluid balance, blood transfusion if anaemic

Adjunctive therapy

- Antispasmodics: induce smooth muscle relaxation (e.g. hyoscine, mebeverine)
- Anti-diarrhoeals: used in patients where diarrhoea is a problem (loperamide is the drug of choice)
- Bulk-forming laxatives: fibre improves constipation (e.g. ispaghula husk is a non-fermenting soluble fibre and tends to cause less bloating than other laxatives).

Management of symptoms

- Pain: antispasmodics; avoid bulking agents, wheat bran
- Diarrhoea: loperamide; avoid bulking agents
- Constipation: ispaghula; avoid anticholinergics
- Bloating/distension: avoid wheat bran

Diverticular disease

- Pouches of mucosa extrude through the muscular wall through weakened areas near blood vessels to form diverticula
- Diagnosis: barium enema
- Symptoms: bleeding, abdominal pain, fever, intestinal obstruction
- Management: increase fibre content in diet; anti-infective agents (ciprofloxacin, metronidazole) are used when the diverticula become infected.

Intestinal malabsorption syndrome: coeliac disease

Symptoms

- Diarrhoea or constipation
- Anaemia
- Mouth ulcers, stomatitis
- Dyspepsia, abdominal pain
- Anxiety, depression, fatigue
- Osteoporosis
- Weakness.

Management plan

- Strict gluten-free diet
- Monitor progress
- Add supplements: iron, folic acid, calcium
- Prednisolone for short term.

Practice summary

- Inflammatory bowel diseases are chronic conditions where the aims of treatment are to achieve and maintain remission.
- During relapse corticosteroid therapy may be required.
- Long-term management of ulcerative colitis and Crohn's disease includes use of aminosalicylates, immunosuppressants, infliximab and adalimumab.

Questions

1 Infliximab is normally recommended for the treatment of severe active Crohn's disease when treatment with immunomodulating drugs and corticosteroids has failed or is not tolerated, and when surgery is inappropriate.
(a) Describe the presentation of active Crohn's disease.
(b) Explain the use of corticosteroids and immunomodulating drugs in Crohn's disease.
(c) Comment on the recommendations to use infliximab in severe active disease.

Answers

1 (a) Active Crohn's disease is the relapse of the inflammatory gastrointestinal tract condition which presents with symptoms of ill-health and abdominal pain. Rectal bleeding, anaemia and obstruction may occur.
(b) Corticosteroids are the mainstay of treatment during the acute attack. If treatment fails, then the use of immuno-modulating drugs such as ciclosporin may be considered. The drugs should be used for the shortest period possible.
(c) Infliximab is an expensive treatment that requires parenteral administration and patient monitoring.

Further reading

Feighery C (1999). Coeliac disease. *BMJ* 319: 236–239.
Mpofu C and Ireland A (2006). Inflammatory bowel disease: The disease and its diagnosis. *Hosp Pharm* 13: 153–158.
St Clair Jones A (2006). Inflammatory bowel disease: Drug treatment and its implications. *Hosp Pharm* 13: 161–166.

18

Emesis

Learning objectives:

- To appreciate pathophysiology of nausea and vomiting and how this reflects on choice of drug therapy
- To develop skills necessary for the use of antiemetics in specific scenarios.

Background

Emesis, also referred to as vomiting, is usually preceded by nausea. Nausea and vomiting occur usually as a result of a natural protective reflex against toxins or as a result of stimuli from the olfactory, visual, vestibular or psychogenic mechanisms. There are a number of aetiological factors related to the occurrence of nausea and vomiting:

- acute infection
- gastroenteritis
- labyrinthitis
- motion sickness
- migraine
- pregnancy
- postoperative occurrence
- cancer treatment.

Clinical manifestations of nausea and vomiting

- Sweating, pallor, tachycardia as a result of response by the autonomic nervous system
- Metabolic consequences (dehydration) as a result of loss of fluid.

Pathogenesis

The vomiting centre in the brain is the main area for coordination of the occurrence of this reflex. The vomiting centre depends on feedback from the vestibular system, the chemoreceptor trigger zone (CTZ), the vagus nerve and higher brain centres. The CTZ is rich in receptors, namely receptors sensitive to serotonin ($5HT_3$) and dopamine (D_2). It is not protected by the blood–brain barrier and therefore it is very sensitive to drugs. The vestibular system is rich in cholinergic and histamine receptors while the vagus nerve reproduces feedback from the gastrointestinal tract.

Non-pharmacological approach to nausea and vomiting

- Rest
- Abstinence from food, alcohol
- Rehydration.

Pharmacotherapy

Antiemetic treatment should be considered either for prophylaxis or for treatment of nausea and vomiting when the cause has been identified. Choice of drug therapy depends on the aetiology of the condition.

- Use antiemetics in anticipation of vomiting.
- Consider routes other than oral route (e.g. suppositories or parenteral administration).

Classification of antiemetics

- $5HT_3$ antagonists: granisetron, ondansetron
- D_2 antagonists: phenothiazines (e.g. prochlorperazine), butyrophenones (e.g. droperidol, haloperidol), benzimidazoles (e.g. domperidone)
- $D_2/5HT_3$ antagonists: metoclopramide, dexamethasone
- Antimuscarinics: hyoscine
- Antihistamines: cinnarizine, dimenhydrinate, promethazine.

Antiemetic drugs of choice are listed in Table 18.1.

In motion sickness, the vomiting centre is triggered by the vestibular system. Antiemetics that have an antihistamine or an anticholinergic activity are effective. Serotonin and dopamine antagonists are not effective (see Chapter 61).

Common side-effects of antiemetics are listed in Table 18.2.

Postoperative nausea and vomiting (PONV)

Risk factors

- Female gender
- History of motion sickness or PONV
- Non-smokers
- Use of postoperative opioids
- Anaesthesia: opioids, nitrous oxide, inhalation anaesthetic (e.g. isoflurane)
- Pain, anxiety, dehydration

Table 18.2 Common side-effects of antiemetics

Drug	Side-effect
Antihistamines	Sedation
Anticholinergics	Dry mouth, blurred vision
Phenothiazines, butyrophenones, metoclopramide	Extrapyramidal symptoms, sedation
Betahistine	Nausea
$5HT_3$ antagonists	Headache, constipation, flushing

Table 18.1 Antiemetic drugs of choice

Motion sickness	Antihistamines, anticholinergics
Labyrinthitis	Phenothiazines, betahistine
Migraine	Metoclopramide, phenothiazines
Post-operative	Butyrophenones, phenothiazines, antihistamines, metoclopramide
Pregnancy[a]	Antihistamines, phenothiazine, metoclopramide
Cytotoxic therapy	Metoclopramide, $5HT_3$ antagonists, benzodiazepines, corticosteroids

[a]Drug therapy should if possible be avoided. Domperidone is contraindicated in pregnancy. When phenothiazines are administered during the third trimester, extrapyramidal effects in neonates have been reported. See also Chapter 51.

- Type of surgery: intra-abdominal, gynaecological and interventions to the middle ear are associated with increased risk
- Duration of surgery: the longer the duration, the higher the risk.

Non-pharmacological measures

- Preoperative fasting measures
- Adequate hydration – assess need for intravenous infusion
- Adequate pain management.

Nausea and vomiting associated with cytotoxic therapy

The occurrence of nausea and vomiting with the administration of cytotoxic therapy may limit drug administration because of patient compliance and due to the metabolic complications associated with the occurrence of vomiting. In patients who are receiving highly emetogenic cytotoxic chemotherapy or in patients susceptible to develop this side-effect, a combination of antiemetics may be used. In addition to the conventional antiemetics, a cannabinoid (nabilone) or a neurokinin receptor antagonist (aprepitant) may be considered in patients who are resistant to the other drugs (see also Chapter 42).

Nabilone

- Used in nausea and vomiting caused by cytotoxic chemotherapy
- Cautions: history of psychiatric diseases, elderly, hypertension, heart disease
- Side-effects: sedation, behavioural disturbance, hypotension
- Available for oral administration.

Aprepitant

- Used as an adjunct with dexamethasone and $5HT_3$ antagonists
- Cautions: hepatic impairment, pregnancy
- Side-effects: hiccups, dyspepsia, diarrhoea, constipation, anorexia, asthenia, headache, dizziness
- Available for oral administration.

Some antiemetic drugs that are used in cytotoxic chemotherapy present with constipation as a side-effect. The occurrence of this side-effect may be further precipitated in patients receiving opioid drugs. Consider use of a laxative that can be administered long term such as lactulose.

Practice summary

- Risk of occurrence of dystonic reactions (facial and muscle spasm) due to metoclopramide is higher in females, and young (less than 20 years) and very old people.
- Compared with metoclopramide and the phenothiazines, domperidone does not readily cross the blood–brain barrier and therefore causes fewer central effects (sedation, dystonic reactions).
- Antihistamines and anticholinergics are the antiemetics of choice in motion sickness.

Questions

1. List the unwanted effects of metoclopramide.
2. Giving examples, discuss therapeutic options in the management of chemotherapy-induced nausea and vomiting.

Answers

1. Sedation and dystonic reactions occur especially in females younger than 20 years old and in older persons.
2. For the acute symptoms: oral metoclopramide, domperidone and prochlorperazine are preferred. During chemotherapy intravenous,

administration, of serotonin antagonists is used. Dexamethasone may be used as an adjuvant drug. For delayed symptoms, occurring a few hours after chemotherapy administration, domperidone is the most effective. For anticipatory nausea metoclopramide with a short-acting benzodiazepine, such as lorazepam, is used.

Further reading

Husband A and Worsley A (2007). Nausea and vomiting: causes and complications. *Hosp Pharm* 14: 185–188.

Husband A and Worsley A (2007). Nausea and vomiting: pharmacological management. *Hosp Pharm* 14: 189–192.

Rahman M H and Beattie J (2004). Post-operative nausea and vomiting. *Pharm J* 273: 786–788.

19

Cardiovascular disorders

Learning objectives:

- To present clinical assessment and parameters (signs, symptoms and laboratory markers) that are monitored in cardiovascular disease management
- To describe pharmacist actions (treatment checks and treatment changes) in cardiovascular disease management and the use of pharmacotherapy.

Background

Cardiovascular disorders are chronic conditions, the most common of which are:

- hypertension
- ischaemic heart disease
- heart failure
- cardiac arrhythmias
- thromboembolism
- cerebrovascular disease.

Factors that predispose to cardiovascular disorders

- Age
- Alcohol
- Diabetes
- Diet
- Ethnicity
- Family history
- High plasma cholesterol level
- Hypertension
- Obesity
- Sedentary occupation
- Smoking
- Stress.

Physical examination

- Signs of impaired cardiac function such as reduced cardiac output and/or valvular dysfunction (from echocardiography), increase in heart size (cardiomegaly seen on echocardiogram or X-ray and indicated by auscultation), impaired renal function
- Symptoms of fluid retention (such as breathlessness, oedema, raised blood pressure)
- Symptoms of circulatory disorder and/or impaired oxygenation (pallor, muscular weakness and pain, paraesthesia and cyanosis)
- Signs of arrhythmia from pulse, auscultation and heart sounds
- Examination of the entire patient: to assess for signs of tiredness, depression, anxiety, diminished mobility and evidence of loss of quality of life or well-being.

Measures of cardiovascular function

- Blood pressure: to identify high blood pressure as a risk factor of ischaemic heart disease and stroke or a low blood pressure associated with heart failure
- Pulse rate and regularity
- Ejection fraction: (%) of left ventricular stroke volume

- Estimation of heart size from echocardiography, X-ray and auscultation.

Other physical signs and symptoms

- Symptoms presented: fainting spells, cough at night, oedema of the ankle, chest pain, dyspnoea. Description of the type of chest pain felt helps to differentiate between chest pain due to cardiovascular disorders and non-cardiac chest pain. In angina and myocardial infarction the pain is described as being compressive in nature, with the patient describing tightness, 'crushing' and heavy pressure.
- Investigation: chest X-ray to detect enlarged heart due to heart failure (left ventricular dilatation due to high pre-load, that is overstretching of the heart in decompensated heart failure).
- Stress test (exercise test): to determine heart response to the stress associated with exercise – muscular activity.

Laboratory tests

- Cardiac enzymes: creatine kinase (CK) and its isoenzyme fraction CK-MB, lactic dehydrogenase and its isoenzymes LDH_1 and LDH_2 are enzymes that are found in the cardiac muscle. Their level in serum rises subsequent to cardiac muscle cell damage and they are used as parameters to identify myocardial infarction. CK-MB rises within 3–5 hours after a myocardial infarction while LDH increases within 12 hours after a myocardial infarction.
- C-reactive protein: a biological marker for systemic inflammation and is increased in patients at risk of myocardial infarction, stroke and peripheral arterial disease.
- Lipid profile: to evaluate occurrence of hyperlipidaemia.
- Troponins: troponin I and T are complexes of proteins that are specific to cardiac muscle involved in the mediation of actin and myosin interaction at the muscular level. Their levels increase within a few hours of a myocardial infarction.

Stress/exercise test

ECG is recorded at rest and during a standard protocol of gradually increasing levels of exercise. This:

- indicates degree of coronary artery disease
- assesses ability to perform daily activities.

Patients taking beta-adrenoceptor blockers and calcium channel blockers tend to have bradycardia and therefore are not able to achieve their maximal heart rates. These patients would be limited from exercising to full capacity during a stress test. Rapid withdrawal of beta-adrenoceptor blockers and calcium channel blockers may cause exacerbation of angina.

It may be undertaken as a screening test or to monitor patient outcomes following a myocardial infarction or to assess therapeutic management.

- Contraindications: unstable angina, physiological limitations (e.g. mobility restrictions, severe respiratory disease).

Echocardiography

Carried out to assess heart valves, septum and cardiac muscle walls. Size, shape and movement during the cardiac cycle are assessed. In Doppler echocardiography, cardiac blood flow patterns are evaluated.

Cardiac catheterisation

A catheter is threaded through the right and left side of the heart to assess pressures in the heart chambers. It is used to evaluate cardiac function.

- In angiography a contrast agent is injected into the coronary arteries for visualisation purposes. Used to assess the size of the artery and extent of occlusion and to plan interventions. Interventions that may be performed during angiography include percutaneous transluminal coronary angioplasty and stent placement.

- In angioplasty a balloon catheter is introduced into coronary arteries to correct for narrowing of the blood vessels.

Contraindications

- Conditions that predispose to a higher risk of bleeding during or after the intervention: cerebrovascular accident, severe anaemia, uncontrolled hypertension, active gastrointestinal bleeding, anticoagulation (warfarin)
- Fever or untreated infection
- Allergy to angiographic contrast dyes.

Coronary artery by-pass surgery (CABG)

Early complications

- Arrhythmias
- Chest pain
- Fever and wound infection
- Neuropsychological change.

Medications considered in post-CABG patients

- Antiplatelet agents (e.g. aspirin)
- Cardioprotective drugs (e.g. perindopril (angioven-converting enzyme or ACE inhibitor))
- Lipid-regulating drugs (statins).

Classification of anti-arrhythmic drugs

- Act on supraventricular arrhythmias (e.g. adenosine, digoxin, verapamil)
- Act on supraventricular and ventricular arrhythmias (e.g. amiodarone, beta blockers such as carvedilol and sotalol, flecainide)
- Act on ventricular arrhythmias (e.g. lidocaine).

Anti-arrhythmic agents have a negative inotropic effect and this tends to be additive if multiple therapy is adopted. The occurrence of hypokalaemia or hyperkalaemia increases the risk of arrhythmias. In post-CABG patients atrial fibrillations are common in the early postoperative days. Unless contraindicated, beta blockers are preferred since following surgery there is a high sympathetic tone. Amiodarone and verapamil may also be considered.

Adenosine

- Used in supraventricular arrhythmias, causes temporary complete sinoatrial and atrioventricular block
- Short duration of action (10–20 seconds), prolonged if patient taking dipyridamole
- Contraindication: asthma (verapamil is preferred)
- Side-effects: unpleasant sensation in the chest, transient facial flush, headache
- Administration by rapid intravenous injection.

Amiodarone

- Used for supraventricular and ventricular arrhythmias, slows heart rate and AV conduction
- Disadvantages: very long half-life (50 days), side-effect profile, drug interactions
- Contraindications: heart sinus bradycardia, thyroid disorders
- Side-effects: corneal microdeposits (interfere with night vision), phototoxicity (requires use of sunscreen continued for a few months after withdrawal), thyroid dysfunction, peripheral neuropathy, pulmonary fibrosis, hepatotoxicity
- Patient monitoring: thyroid function, liver function, ECG, eye examination since drug should be stopped to prevent blindness if optic neuritis or optic neuropathy occurs
- Drug interactions: increased risk of arrhythmias (e.g. with moxifloxacin, co-trimoxazole, antipsychotics, tricyclic antidepressants), increased anticoagulant effect (e.g. with warfarin), increased risk of myopathy (e.g. with

simvastatin), increased risk of bradycardia (e.g. with beta-blockers)
- Administration as intravenous infusion or orally (tablets).

Flecainide

- Used for supraventricular and ventricular arrhythmias especially management of acute arrhythmias
- Contraindications: heart failure, history of myocardial infarction
- Caution: hypokalaemia reduces efficacy of flecainide and increases risk of precipitating serious arrhythmias
- Side-effects: nausea, vomiting, dyspnoea, visual disturbances
- Patient monitoring: plasma potassium concentration
- Drug interactions: increased risk of bradycardia (e.g. with beta-blockers), increased risk of arrhythmias (e.g. with antipsychotics, tricyclic antidepressants)
- Administration as intravenous infusion or orally (tablets).

Lidocaine

- Used in ventricular arrhythmias especially in emergency use and after myocardial infarction
- Contraindications: atrioventricular (AV) block
- Side-effects: dizziness, paraesthesia or drowsiness (reduced by administering intravenous injection slowly)
- Administration: parenteral (injection or infusion). With intravenous injection, duration of action is short (about 15–20 minutes).

Cardiac transplantation

Risk factors

- Type 1 diabetes
- Hyperlipidaemia.

Postoperative management

- Positive inotropic drugs to stimulate heart muscle contraction and increase heart rate
- Immunosuppression to prevent organ rejection.

Managing cardiac emergencies

- Ventricular fibrillations may cause cardiac arrest and they can be detected from the ECG. Electrolyte imbalance, hypoxia and acidosis may predispose a patient to develop ventricular fibrillations. Patient is defibrillated using a defibrillator.
- AV blocks (heart blocks) may occur after heart surgery or myocardial infarction or damage to the AV node.
- In ventricular fibrillations, adrenaline is administered through an intravenous line to induce heart beats and increase blood flow.
- In AV blocks, atropine is used and the degree of heart block is assessed to identify need for a pacemaker.

Sympathomimetic drugs

The clinical effects of sympathomimetic drugs depend on the extent of activity at the different receptors within the sympathetic nervous system (alpha, $beta_1$ and $beta_2$) (see also Chapter 13).

Adrenaline

- Adrenaline is a potent stimulator of alpha and beta receptors
- Common side-effect: tachycardia
- Administration and uses:
  - anaphylactic shock – administered by intramuscular injection; pen device for patient self-administration for management of severe allergy
  - cardiac arrest – intravenous administration preferably through a central line; if injected through a peripheral line, drug must be

flushed with saline to aid entry into central circulation.

Noradrenaline

- Compared with adrenaline, noradrenaline lacks the methyl substitution in the amino group. Noradrenaline is a potent agonist at alpha receptors. Compared with adrenaline it has equipotent activity at $beta_1$ receptors but little action on $beta_2$ receptors.
- Common side-effects: bradycardia, hypertension
- Administration and uses:
  - acute hypotension: intravenous infusion via central venous catheter
  - cardiac arrest: rapid intravenous or intra-cardiac injection.

Noradrenaline and adrenaline are compared in Table 19.1.

Dopamine

- Dopamine is a precursor of noradrenaline and adrenaline. It is a cardiac stimulant through its interaction with the $beta_1$ receptors in the cardiac muscle. It also causes the release of norepinephrine from nerve terminals.
- When given at low doses, it increases systolic blood pressure with minimal effect on peripheral resistance.
- Side-effects: nausea, vomiting, peripheral vasoconstriction, tachycardia.
- Administration: intravenous infusion.

Clinical uses of sympathomimetics

The clinical use of noradrenaline, adrenaline and dopamine are listed in Table 19.2.

Onset of action of sympathomimetics

- Noradrenaline: immediate
- Adrenaline: 3–5 minutes
- Dopamine: 2–5 minutes.

Table 19.2 Clinical uses of sympathomimetics

Drug	Clinical use
Noradrenaline	Acute hypotension Cardiac arrest
Adrenaline	Acute anaphylaxis Angioedema Cardiopulmonary resuscitation
Dopamine	Cardiogenic shock in infarction or cardiac surgery

Table 19.1 Comparing noradrenaline and adrenaline

	Noradrenaline	Adrenaline
Structure	HO, HO, OH, NH_2	HO, HO, OH, H, N, CH_3
Pulse rate	Decreased, cardiac output is unchanged or decreased	Increased, cardiac output is enhanced
Blood pressure	Increased, increased systolic and diastolic blood pressure	Increased for systolic blood pressure, diastolic blood pressure increased at higher doses
Peripheral resistance	Increased due to activity on alpha receptors, results in decreased blood flow to kidneys and liver	Decreased
Respiratory effects	Bronchodilator effect	Bronchodilator effect

Atropine

- Atropine is a tertiary amine antimuscarinic agent which increases the heart rate.
- It inhibits parasympathetic system and results in blockage or slowing down of the sinoatrial node.
- It is used in bradycardia and in occurrences of bradyarrhythmias such as prevention and management of bradyarrhythmias in anaesthesia and in cardiac arrest.
- It is administered intravenously as a single dose in cardiopulmonary resuscitation.
- Common side-effects: bradycardia (low doses), tachycardia (high doses).
- See also Chapter 13.

Practice summary

- Patients with a cardiovascular condition may have other cardiac comorbidities which need to be taken into consideration when identifying drug therapy and planning patient monitoring.
- Drug therapy and lifestyle modifications are for the long term. Patient needs to receive information on the medication, and drug-related problems should be identified so as to achieve patient compliance.
- Parameters of cardiovascular function, physical examination and laboratory tests could be used routinely to assess patient condition and monitor treatment outcomes.

Question

1 Describe the use of sympathomimetic agents in anaphylactic shock.

Answer

1 Sympathomimetic agents such as adrenaline are used in acute anaphylaxis. Adrenaline is a potent $beta_2$ agonist which increases heart rate and force of contraction. A common side-effect is tachycardia. It stimulates alpha receptors at higher concentrations. Onset of action is 3–5 minutes. Administered as an intramuscular injection or as a pen device for patient self-administration for management of severe allergy.

Further reading

Chernecky C, Alichnie M C, Garrett K, George-Gay B, Hodges R K and Terry C (2002). *ECGs and the Heart.* Philadelphia: WB Saunders Co.

Longe R L, Calvert J C and Young L Y, eds (1996). *Physical Assessment: A guide for evaluating drug therapy.* Vancouver: Applied Therapeutics Inc.

Tietze K J (2004). *Clinical Skills for Pharmacists: A patient-focused approach*, 2nd edn. St Louis: Mosby.

Acknowledgements

Bernard Coleiro, Consultant Physician, Department of Medicine, Mater Dei Hospital, Malta.

20

Hypertension

Learning objectives:

- To understand regulation of blood pressure and significance of hypertension
- To familiarise oneself with blood pressure monitoring
- To identify drugs used in hypertension and appreciate their characteristics
- To review current guidelines for the management of hypertension
- To understand management goals
- To appreciate use of drug therapy, patient monitoring and follow-up required
- To identify principles of drug therapy in hypertensive emergency.

Background

Hypertension is a chronic condition characterised by a sustained diastolic reading greater than or equal to 80 mmHg and a systolic reading greater than or equal to 120 mmHg (120/80 mmHg). Occurrence can damage blood vessels and increase probability of development of atheromatous disease. Treatment is aimed to decrease morbidity and mortality.

Factors implicated in primary hypertension include:

- age
- genetics
- environment
- weight
- race.

Causes of secondary hypertension include:

- renal disease
- pregnancy
- hormonal factors
- drug-induced factors (e.g. oral contraceptives, corticosteroids).

Regulation of blood pressure

- Peripheral vascular resistance (depends on arteriolar volume)
- Cardiac output (depends on heart rate, contractility, filling pressure, blood volume)
- Blood pressure = cardiac output × peripheral vascular resistance.

Sympathetic nervous system

Baroreceptors present in the aorta and carotid sinus:

- increase cardiac output
- increase peripheral resistance.

The renin–angiotensin–aldosterone system is shown in Figure 20.1.

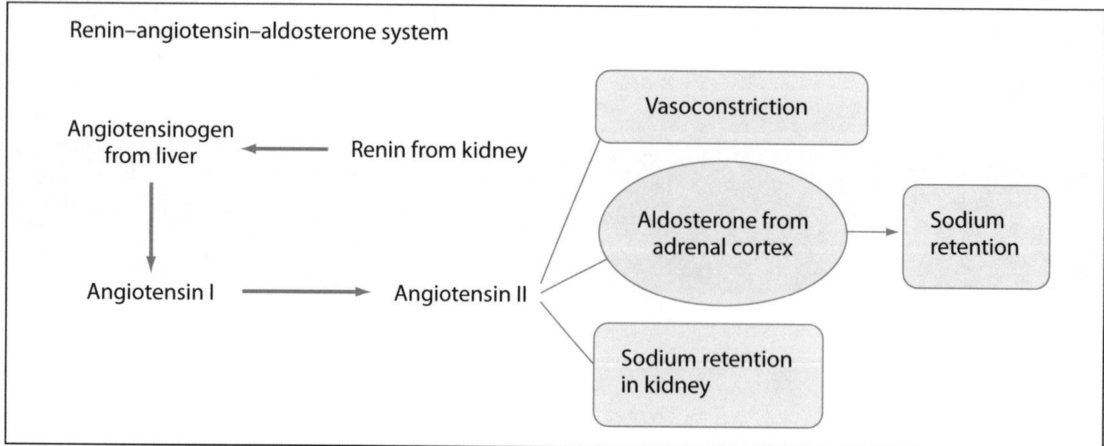

Figure 20.1 Renin–angiotensin–aldosterone system.

Risk factors

- Family history
- Age
- Obesity
- Smoking
- Lifestyle: stress, sedentary, diet
- Diabetes mellitus
- Hyperlipidaemia.

Target organ damage due to hypertension

- Cardiovascular: constriction of arterioles and insufficient blood flow to coronary vasculature leads to angina, myocardial infarction; left ventricular hypertrophy may occur due to increased cardiac output leading to heart failure.
- Renal: arteriolar nephrosclerosis leads to polyuria, nocturia, protein and red blood cells in urine, elevated serum creatinine, renal insufficiency.
- Cerebral: decreased blood flow and decreased oxygen supply lead to transient ischaemic attacks, cerebral thromboses, haemorrhage.
- Retinal: damage to arterioles of retina leads to haemorrhage, visual disturbances.

Occurrence of hypertension may exacerbate:

- atherosclerosis
- coronary artery disease
- congestive heart failure
- diabetes mellitus
- insulin resistance
- stroke
- renal disease
- retinal disease.

Blood pressure measurement

Using a sphygmomanometer (see also Chapter 11)

- Patient should be relaxed, sitting down with arm at about the level of the heart; check pressure in both arms.
- Three consecutive elevated readings taken on three separate occasions should be documented before the diagnosis of 'hypertension' is applied to a patient.
- Interpretation of results: systolic reading is more important than diastolic reading; patient history and family history are taken into consideration when deciding on line of action.

Management goals

- European Guidelines for the management of hypertension were issued in June 2007 by the European Society of Hypertension jointly with the European Society of Cardiology.[1]
- Overall goal to achieve blood pressure (BP) of 140/90 mmHg.
- Goal takes into consideration comorbidities (e.g. in diabetes the goal is to achieve 130/80 mmHg).
- Pharmacotherapy should consider the five important drug classes: ACE inhibitors, angiotensin receptor antagonists, beta-blockers, calcium channel blockers and diuretics.
- Choice of drug therapy should depend on:
  - comorbidities (e.g. diabetes mellitus – ACE inhibitors or angiotensin receptor antagonists; metabolic syndrome – angiotensin-converting enzyme (ACE) inhibitors, angiotensin receptor antagonists, calcium antagonists)
  - history of clinical events (e.g. myocardial infarction – beta-blockers, ACE inhibitors, angiotensin receptor antagonists; angina pectoris – beta-blockers, calcium channel blockers (avoiding short-acting dihydropyridines); heart failure – diuretics, beta-blockers (particularly carvedilol), ACE inhibitors, angiotensin receptor antagonists)
  - organ damage (e.g. renal dysfunction – ACE inhibitors, angiotensin receptor antagonists; left ventricular hypertrophy – ACE inhibitors, angiotensin receptor antagonists, calcium channel blockers).
- Regardless of which drug therapy is used, monotherapy achieves blood pressure goal in only a limited number of patients. Majority of patients require multiple drug therapy.
- Lifestyle measures are relevant for all patients: smoking cessation, weight reduction and maintenance, reduction of excessive alcohol intake, physical exercise, reduction of salt intake, increased fruit and vegetable intake, decreased saturated and total fat intake.

When to refer

- High blood pressure (more than 180/110 mmHg with signs of papilloedema and/or retinal haemorrhage)
- Suspected phaeochromocytoma (signs include labile or postural hypotension, headache, palpitations, pallor and diaphoresis)
- Unusual signs and symptoms or symptoms that suggest a secondary cause of high blood pressure.

Management of hypertension

- Confirm diagnosis through repeated blood pressure measurement
- Patient assessment for underlying cause(s) and comorbidities
- Assess occurrence of target organ damage
- Review treatment options
- Establish treatment goals
- Identify and manage other risk factors (e.g. hyperlipidaemia)
- Patient follow-up.

Reviewing treatment options

- Pharmacotherapy or non-pharmacological measures only?
- Which drug(s)?

Diagnosis and management of hypertension are shown in Figure 20.2.

Cardiovascular risk assessment

- Urine test for proteinuria and albuminuria
- Blood tests: glucose, electrolytes, creatinine, serum total cholesterol and high-density lipoprotein (HDL) cholesterol
- ECG.

Lifestyle changes

- Weight reduction
- Exercise

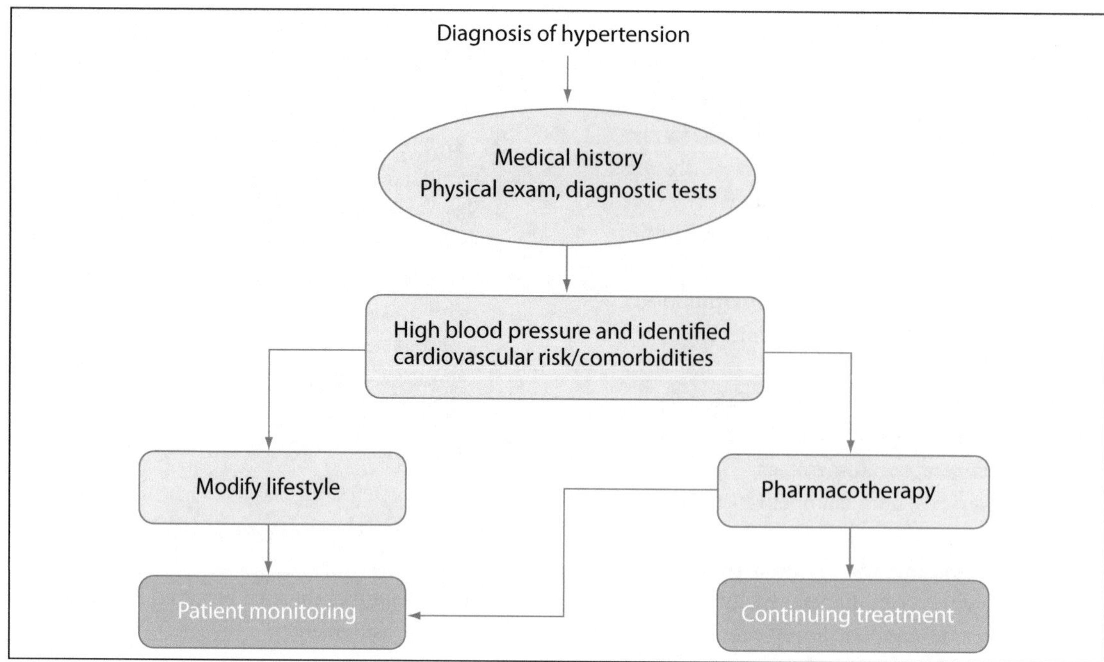

Figure 20.2 Diagnosis and management of hypertension.

- Diet (low-salt diet)
- Smoking cessation
- Alcohol restriction.

Factors influencing choice of drug

- Contraindications to drug
- Presence of target organ damage, renal disease, diabetes or cardiovascular disease
- Other coexisting disorders
- Interactions with drugs used for other conditions by the patient
- Age
- Occupation
- Lifestyle.

Use of antihypertensive drugs

- Initiate drug therapy at a low dose
- Consider multiple drug therapy
- Change to different class of drugs if drug is not producing effect on blood pressure levels or if side-effects are a significant problem
- Use formulations that provide a 24-hour control: better adherence and ensure control of blood pressure in early morning when there is surge of blood pressure. (Note use of ambulatory blood pressure monitors to detect variation of blood pressure control.)

See Figure 20.3 for decision-making in management of hypertension.

Potential indications for the use of ambulatory blood pressure monitor

- Unusual blood pressure variability
- White coat hypertension
- Evaluation of nocturnal or drug-resistant hypertension
- Determining efficacy of treatment over 24 hours
- Diagnoses and treatment of hypertension in pregnancy.

Drug therapy

- Diuretics: reduce blood volume
- Sympatholytics: reduce ability of sympathetic system to raise blood pressure

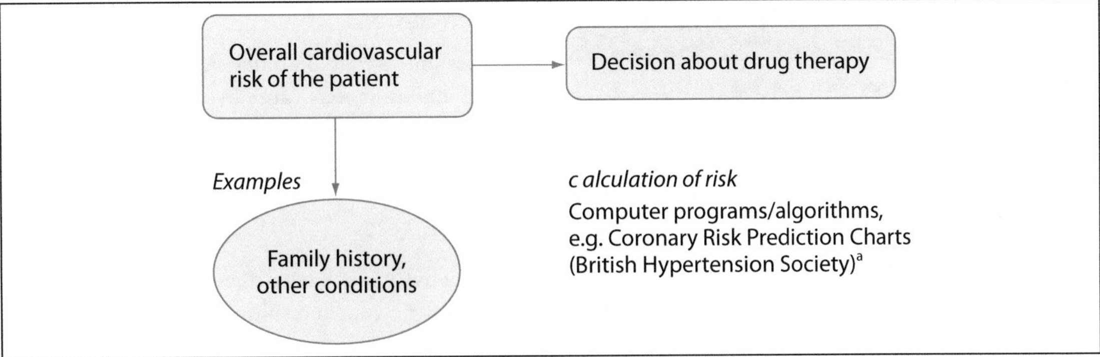

Figure 20.3 Decision-making in management of hypertension. [a]To be found in the BNF.[2]

- Calcium channel blockers: reduce peripheral resistance
- ACE inhibitors, angiotensin II antagonists: reduce peripheral resistance

Diuretics

- Create a negative sodium balance resulting in a reduction of blood volume
- Thiazides (e.g. bendroflumethiazide, indapamide)
- Loop diuretics (e.g. furosemide) are used mainly in pulmonary oedema due to ventricular failure, chronic heart failure (see also Chapter 22).
- Potassium-sparing diuretics (e.g. amiloride (+ hydrochlorthiazide), spironolactone)
- Caution: hypokalaemia.

Thiazide diuretics

- Reduce sodium and water retention in the distal convoluted tubule in the kidney resulting in a reduction of the peripheral resistance
- Cause loss of potassium and magnesium salts
- Potassium supplementation should be considered
- Maximal hypotensive effect is reached at relatively low doses.

Bendroflumethiazide and indapamide are compared in Table 20.1 and their chemical structures shown in Figure 20.4.

Potassium-sparing diuretics

- Retain potassium and therefore no need to consider potassium supplementation
- Act in the distal convoluted tubule
- Are weak diuretics and in fact may be found in combination products with thiazides.

Table 20.1 Comparison of bendroflumethiazide and indapamide

	Bendroflumethiazide	Indapamide
Half-life (hours)	3–4	14
Duration of effect (hours)	6–12	24–36
Dose (mg)[a]	2.5	2.5

[a]To be administered in the morning to reduce nocturnal need for urination.

Figure 20.4 Chemical structures of bendroflumethiazide and indapamide.

Table 20.2 Side-effects of diuretics

Side-effect	Key monitoring parameters
Hypokalaemia	Fatigue, weakness, bilateral calf pain, palpitations, gastrointestinal upset
Dehydration	Tachycardia, dizziness upon standing up, thirst, postural hypotension, decreased skin turgor
Hyperuricaemia	Feeling of fullness in arch of foot, occasionally painful joint – development of gout (usually big toe), high serum uric acid
Hyperlipidaemia	High serum cholesterol and triglycerides
Impaired glucose tolerance	High serum glucose

Side-effects of diuretics

The side-effects of diuretics are listed in Table 20.2.

Hypercalcaemia and impotence may also be reported as side-effects.

For potassium-sparing diuretics, hyperkalaemia rather than hypokalaemia may occur. Key monitoring parameters to identify occurrence of hyperkalaemia include gastrointestinal hyperactivity, muscle weakness and cramps.

Patients at risk of developing electrolyte imbalance

- Patients with vomiting
- Patients with diarrhoea
- Elderly patients
- Patients with ascites due to liver cirrhosis
- Patients with oedema due to nephritic syndrome
- Patients receiving parenteral fluid therapy.

Cautions and contraindications of diuretics

- Gout
- Renal disease
- Diabetes
- Electrolyte imbalance.

Drug interactions

- Potassium-sparing diuretics: ACE inhibitors since ACE inhibitors may cause hyperkalaemia
- With NSAIDs: hypotensive effect is inhibited.

Beta-blockers

- Competively block beta receptors of the sympathetic system resulting in slowing of the heart, reduction in the force of contractions and lengthening of diastole.
- Side-effects: bradycardia, heart failure, hypotension, bronchospasm, peripheral vasoconstriction, fatigue, depression, vivid dreams.
- Cautions/contraindications: asthma, COPD, peripheral vascular disease, Raynaud's phenomenon, heart block, diabetes mellitus (they may mask symptoms of hypoglycaemic attacks).

Various beta-blockers are compared in Table 20.3 (see also Chapter 21) and their chemical structures are shown in Figure 20.5.

Propranolol has a high octanol/buffer partition coefficient indicating a high lipophilicity. It enters the central nervous system better than other beta-blockers. Its primary clearance route is through the liver while more hydrophilic agents such as atenolol are cleared primarily through the kidneys. This should be kept in mind when selecting a drug in patients with renal or liver disease.

Intrinsic sympathomimetic activity

Beta-blockers act by stimulating beta receptors when background sympathetic activity is low and blocking them when activity is high.

- Less resting bradycardia and possibly less cold extremities
- Extrapolation in practice: limited.

Side-effects

The side-effects of beta-blockers are summarised in Table 20.4.

Table 20.3 Comparison of beta-blockers

Drug	Cardioselectivity[a]	Lipid solubility	Intrinsic sympathomimetic activity	Half-life (hours)	Starting dose
Atenolol	+	Low	0/low	6–7	50 mg once daily
Carvedilol	–	High	0/low	6–10	12.5 mg once daily
Labetalol	–	Low	0/low	8	100 mg twice daily with food
Propranolol	–	High	0/low	3–6	80 mg twice daily

[a]Implying lesser effects on airways and lower risk of precipitating bronchospasm.

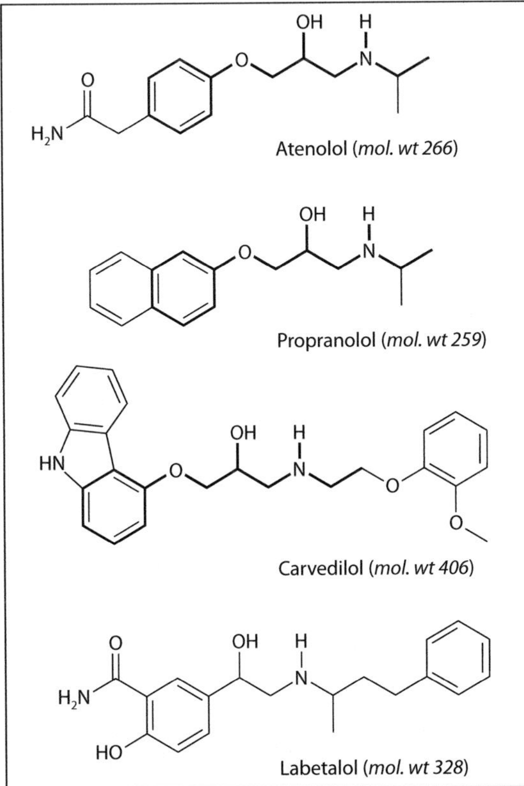

Figure 20.5 Chemical structures of atenolol, propanolol, carvedilol and labetalol.

Angiotensin-converting enzyme inhibitors

ACE inhibitors decrease formation of angiotensin II, resulting in decreased vasoconstriction and decrease in aldosterone production, which in turn results in decreased fluid retention.

Table 20.4 Side-effects of beta-blockers

Side-effect	Key monitoring parameters
Coldness of extremities	
Central nervous system	Nightmares, sedation, hallucinations
Congestive heart failure	Dyspnoea, orthopnoea, weight gain, ankle oedema, tachycardia
Bronchospasm	Wheezing
Hyperglycaemia	Polyuria, polydipsia
Hypoglycaemia	Increased sweating

- Rapid onset of action
- Side-effects: hypotension (especially first dose), hyperkalaemia, cough, renal impairment
- Cautions: patients receiving diuretics, peripheral vascular disease, renovascular disease, severe or symptomatic aortic stenosis, hypertrophic cardiomyopathy
- Check renal function prior to initiating therapy
- Monitor renal function during therapy
- Care in elderly patients since they are at risk of renal side-effects
- Avoid concomitant NSAID use in patients at risk of renal side-effects since concomitant use increases risk and antagonises hypotensive effect of ACE inhibitors.

Some ACE inhibitors are compared in Table 20.5.

Captopril (see Figure 20.6) contains a sulphhydryl group which serves as the zinc-binding group

Table 20.5 Some ACE inhibitors compared

Drug	Half-life (hours)	Starting dose
Captopril	2–3	12.5 mg twice daily
Enalapril	11	5 mg once daily
Lisinopril	12	10 mg once daily
Perindopril	25–20	4 mg once daily
Ramipril (for active metabolite, ramiprilat)	13–17	1.25 mg once daily

ACE, angiotensin-converting enzyme.

Captopril (*mol. wt 266*)

Figure 20.6 Chemical structure of captopril.

that is required for ACE inhibitory effects. The presence of the sulphhydryl group is associated with a higher incidence of skin rashes and taste disturbances. Also the sulphhydryl component may form a disulphide which results in a short half-life for the product.

Enalapril, lisinopril, perindopril and ramipril (see Figure 20.7) are dicarboxylate-containing ACE inhibitors that do not feature a sulphhydryl group. The presence of large hydrophobic heterocyclic rings in the N-ring of perindopril, ramipril, moexipril, quinapril and trandolapril result in increased potency and longer half-life when compared with enalapril and lisinopril. This feature also results in enalapril and lisinopril lacking lipid solubility. Perindopril shows the highest oral bioavailability, followed by trandolapril.

Side-effects

The side-effects of ACE inhibitors are summarised in Table 20.6.

Patients at risk of hypotension with ACE inhibitors

- Those on concomitant diuretics
- Patients with heart failure
- Dehydrated patients
- Patients on a low-sodium diet
- Dialysis patients
- Elderly patients.

Patients are advised to start first dose at night to avoid consequences of hypotension.

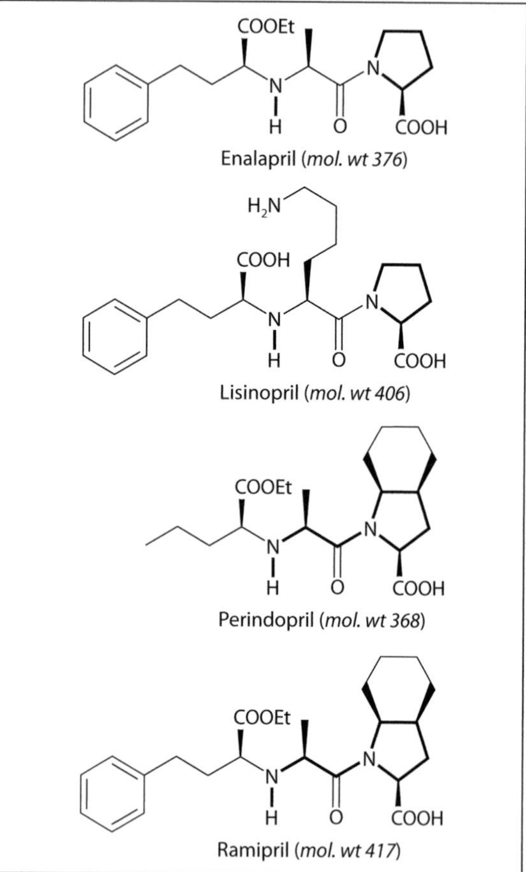

Figure 20.7 Chemical structures of enalapril, lisinopril, perindopril and ramipril.

Angiotensin II receptor antagonists (ARBs)

These are specific angiotensin II receptor antagonists, which thus block the vasoconstrictor and aldosterone-secreting effects of angiotensin II.

Table 20.6 Side-effects of ACE inhibitors

Side-effect	Key monitoring parameters
Hypotension	Usually occurs in volume-depleted patients
Hyperkalaemia	Usually occurs if concomitant use of potassium supplement or potassium-sparing diuretic
Renal effects	Cough

ACE, angiotensin-converting enzyme.

- Do not inhibit breakdown of bradykinin, so less likely to cause cough as a side-effect
- Used as an alternative therapy to ACE inhibitors
- Side-effects: hypotension, dizziness, hyperkalaemia
- Caution: renal artery stenosis.

ARB half-lives and starting dosages are listed in Table 20.7 and their chemical structures in Figure 20.8.

Calcium channel blockers

- Examples: dihydropyridines: nifedipine, amlodipine
- Interfere with the opening/closing of calcium channels in cardiac, vascular and smooth muscle cells
- The dihydropyridines (e.g. nifedipine, amlodipine) cause peripheral vasodilatation and have little direct effect on heart compared with verapamil and diltiazem (which are other types of calcium channel blockers)
- Rapid onset of action
- Should be avoided in heart failure
- Upon withdrawal may exacerbate angina

Table 20.7 Angiotensin II receptor antagonist half-lives and starting dosages

	Half-life (hours)	Starting dose
Losartan	2	50 mg daily
Telmisartan	>20	40 mg daily
Valsartan	5–9	80 mg daily

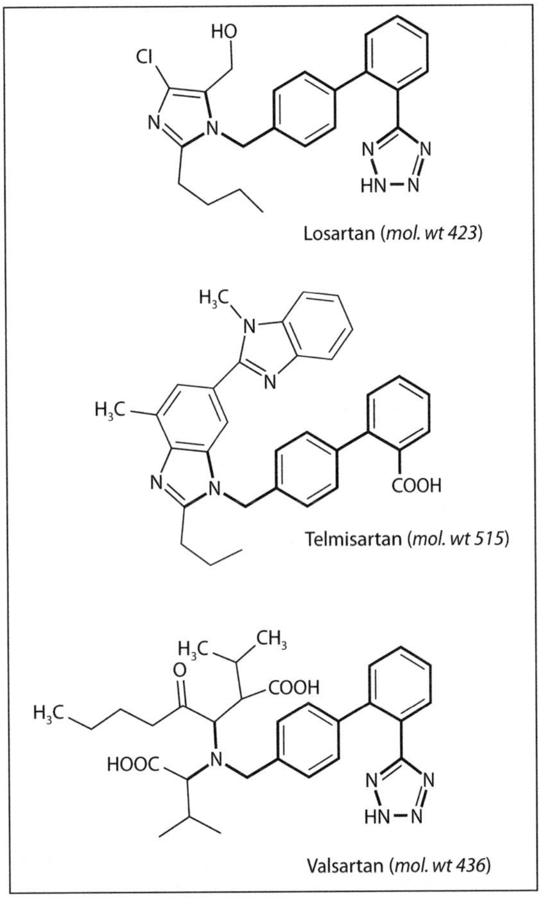

Losartan (*mol. wt 423*)

Telmisartan (*mol. wt 515*)

Valsartan (*mol. wt 436*)

Figure 20.8 Chemical structures of losartan, telmisartan and valsartan.

- Side-effects: palpitations, flushing, oedema, headache, dizziness
- Sustained-release preparations or long-acting drugs such as amlodipine are preferred to decrease risk of myocardial infarction
- See also Chapter 21.

Last line drugs

These are summarised in Table 20.8.

Rilmenidine

This drug selectively binds to I_1-imidazoline receptors in the brainstem. The receptors influence adrenergic vasomotor tone involved in blood pressure regulation. I_1-imidazoline receptors are also available in the kidneys.

Table 20.8 Last line drugs

Drug	Side-effects
Centrally acting drugs Methyldopa, moxonidine	Depression Vasodilatation
Vasodilator antihypertensive drugs Minoxidil	Potent vasodilator Marked fluid retention Hirsutism Reflex tachycardia
Adrenergic neuron blockers Guanethidine	Severe postural hypotension Diarrhoea
Alpha-adrenoceptor blockers Doxazosin (see also Chapter 41)	Postural hypotension Dizziness Vertigo

Rilmenidine is an antihypertensive agent with a central action on the brainstem and a peripheral activity in the kidney. Its characteristic is that it is selective for the I_1-imidazoline receptors rather than also interacting with cerebral alpha$_2$-adrenergic receptors.

- Available as tablets 1 mg, dosage regimen: one tablet per day
- Contraindications: severe depression, renal insufficiency (creatinine clearance <15 mL/min)
- Side-effects: rare; asthenia, palpitations, insomnia.

Contraindications and cautions

The contraindications and cautions to use of drug therapy are summarised in Tables 20.9 and 20.10.

Drug interactions

Some of the common drug interactions with antihypertensive drugs are listed in Table 20.11.

Table 20.9 Contraindications to drug therapy

Drug class	Contraindications
ACE inhibitors	Renovascular disease
Angiotensin II receptor antagonists	Renovascular disease
Beta-blockers	Asthma, chronic obstructive pulmonary disease, heart block
Calcium channel blockers	Heart block, heart failure
Thiazide diuretics	Gout

Table 20.10 Cautions to use of drug therapy

Drug	Caution
Beta-blockers	Heart failure, peripheral vascular disease, diabetes
ACE inhibitors/ARBs	Renal impairment, peripheral vascular disease

ACE, angiotensin-converting enzyme; ARBs, angiotensin II receptor antagonists.

Potential problems with non-prescription medicines in hypertension

- Antacids (high sodium content)
- Cold preparations for systemic use containing sympathomimetics
- NSAIDs
- Potassium-containing preparations (e.g. salt substitutes, potassium citrate indicated for cystitis).

Pharmacist patient review

- To monitor blood pressure
- To provide patient support with drug therapy and lifestyle modifications

Table 20.11 Common drug interactions with antihypertensive drugs

Drug class	Interacting drug	Interaction
Thiazide diuretics	NSAIDs Digoxin	Decreased hypotensive effect Digoxin toxicity if hypokalaemia occurs
Beta-blockers	Antiarrhythmics Sympathomimetics NSAIDs	Bradycardia Severe hypertension Decreased hypotensive effect
ACE inhibitors	NSAIDs	Hyperkalaemia
ACE inhibitors and angiotensin II receptor blockers	K^+ supplementation K^+-sparing diuretics	Hyperkalaemia Hyperkalaemia

ACE, angiotensin-converting enzyme; NSAIDs, non-steroidal anti-inflammatory drugs.

- To discuss symptoms and medication (identify unwanted drug effects, any other drugs taken by patient for other disease states)
- To evaluate need for patient referral to prescriber (based on laboratory test results and/or the presence of other symptoms)
- To consider use of other drugs that reduce cardiovascular risk (aspirin and statin therapy).

Drug therapy in the elderly

- Calcium channel blockers indicated as first-line agents
- Diuretics less effective when there is compromised renal function
- Beta-blockers less potent in the elderly
- Effect of ACE inhibitors may be decreased due to lower renin levels.

Hypertension in pregnancy

Two conditions associated with hypertension in pregnancy are *pre-eclampsia* – pregnancy-induced hypertension, 140/90 mmHg developing during pregnancy in a woman whose blood pressure was previously normal – and *eclampsia* – occurrence of convulsions caused by hypertension.

- Methyldopa is the drug of choice.
- Calcium channel blockers (amlodipine and nifedipine): manufacturer advises avoidance but risk of uncontrolled maternal hypertension should be balanced against risk of use of drug.
- Beta-blockers tend to cause birth of smaller babies.
- ACE inhibitors and angiotensin II receptor blockers cannot be used – they may damage the fetus and cause problems in the neonate.
- Diuretics avoided because of decreased intravascular volume.

Phaeochromocytoma

Phaeochromocytoma is a tumour of chromaffin tissue of the adrenal medulla or sympathetic paraganglia.

- Leads to uncontrolled and irregular secretion of adrenaline and noradrenaline
- Causes raised blood pressure, increased heart rate, palpitations, headache
- Use phenoxybenzamine, alpha-blockers or beta-blockers.

Hypertensive emergency

This is a severe elevation in blood pressure with a diastolic above 120–130 mmHg and the presence of acute or on-going end-organ damage, with cerebral infarction and pulmonary oedema being the most common occurrences of end-organ damage.

- This may be a medical emergency and requires prompt reduction of blood pressure within minutes to 1 hour
- Conditions that predispose to hypertensive emergency include phaeochomocytoma, renal vascular disease, head injury, severe burns, eclampsia
- Goal of treatment: diastolic pressure 100–119 mmHg.

Major complications that occur in a hypertensive emergency include:

- angina
- myocardial infarction
- congestive heart failure
- cerebral infarction
- intracranial haemorrhage.

Management of hypertensive crisis

- Very rapid fall in blood pressure can cause reduced cerebral perfusion leading to: cerebral infarction, blindness, renal function deterioration, myocardial ischaemia
- Oral antihypertensive drugs are used to decrease blood pressure slowly
- Parenteral treatment: rarely adopted; drug of choice is nitroprusside.

Nitroprusside

- Direct-acting arterial and venous vasodilator that is available for parenteral administration
- Immediate onset of action
- Antihypertensive effect disappears within 2–5 minutes after discontinuation
- Starting dose: 0.5–10 micrograms/kg per min via continuous infusion
- Caution: hypothyroidism, hyponatraemia, ischaemic heart disease, impaired cerebral circulation, elderly, hypothermia
- Side-effects: hypotension, nausea and vomiting; if treatment is for more than 24–28 hours, thiocyanate toxicity (it reacts with sulphhydryl groups in blood and tissue producing thiocyanate).

Labetalol

- An alpha- and beta-adrenergic blocking drug.
- Produces a reduction in peripheral vascular resistance, blood pressure and heart rate
- Rapid onset of action: 5 minutes
- Duration of effect: 6 hours or longer
- Dose: 0.5–2 mg/min continuous infusion
- Advantage: available for parenteral and oral administration and so allows easy conversion from intravenous administration to oral therapy
- Side-effects: orthostatic hypotension, nausea and vomiting, dizziness, flushing, headache
- Contraindications: asthma, congestive heart failure, bradycardia.

Diazoxide

- Causes a vasodilator effect on the arterioles resulting in decreased peripheral resistance. It also inhibits the secretion of insulin by the beta cells of the pancreas
- Available for parenteral administration
- Onset of action within 2–5 minutes with a preliminary rise in blood pressure immediately after administration
- Caution: ischaemic heart disease, renal impairment
- Side-effects: tachycardia, hypotension, hyperglycaemia, sodium and water retention
- Patient monitoring: blood pressure, blood glucose levels particularly in patients with diabetes.

Practice summary

- The regulation of blood pressure depends on the peripheral resistance and the cardiac output. These factors are affected by the sympathetic nervous system and the renin–angiotensin–aldosterone system.

- Drugs that are used as antihypertensives aim to reduce blood volume (diuretics), decrease sympathetic activity (beta-adrenoceptor blockers), reduce peripheral resistance (calcium channel blockers) and affect the renin–angiotensin–aldosterone system (ACE inhibitors, angiotensin II antagonists).
- Antihypertensives may be used in monotherapy or as combination therapy.

Questions

1. Compare atenolol and enalapril considering indications, dosage regimen, side-effects and contraindications.
2. Name two conditions when thiazide diuretics should be used with caution or are contraindicated.
3. What is the clinical implication when a patient who is receiving a thiazide diuretic is also started on naproxen?
4. Giving reasons for your answer, explain when bendroflumethiazide is indicated.
5. Describe drug therapy that should be considered as first line in a 58-year-old patient diagnosed with hypertension who has a history of diabetes mellitus. What other preventive drug therapy could be considered?

Answers

1. Atenolol and enalapril are compared in Table 20.12.
2. Gout, renal disease, diabetes, electrolyte imbalance.
3. Naproxen is a non-steroidal anti-inflammatory drug that causes salt and fluid retention, thus decreasing the hypotensive effect of thiazide diuretics.
4. Bendroflumethiazide is a thiazide diuretic that reduces sodium and water retention in the distal convoluted tubule in the kidney, creating a negative sodium balance, resulting in a reduced blood volume and a reduced peripheral resistance. It is indicated in hypertension and oedema.
5. In a 58-year-old patient diagnosed with hypertension and with a history of diabetes mellitus an angiotensin-converting enzyme (ACE) inhibitor is indicated as first-line treatment. ACE inhibitors should be used with caution in renovascular disease; however, in diabetes they have a renoprotective effect. Renal function should be checked prior to initiating therapy and monitored during therapy. ACE inhibitors may cause profound first-dose hypotension, so first doses should be given at night. Potassium levels must be monitored.

Table 20.12 Comparison between atenolol and enalapril

Generic name	Atenolol	Enalapril
Mode of action	Cardioselective beta-blocker. Works by selectively blocking the beta receptors in the sympathetic nervous system	ACE inhibitor which decreases the production of angiotensin II, a potent vasoconstrictor, and also decreases aldosterone production and hence fluid retention. These actions lower the blood pressure
Indications	Hypertension, angina, myocardial infarction, arrhythmia	Hypertension, heart failure
Dosage regimen	Once daily	Once daily
Side-effects	Bronchospasm, bradycardia, heart failure, hypotension, peripheral vasoconstriction, fatigue, depression, vivid dreams	Profound first-dose hypotension, persistent dry cough, renal impairment, hyperkalaemia, skin rashes
Contraindications	Asthma and chronic obstructive pulmonary disease, heart block, peripheral vascular disease, diabetes	Pregnancy, renovascular disease, hypersensitivity

ACE, angiotensin-converting enzyme.

Persistent cough may be a problematic side-effect. Angiotensin II receptor antagonists do not inhibit bradykinin, have fewer side-effects than ACE inhibitors and are indicated when patients are intolerant to ACE inhibitors due to the cough side-effect. Other preventive drug therapy that can be considered to reduce cardiovascular risk includes low-dose aspirin and statin therapy.

Further reading

Williams B, Poulter N R, Brown M J, Davis M, McInnes G T, Potter J F *et al.* (2004). Guidelines for management of hypertension: report of the fourth working party of the British Hypertension Society, 2004–BHS IV. *J Hum Hypertens* 18: 139–185.

National Institute for Health and Clinical Excellence (2006). Hypertension. http://www.nice.org.uk/CG034.

References

1 Mancia G, de Backer G, Dominiczak A *et al.*, guidelines for the management of arterial hypertension. *J Hypertens* 2007; 25: 1105–1187.

2 Joint Formulary Committee. *British National Formulary*, 57th edn. London: British Medical Association and Royal Pharmaceutical Society of Great Britain, 2009.

Acknowledgements

Bernard Coleiro, Consultant Physician, Department of Medicine, Mater Dei Hospital, Malta

21

Ischaemic heart disease

Learning objectives:

- To describe clinical presentation of ischaemic heart disease
- To identify goals of therapy and review pharmacotherapy
- To develop skills to be able to assess effectiveness of pharmacotherapy and monitor patient progress.

Background

Ischaemic heart disease is a condition characterised by a reduced supply of oxygenated blood to cardiac tissue. This occurs as a result of:

- oxygen demand exceeding supply when vascular supply to the heart is impeded (e.g. atheroma, thrombosis)
- oxygen demand is increased (e.g. severe ventricular hypertrophy as a result of hypertension, iron-deficiency anaemia).

Clinical manifestations

- Death of cardiac tissue results in myocardial infarction
- Reversible coronary artery ischaemia results in angina pectoris, which may present as:
  - unstable angina
  - chronic stable/exercise-induced angina – patient presents with a reproducible pattern of angina that is precipitated by a certain level of emotional stress or physical activity
  - variant/Prinzmetal's angina – occurs due to coronary artery spasm.

Prognosis

Mortality is related to:

- history of previous infarction
- hypertension
- heart failure
- tachycardia.

The first few hours after a myocardial infarction are the most critical and ventricular fibrillation is most likely to occur.

Diagnosis

- Pain: gripping or tight in nature occurring in the retrosternal region of the chest; pain may radiate to neck, back, left shoulder with possible involvement of jaw, teeth or epigastrum
- Sweating, pallor

- Fever after myocardial infarction may occur within 12 hours.

Differential diagnosis when symptoms are presented

Symptoms of ischaemic heart disease may be very similar to chest pain that is related to other conditions such as:

- gastrointestinal problems: dyspepsia, gastro-oesophageal reflux disease, ulceration, carcinoma
- musculoskeletal pains
- panic attack
- pulmonary embolism.

Diagnostic tests

- ECG: ST-segment depression, T-wave inversion indicating angina and ST-segment elevation indicating myocardial infarction
- Exercise tolerance test
- Blood tests: elevation of cardiac-specific troponin I and T, creatine kinase.

Lifestyle changes and reduction of risk of myocardial infarction

Lifestyle modifications are very important in the management of patients with ischaemic heart disease. Table 21.1 presents an estimate of the percentage lowering of the risk of myocardial infarction per intervention. Combining multiple interventions will have an additive effect.

Table 21.1 Lifestyle modifications and risk reduction of myocardial infarction

Intervention	Percentage lower risk
Stopping smoking for >5 years	50–70%
Reducing plasma cholesterol	2% for each 1% reduction
Control of hypertension	2–3%/1 mmHg decrease in diastolic pressure
Active lifestyle	45%
Low-dose aspirin	33%

Goals of treatment

- To prevent myocardial infarction and associated mortality
- To increase length of pain-free survival with a good quality of life.

Rationale of drug treatment in angina

- Decrease workload of the heart
- Improve coronary blood supply.

Rationale of drug treatment in myocardial infarction

- Immediate care: remove pain, prevent deterioration, limit infarct size
- Management of complications: heart failure, arrhythmias
- Prevention of second infarction.

Treatment of angina

An acute attack in chronic stable angina

- Glyceryl trinitrate (Figure 21.1)
- Isosorbide mononitrate/ dinitrate.

Prevention of acute attack, treatment of unstable angina

- Aspirin
- Glyceryl trinitrate

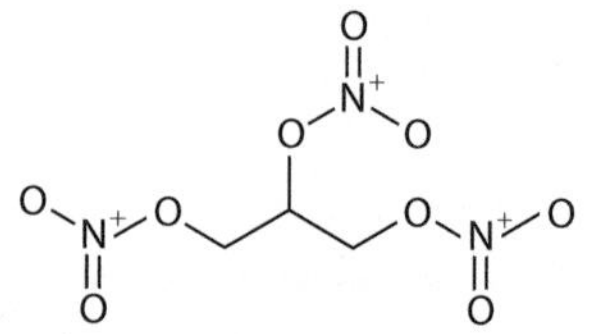

Glyceryl trinitrate (propane-1,2,3-triol trinitrate)

Figure 21.1 Chemical structure of glyceryl trinitrate.

- Isosorbide mononitrate/dinitrate
- Beta-blockers
- Calcium channel blockers
- Nicorandil
- Ivabradine
- Trimetazidine.

Nitrates

- These are converted to nitric oxide, which in turn combines with sulphhydryl groups to form nitrosothiols. These activate production of cyclic GMP which causes smooth muscle relaxation and vasodilatation.
- Nitrate esters are volatile and explosive. These characteristics create problems during production of the dosage forms. They are labile to moisture since moisture will lead to hydrolysis of the ester bond in turn leading to a decreased therapeutic effect.
- Nitrates cause vasodilatation and venodilatation, leading to a decrease in preload and a reduction in cardiac work and may also cause coronary vasodilatation to improve coronary blood supply.
- A disadvantage is that tolerance may occur. For this reason plan a nitrate-free period for 4–8 hours per day. This nitrate-free period should be undertaken when there is least risk of infarction (e.g. during the night). During the nitrate-free period, angina protection is received from concomitant therapy with beta-blockers or calcium channel blockers.
- Side-effects: throbbing headache, flushing, postural hypotension (prevented by sitting down), dizziness, fainting. Care should be taken to avoid falls due to postural hypotension.

Dosage forms

- Sublingual tablets: cheap, deteriorate rapidly, storage in dark container without cotton-wool wadding required; administered sublingually since drug is metabolised due to first-pass effect
- Sublingual sprays: more expensive than sublingual tablets, sprayed under or on the tongue
- Ointments: messy
- Patches: expensive
- Parenteral preparations: used in patients with chest pain due to myocardial infarction or severe ischaemia (unstable angina) and in the treatment of left ventricular failure.

Glyceryl trinitrate is used for symptomatic relief of angina. Sublingual tablets and the aerosol spray provide rapid (1–2 minutes) symptomatic effect that lasts for about 20–30 minutes. If first dose does not relieve pain the patient can repeat dose within 5 minutes. If the use of nitrates for symptomatic relief is required regularly, the patient should seek professional advice.

Isosorbide mononitrate

- Formulation for once-daily oral administration available
- Preferred to glyceryl trinitrate because therapeutic response more predictable.

Isosorbide dinitrate

- Metabolised into the mononitrate component
- Administration requires divided daily doses which may have a negative impact on compliance.

Beta-blockers

These cause a decrease in heart rate, blood pressure and force of ejection in systole. The use of beta-blockers in chronic angina has been shown to decrease incidence of angina attacks and lower morbidity and mortality in patients with other cardiovascular disorders.

Cardioselective agents and agents with low lipophilicity are preferred. Cardioselective agents include atenolol, bisoprolol, metoprolol and nebivolol. Agents that are mostly water soluble are less likely to enter the brain and cause sleep disturbances. Such products include atenolol, nadolol and sotalol.

- Contraindications: asthma, COPD, peripheral vascular disease, heart failure, bradycardia, heart block
- Cautions: diabetes – may cause deterioration in glucose control and interfere with signs of hypoglycaemia

- Care: should not be stopped abruptly especially in patients with ischaemic heart disease since abrupt withdrawal may precipitate angina due to rebound receptor hypersensitivity
- See also Chapter 20.

Calcium channel blockers

These act as arterial vasodilators. The dihydropyridine calcium channel blockers such as amlodipine, felodipine, nicardipine and nifedipine have more influence on the blood vessels and less on the myocardium compared with verapamil.

Modified-release formulations of nifedipine are preferred to avoid large fluctuations in blood pressure and occurrence of tachycardia. Amlodipine and felodipine have a longer duration of action and are given once a day.

Verapamil has more influence on heart rate. It is indicated when beta-blockers are contraindicated. A characteristic side-effect is marked constipation. It should not to be used with beta-blockers (additive effect leading to bradycardia).

- Side-effects: flushing, headache, reflex tachycardia (may warrant the use of beta-blockers) and ankle swelling
- Contraindications: severe hypotension, severe aortic stenosis, extreme bradycardia, moderate-to-severe heart failure, cardiogenic shock
- See also Chapter 20.

Nicorandil

This is a potassium channel activator with a nitrate component.

- Causes arterial and venous vasodilatation
- Similar efficacy to other anti-anginal drugs in the prevention and long-term use in the management of angina. Used with other anti-anginal drugs
- Side-effects: headache, flushing, nausea and vomiting, dizziness
- Caution: hypotension, left ventricular failure, acute pulmonary oedema.

Ivabradine

This is used for chronic stable angina.

- Selective inhibitor of the sinus node I_f, resulting in a decrease in heart rate
- Maintains myocardial contractility, atrioventricular conduction and ventricular repolarisation
- Particularly indicated in patients who have a contraindication or intolerance to beta-blockers.

Trimetazidine

This is a 3-ketoacyl-CoA thiolase (KAT) inhibitor which results in decreased fatty acid oxidation in the myocardium, thus decreasing metabolic damage due to ischaemia. It can be used in combination therapy with other anti-anginal drugs.

ACE inhibitors and management of angina

The HOPE (Heart Outcomes Prevention Evaluation) study (2000)[1] demonstrated the benefits of ACE inhibitors in patients aged 55 years or older at high risk of cardiovascular complications, characterised by a high prevalence of diabetes, hypertension, stroke and obstructive peripheral vascular disease.

The EUROPA (European Trial on Reduction of Cardiac Events with Perindopril in Stable Coronary Artery Disease) study (2003)[1] has demonstrated the positive outcomes with the use of perindopril in patients with stable coronary heart disease. Among patients with stable coronary heart disease without apparent heart failure, perindopril can significantly improve the outcome. Treatment with perindopril together with other preventive medications should be considered.

Drugs that may worsen symptoms of angina

- Short-acting preparations of nifedipine
- Sumatriptan

- Sildenafil
- Thyroxine
- Sympathomimetics.

Patients should be advised to avoid drugs containing sympathomimetics such as systemic use of cold preparations.

Treatment of myocardial infarction

- Oxygen to counteract the occurrence of hypoxia, pulmonary oedema or continuing myocardial ischaemia
- Intravenous diamorphine, sublingual glyceryl trinitrate or intraveneous glyceryl trinitrate or isosorbide dinitrate against pain and distress
- Intravenous metoclopramide or prochlorperazine as antiemetics
- Drugs used to limit infarct size: thrombolytics + aspirin + heparin, beta-blockers, ACE (angiotensin-converting enzyme) inhibitors or angiotensin II receptor antagonists.

Thrombolytics

These activate plasminogen to form plasmin which degrades fibrin and so breaks up thrombi. Studies have confirmed that the use of streptokinase and alteplase reduce mortality. Other thrombolytics are also available (e.g. reteplase, tenecteplase). They have to be administered parenterally within 12 hours of symptom onset. The earlier the treatment is started the better.

- Cautions: risk of bleeding (e.g. patient has undergone invasive procedures), hypertension (blood pressure should be reduced below 180/100 mmHg before initiating therapy), elderly, diabetic nephropathy, and recent or concurrent use of drugs that increase risk of bleeding
- Antibodies to streptokinase occur after 4 days and therefore it should not be used again beyond 4 days of first administration
- Contraindications: conditions that increase risk of bleeding (e.g. trauma, recent surgery, aneurysm, recent symptoms of peptic ulceration, heavy vaginal bleeding)
- Side-effects: nausea, vomiting, bleeding, reperfusion arrhythmias and recurrent ischaemia and angina, hypotension.

Prevention of myocardial infarction

- Antiplatelet drugs (aspirin, clopidogrel)
- Beta-blockers (established that they reduce re-infarction rate)
- Statins
- ACE inhibitors
- Take into consideration other disease states (e.g. diabetics need to achieve optimum blood glucose level control).

Practice summary

Continuous preventive treatment in angina

- Beta-blockers and oral long-acting nitrates
- Verapamil: highly negative inotropic calcium channel blocker which reduces cardiac output and slows heart rate. May precipitate heart failure, not to be used in conjunction with beta-blockers
- Beta-blocker + amlodipine/nifedipine + nicorandil.

Patient monitoring

- Monitor blood pressure
- Target total cholesterol level <5 mmol/L, low-density lipoprotein (LDL) <3 mmol/L
- Monitor occurrence of diabetes.

Concomitant disease states and choice of preventive treatment

Disease states that occur with ischaemic heart disease and preventive treatments are summarised in Table 21.2.

Table 21.1 Lifestyle modifications and risk reduction of myocardial infarction

	Cautions	Suggested therapy
Heart failure	Beta-blockers to be used with caution; verapamil is contraindicated	Calcium channel blockers of the dihydropyridine group
Diabetes mellitus	Avoid beta-blockers since these may reduce warning signs of hypoglycaemia	Calcium channel blockers
Migraine		Beta-blockers since also effective in migraine prophylaxis
COPD/asthma	Beta-blockers may lead to bronchospasm – avoid	Calcium channel blockers
Hyperthyroidism		Beta-blockers since these reduce cardiac effects in hyperthyroidism
Glaucoma	Note: concomitant use of beta-blocker eye drops to be avoided	Beta-blockers

COPD, chronic obstructive pulmonary disease.

Questions

1. Giving reasons for your answer, explain when glyceryl trinitrate is indicated.
2. Describe drug therapy that should be considered as first line in a 52-year-old patient diagnosed with ischaemic heart disease who has a history of hyperthyroidism. What other preventive drug therapy could be considered?

Answers

1. Glyceryl trinitrate is used in the prophylaxis and treatment of angina. It is converted to nitric oxide which in turn combines with sulphhydryl groups to form nitrosothiols. These activate the production of cyclic GMP which causes smooth muscle relaxation and vasodilatation.
2. Use a beta-blocker such as atenolol: it decreases heart rate, blood pressure and force of ejection in systole, and reduces morbidity and mortality in ischaemic heart disease. It also has symptomatic control of tachycardia and tremor associated with hyperthyroidism. Many of the common symptoms of hyperthyroidism such as palpitations, trembling and anxiety are mediated by increases in beta-adrenergic receptors on cell surfaces. Beta-blockers reduce rapid pulse associated with the sensation of palpitations and decrease tremor and anxiety.

Further reading

Briffa T, Hickling S, Knuiman M, Hobbs M, Hung J, Sanfilippo F M *et al.* (2009). Long term survival after evidence based treatment of acute myocardial infarction and revascularisation: follow-up of population based Perth MONICA cohort, 1984–2005. *BMJ* 338: b36.

Hippisley-Cox J and Coupland C (2005). Effect of combinations of drugs on all cause mortality in patients with ischaemic heart disease: nested case-control analysis. *BMJ* 330: 1059–1063.

Reference

1 EUROPA (European Trial on Reduction of Cardiac Events with Perindopril in Stable Coronary Artery Disease) Investigators. Efficacy of perindopril in reduction of cardiovascular events among patients with stable coronary artery disease: randomized, double-blind placebo-controlled, multicentre trial (the EUROPA study). *Lancet* 2003; 362: 782–788.

Acknowledgements

Bernard Coleiro, Consultant Physician, Department of Medicine, Mater Dei Hospital, Malta.

22

Congestive heart failure

Learning objectives:

- To review characteristics of congestive heart failure
- To highlight pharmacotherapeutic management of congestive heart failure
- To identify pharmacist intervention in patient care and patient monitoring.

Background

Congestive heart failure (CHF) occurs when the heart fails to sustain an adequate delivery of blood to tissues. It is a common condition progressing to early death and affecting quality of life (fatigue, breathlessness, oedema).

Signs and symptoms of heart failure

- Dyspnoea, orthopnea
- Inspiratory crackles
- Lower extremity oedema
- Arrhythmias
- Tachycardia
- Decreased exercise tolerance
- Fatigue
- Abdominal symptoms: nausea, abdominal pain.

Classification

New York Heart Association (NYHA) Functional Classification of Congestive Heart Failure

- Class I: no symptoms (dyspnoea, fatigue, palpitations) associated with ordinary activity. Physical activity not limited
- Class II: asymptomatic at rest, but symptoms occur with ordinary activity. Physical activity minimally limited
- Class III: asymptomatic at rest, but symptoms occur with less than ordinary activity. Physical activity markedly limited interfering with daily lifestyle
- Class IV: symptoms at rest. Physical activity worsens symptoms.

Investigations

- Echocardiography: to assess haemodynamic factors and identify structural changes.

Lifestyle modifications

- Sodium restriction – very critical in treatment of heart failure
- Avoidance of excessive fluid intake
- Smoking cessation
- Decreased alcohol consumption or abstinence
- Regular exercise – walking
- Self-monitoring by patient of body weight – to assess fluid retention.

Goals of therapy

- Improvement in survival
- Alleviation of symptoms and improvement in quality of life
- Improvement in exercise capacity
- Prevention of treatment-associated hypotension and electrolyte changes.

Treatment

- ACE (angiotensin-converting enzyme) inhibitors: standard of care unless there is a contraindication to their use
- Diuretics: thiazides, loop diuretics
- Aldosterone antagonists: spironolactone
- Beta-blockers: carvedilol
- Cardiac glycosides: digoxin
- Vasodilators: isosorbide dinitrate+hydralazine.

ACE inhibitors

- Relieve symptoms and improve exercise tolerance, improve prognosis
- Significant contraindications:
  - history of intolerance or severe adverse reactions
  - serum potassium concentration >5.5 mol/L
  - renal disorders
  - symptomatic hypotension
  - aortic valve stenosis
- Action: block vasoconstriction, increase cardiac output
- Useful in preventing progression of heart failure
- See also Chapter 20.

ACE inhibitors used in the treatment of heart failure are listed in Table 22.1.

Diuretics

- Provide effective symptomatic control in patients with oedema with little long-term impact on prognosis
- If gradual diuresis is aimed at or symptoms are mild a thiazide diuretic (e.g. bendroflumethiazide) is preferred
- If there is persistent volume overload despite the use of thiazides, severe volume overload, or decreased renal function, a loop diuretic (e.g. furosemide) is preferred
- Monitor renal function
- See also Chapter 20.

Table 22.1 ACE inhibitors in the treatment of heart failure

Drug	Initial dose	Max. dose	Side-effects
Captopril	6.25–12.5 mg three times daily	50 mg three times daily	Hypotension, hyperkalaemia, cough, skin rash, renal failure
Enalapril	2.5 mg daily	20 mg twice daily	
Lisinopril	2.5 mg daily	35 mg daily	
Perindopril[a]	2 mg daily	4 mg daily	

[a]Bioavailability affected by food; take on an empty stomach.

Table 22.2 Diuretics in the treatment of heart failure

Drug	Initial dose (oral dose)	Max. dose (oral dose)	Side-effects of all drugs
Bendroflumethiazide	5 mg morning	10 mg daily	Postural hypotension,
Furosemide	40 mg morning	80 mg daily	Hypokalaemia,
Bumetanide	1 mg morning	5 mg daily increased by 5 mg every 12–24 hours according to response	Hyperuricaemia
Metolazone[a]	5 mg morning	80 mg daily	

[a]Profound diuresis may occur; preferred for short-term use during acute period.

Diuretics used in the treatment of heart failure are listed in Table 22.2.

Aldosterone antagonists: spironolactone

- A potassium-sparing diuretic which potentiates thiazide or loop diuretics by antagonising aldosterone
- Used in patients with severe heart failure who are receiving an ACE inhibitor and a diuretic with insufficient response
- 25 mg daily dose reduces symptoms and mortality
- Monitor serum creatinine and electrolyte levels (potassium)
- Drug interaction with digoxin: spironolactone increases plasma concentration of digoxin.

Beta-blockers

- Carvedilol, bisoprolol and metoprolol have shown positive effects on prognosis
- Used in combination with ACE inhibitors, diuretics, and digoxin to reduce the morbidity of heart failure
- Caution: may initially worsen heart failure – titrate dose and monitor patient, avoid abrupt withdrawal of beta-blockers
- Oral administration: give with food to slow absorption and minimise risk of orthostatic hypotension
- Monitor digoxin levels with concurrent use, increased risk of atrioventricular (AV) block and bradycardia when given with digoxin
- For carvedilol: initial dose – 3.125 mg twice daily; maximum dose 25 mg twice daily in patients with body weight less than 85 kg and 50 mg twice daily in patients over 85 kg.
- See also Chapter 20.

Cardiac glycosides: digoxin

- A positive inotropic agent indicated in patients at highest risk for clinical deterioration or patients who cannot tolerate ACE inhibitors or remain asymptomatic
- Narrow therapeutic index
- Monitor serum concentrations, renal functions and electrolytes
- Side-effects: arrhythmias, confusion, nausea, anorexia, visual disturbances.

Vasodilators: isosorbide dinitrate ± hydralazine

- Occurrence of significant adverse effects: headache, palpitations, nasal congestion
- Nitrate-free period each day of about 10 hours: in heart failure the nitrate-free period should occur during the day when dyspnoea can be managed with diuretics while nitrate is used at night to manage paroxysmal nocturnal dyspnoea
- Used in combination since nitrates produce mainly venous dilatation and hydralazine produces arterial vasodilatation.

Angiotensin II receptor antagonists (ARBs)

- May be considered in patients who cannot tolerate ACE inhibitors
- CHARM[1] (Candesartan in Heart Failure: Assessment of Reduction in Mortality and Morbidity) study (1999) showed that candesartan reduced cardiovascular deaths and hospital admissions for symptomatic heart failure.

Use of calcium channel blockers in patients with heart failure

Studies have indicated that the negative inotropic effects of calcium channel blockers may result in worsening of heart failure. This is particularly relevant for verapamil and diltiazem. There is a possibility that amlodipine and felodipine have minimal negative inotropic effects but their use is not implicated in adverse effects on morbidity and mortality.

Common management mistakes in heart failure

- Improper dosage of diuretics
- Failure to assess quality of life
- Failure to consider long-term therapeutic goals
- Inadequate dose of ACE inhibitors
- Failure to use hydralazine and isosorbide dinitrate
- Use of potentially harmful drugs
- Inadequate monitoring of renal function.

Identification of precipitating factors

- Respiratory infection
- Pulmonary embolism
- Anaemia
- Uncontrolled cardiovascular disease: hypertension, arrhythmias, ischaemia
- Uncontrolled endocrine disease: diabetes, thyroid disease
- Drugs with negative inotropic effect (e.g. verapamil)
- Antacids with high sodium content, NSAIDs: renal retention of sodium and water
- Non-compliance with treatment particularly the diuretic therapy (patients receiving diuretics should be advised about timing of administration to avoid inconvenient micturition).

Practice summary

- Goals of treatment: relieve symptoms and signs, decrease hospitalisation and prolong survival.
- A number of factors may precipitate the condition. Patient should be monitored regularly to identify factors that may have a negative impact on the progress of the condition.
- Drug therapy management requires titrating diuretic dose according to patient need and considering preventive therapy for cardiovascular disease (e.g. aspirin, statins).
- Patient should be monitored for signs of effective control (e.g. improvement in exercise tolerance, decreased oedema) and for signs of toxicity (e.g. digoxin toxicity), and signs of chronic excess of diuretics which may lead to dehydration, fatigue or fainting.

Questions

1. What is the relevance of using a diuretic in congestive heart failure?
2. Give two examples of diuretics that may be used in heart failure. For each example state dose and side-effects to be expected.

Answers

1. Congestive heart failure is a disorder in which the heart loses its ability to pump blood

Table 22.3 Doses and side-effects of two diuretics that may be used in heart failure

Active ingredient	Dose	Side-effects
Bumetanide	1 mg in the morning repeated after 6–8 hours, severe cases 5 mg daily, maximum dose 10 mg	Hyponatraemia, hypokalaemia, hypomagnesaemia, increased calcium excretion, hypotension, hyperuricaemia, hyperglycaemia
Sprionolactone	25–50 mg daily	Gastrointestinal disturbances, impotence, gynaecomastia, menstrual irregularities, lethargy, headache, confusion, rashes, hyperkalaemia

efficiently throughout the body. Heart failure may affect the left, right or both sides of the heart. If the left half of the heart fails (left ventricular failure), fluid will build up in the lungs due to congestion of the veins of the lungs. If the right half of the heart fails (right ventricular failure), general body vein pressure will increase and fluid will accumulate in the body, especially the tissues of the legs and abdominal organs. Fluid may build up in the lungs and legs. Diuretics are important as they relieve symptoms quickly and control fluid retention. Diuretics provide effective symptomatic control in patients with oedema with little long-term impact on prognosis.

2 Bumetanide and spironolactone doses and side-effects are summarised in Table 22.3.

Further reading

Ahmed A, Aronow W S and Fleg J L (2006). Higher New York Heart Association classes and increased mortality and hospitalization in patients with heart failure and preserved left ventricular function. *Am Heart J* 151: 444–450.

Jessup M, Abraham W T, Casey D E, Feldman A M, Francis G S, Ganiats T G *et al.* (2009). Focused update: ACCF/AHA Guidelines for the diagnosis and management of heart failure in adults. *J Am Coll Cardiol* 53: 1343–1382.

Lock J (2003). The benefit of adding a pharmacist to the heart failure team. *Hosp Pharm* 10: 81–83.

Micale Foody J, Farrell M H and Krumholz H M (2002). β-blocker therapy in heart failure. *JAMA* 287: 883–887.

Poole-Wilson P (2004). NICE guidance on heart failure: a challenge for primary care. *Prescriber* 5 January: 8–16.

Reference

1 Pfeffer M A, Swedberg K, Granger C B, Held P, McMurray J J V, Michelson E L *et al.* for the CHARM investigators and committees. Effects of candesartan on mortality and morbidity in patients with chronic heart failure: the CHARM-Overall programme. *Lancet* 2003; 362: 759–766.

Acknowledgements

Bernard Coleiro, Consultant Physician, Department of Medicine, Mater Dei Hospital, Malta.

23

Hyperlipidaemia

Learning objectives:

- To review lifestyle modifications to be recommended
- To appreciate side-effect profile of the drugs
- To develop skills to be able to participate in patient monitoring and identify patients eligible for drug therapy.

Background

Levels of serum cholesterol or triglycerides or both denote increased risk of coronary artery disease. Cholesterol, triglycerides and phospholipids are transported as lipoproteins:

- very low-density lipoproteins (VLDLs)
- intermediate density lipoproteins (IDLs)
- high-density lipoproteins (HDLs)
- chylomicrons
- chylomicron remnants.

Of these, VLDLs and LDLs are undesired lipoproteins and HDLs are desirable to maintain levels of protective HDLs.

Lipid profile

Optimal levels of lipoproteins are listed in Table 23.1. Ideally the LDL:HDL ratio should be less than 3. If the ratio is higher than 4 risk of atherogenesis is high (see also Chapter 11).

Table 23.1 Lipid profile

Parameter	Optimal levels
Total cholesterol	<5.17 mmol/L
Triglycerides	<1.69 mmol/L
LDL-cholesterol	<2.58 mmol/L
HDL-cholesterol	Low >1.03 mmol/L High ≥1.55 mmol/L

In the management of hyperlipidaemia, the primary outcome of therapy should be to lower low-density lipoprotein-cholesterol.

Combined hyperlipidaemia

A condition characterised by fasting plasma triglycerides >2 mmol/L (hypertriglyceridaemia) and low-density lipoprotein >3 mmol/L.

- Usually occurs as a result of metabolic disorders (e.g. insulin resistance)
- Fibrates are mainstay of treatment to reduce serum triglycerides
- Statins are more effective in lowering LDL-cholesterol than fibrates and also exert a reduction in serum triglycerides though the latter effect occurs to a lesser extent when compared with fibrates.

Conditions that cause secondary hyperlipidaemia

- Diabetes mellitus
- Hypothyroidism: correct hypothyroid state before initiating lipid-lowering drugs
- Pregnancy
- Alcohol abuse
- Chronic renal failure especially nephrotic syndrome
- Hepatocellular disease
- Systemic lupus erythematosus.

Drugs that adversely affect the lipoprotein profile

- Amiodarone
- Antipsychotics: particularly the atypical ones
- Corticosteroids
- Beta-blockers
- Diuretics
- Oral contraceptives
- Tamoxifen.

Lifestyle modifications

- Limited daily cholesterol intake
- Limited saturated fat intake: reduced intake of red meats, milk
- Replace saturated fats with monosaturated fats and fish oils
- Increase intake of fruit, cereals and vegetables
- Exercise
- Monitor body weight.

- Lifestyle modifications should be considered as a primary prevention approach adopted even when patient has no previous coronary heart disease and no atherosclerotic vascular disease.
- Screening of adults over 20 years of age or older once every 5 years is indicated to identify patients at risk and recommend lifestyle modifications as appropriate.

Familial hypercholesterolaemia

This is a condition in which high cholesterol concentrations occur due to a genetic risk. The condition may lead to early onset of coronary heart disease and atherosclerosis. Patients at risk of developing familial hypercholesterolaemia including children should be monitored and use of high-dose lipid-regulating drugs considered.

Lipid-regulating drugs are indicated in:

- coronary heart disease
- patients at high risk of developing cardiac disease because of multiple risk factors (smoking, hypertension, diabetes, family history)
- total serum cholesterol concentration >5 mmol/L.

Statins

These are 7-substituted-3,5-dihydroxyheptanoic acids which can feature either a bicyclic ring structure (natural products), such as in simvastatin (Figure

23.1), or a structure where the bicyclic ring has been substituted with aromatic ring systems (synthetic structure), such as in fluvastatin (Figure 23.1).

- Inhibit 5-hydroxy-3-methylglutaryl-CoA (HMG-CoA) reductase which controls the rate-limiting step in the synthesis of cholesterol in liver. Reduce LDL-cholesterol
- Significantly reduce the incidence of myocardial infarction and improve survival in patients with hypercholesterolaemia with or without coronary heart disease. Reduce myocardial infarction and overall mortality. High doses of statins are supported
- Drugs of choice, combined with dietary and lifestyle measures, monitoring of blood pressure, and aspirin where appropriate
- LDL-lowering activity is: rosuvastatin > atorvastatin > simvastatin > pravastatin > fluvastatin
- Dose administered in the evening because cholesterol biosynthesis reaches a peak during the night. This is not so relevant for rosuvastatin and atorvastatin since they have longer half-lives
- Patient monitoring: liver function tests have to be carried out routinely, creatine kinase levels
- Cautions: history of liver disease or high alcohol intake

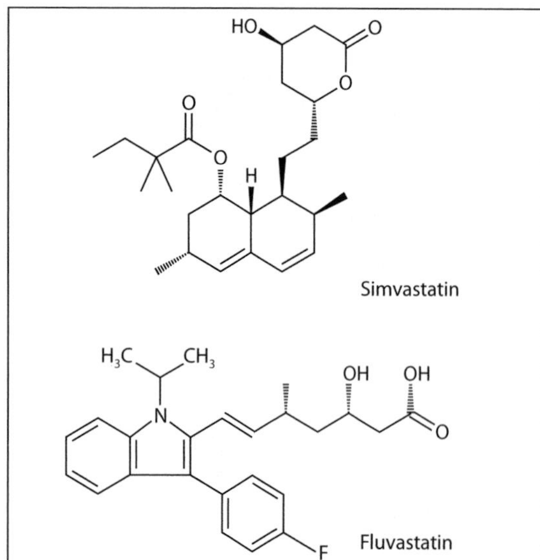

Figure 23.1 Chemical structures of simvastatin and fluvastatin.

- Contraindications: active liver disease, pregnancy, breast-feeding
- Risk of rhabdomyolysis (fatal skeletal muscle disease) which increases when statins are combined with other lipid-regulating drugs
- Patient advice: to report immediately unexplained muscle pain, tenderness or weakness since these are signs of myalgia, myositis and myopathy that warrant cessation of therapy.

Doses for some commonly used statins are summarised in Table 23.2.

Side-effects

Reversible myositis is a rare but significant side-effect of statins. Statins also cause headache, altered liver function tests (rarely hepatitis), paraesthesia and gastrointestinal effects including abdominal pain, flatulence, diarrhoea, nausea and vomiting. Rash and hypersensitivity reactions (including angioedema and anaphylaxis) have been reported rarely.

The side-effect profiles of some statins are compared in Table 23.3.

Muscle effects and statins

Myalgia, myositis and myopathy have been reported with the statins. If myopathy is suspected, creatinine kinase should be measured and if it is markedly elevated (more than five times upper limit of normal), treatment should be discontinued. In patients at high risk of muscle effects, a statin should not be started if creatine kinase is elevated. Rhabdomyolysis with acute renal impairment secondary to myoglobinuria has also been reported.

Table 23.2 Summary of statin doses

Drug	Initial daily dose	Maximum daily dose
Atorvastatin	10 mg	80 mg
Fluvastatin	20–40 mg	80 mg
Pravastatin	10 mg	40 mg
Rosuvastatin	5–10 mg	40 mg
Simvastatin	10–20 mg	80 mg

Table 23.3 Comparison of side-effect profiles of statins

Drug	Common characteristic side-effects
Atorvastatin	Chest pain, fatigue, asthenia, insomnia, dizziness, hypoesthesia, arthralgia, back pain
Fluvastatin	Insomnia
Pravastatin	Fatigue, dizziness, sleep disturbances, abnormal urination, sexual dysfunction, visual disturbances, alopecia
Rosuvastatin	Dizziness, asthenia, proteinuria
Simvastatin	Alopecia, anaemia, dizziness, peripheral neuropathy, asthenia, jaundice, pancreatitis Also note interaction with grapefruit juice (increased risk of rhabdomyolysis)

Risk of myopathy increases in patients:

- with renal impairment
- with hypothyroidism
- receiving other drugs, namely fibrates, lipid-lowering doses of nicotinic acid and immunosuppressants such as ciclosporin.

Table 23.4 Drug interactions with statins and fibrates

Drug class	Drug interactions
Statins	Gemfibrozil, macrolides and telithromycin, azole antifungals, warfarin
Gemfibrozil	Statins, warfarin, antidiabetics – rosiglitazone, repaglinide
Fibrates	Statins, warfarin

Fibrates

These act mainly by decreasing serum triglycerides. They may be used in combination with statins when triglycerides remain high despite statin therapy.

- Patient advice: bezafibrate, fenofibrate to be taken with food, gemfibrozil to be taken half to one hour before food
- Cautions: correct hypothyroidism, hepatic impairment, renal impairment, combination with statins increases risk of muscle effects especially with gemfibrozil (avoid concomitant use with statins)
- Contraindications: severe hepatic and renal impairment, hypoalbuminaemia, primary biliary cirrhosis, gallbladder disease, nephrotic syndrome, pregnancy, breast-feeding
- Common side-effects: gastrointestinal disturbances, anorexia
- Monitoring: liver function tests, creatine kinase.

Drug interactions with statins and fibrates are shown in Table 23.4.

Other pharmacological treatment

Ezetimibe

- Inhibits intestinal absorption of cholesterol
- May be used as an adjunct to statins and the combination exhibits an additive effect but risk of rhabdomyolysis is increased
- Cautions: hepatic impairment, pregnancy, breast-feeding
- Side-effects: gastrointestinal disturbances, headache, fatigue and myalgia
- Given as a once-daily dose.

Bile acid sequestrants: colesevelam, colestyramine and colestipol

- Bind to bile acids resulting in the prevention of their reabsorption and hence in increased clearance of LDL-cholesterol
- Interfere with absorption of fat-soluble vitamins and other drugs

- May cause a rise in triglyceride level especially in patients with already high levels; this occurs to a lesser extent with colesevelam
- Patient advice: to take other drugs at least 1 hour before or 4–6 hours after bile acid sequestrants
- Side-effects: gastrointestinal (constipation, diarrhoea, nausea, vomiting); colesevelam is associated with a lower incidence of gastrointestinal side-effects

Nicotinic acid group: nicotinic acid, acipimox

- These drugs lower both cholesterol and triglyceride concentrations by interfering with the biosynthesis pathway. They increase HDL-cholesterol
- Use of nicotinic acid limited by occurrence of side-effects particularly vasodilatation. Acipimox tends to be associated with a lower occurrence of side-effects but may be less effective as a lipid-lowering agent than nicotinic acid
- Side-effects: diarrhoea, nausea, vomiting, abdominal pain, dyspepsia, flushing, pruritus, rash.

Fish oils: omega-3 fatty acid compounds

- May be used to reduce triglycerides in combination with statins in combined hyperlipidaemia.

Practice summary

- Identify patients including elderly at high risk of atherosclerosis. Commence drug therapy early.
- Pharmacists should participate in the screening of patients at risk, in preparing a treatment plan and in ensuring patient compliance with lipid-regulating drugs which require chronic use.
- Consideration of side-effect profile: hepatotoxicity, myopathy (dose related). Patients should be advised to report immediately any muscle pain.
- Lifestyle modifications and relevant parameters (lipid profile, blood pressure, blood glucose level, body weight) should be monitored regularly.

Questions

1. List four side-effects that could occur with the use of statins.
2. What patient monitoring is required in patients receiving statins? What advice should be given to patients?
3. When is the risk of rhabdomyolysis associated with statins increased?

Answers

1. Headache, gastrointestinal disturbances, paraesthesia, altered liver function tests.
2. Blood cholesterol and lipid levels, liver function tests, creatine kinase and renal function should all be monitored in patients receiving statins. Due to the risk of myositis, myalgia and myopathy, patients should be advised to report immediately any unexplained muscle pain, tenderness and weakness. Patients should be advised to take statins at night.
3. Rhabdomyolysis is a rare fatal skeletal muscle disease which increases when statins are combined with other lipid-regulating drugs such as fibrates. Risk is increased in patients with renal impairment and possibly in those with hypothyroidism. Concomitant treatment with immunosuppressants such as ciclosporin may increase plasma statin concentration and the risk of muscle toxicity.

Further reading

Briel M, Ferreira-Gonzalez I, You J J, Karanicolas P J, Akl E A, Wu P *et al.* (2009). Association between change in high density lipoprotein cholesterol and cardiovascular disease morbidity and mortality: systematic review and meta-regression analysis. *BMJ* 338: b92.

Lopez L M (2002). Managing hyperlipidemia: current and future roles of HMG-CoA reductase inhibitors. *Am J Health-Syst Pharm* 59: 1173–1182.

National Institute for Health and Clinical Excellence (2008). Familial hypercholesterolaemia: identification and management of familial hypercholesterolaemia. http://www.nice.org.uk/CG71.

Paulsen T (2009). Pharmacy's role in the treatment of dyslipidaemias. *Hosp Pharm Eur* July/August: 78–79.

Thompson P D, Clarkson P and Karas R H (2003). Statin-associated myopathy. *JAMA* 289: 1681–1690.

Ye X, Gross C R, Schommer J, Cline R, Xuan J and St Peter W L (2007). Initiation of statins after hospitalization for coronary heart disease. *J Manag Care Pharm* 13: 385–396.

Acknowledgements

Bernard Coleiro, Consultant Physician, Department of Medicine, Mater Dei Hospital, Malta

24

Thrombosis

Learning objectives:

- To appreciate prophylaxis of venous and arterial thromboembolism
- To understand use of pharmacological agents in the prophylaxis and management of thrombosis
- To develop skills to monitor and handle chronic drug therapy.

Background

Thrombosis describes the pathological formation of a clot known as a thrombus consisting of platelets, fibrin, red cells and white cells, which may cause occlusion within blood vessels of the heart.

- *Arterial occlusion:* may lead to myocardial infarction, stroke
- *Venous occlusion:* may lead to deep venous thrombosis, pulmonary embolism
- *Embolus:* part of a clot becomes dislodged and travels to other areas.

Venous thromboembolism (VTE)

- Increase in prevalence in patients over 50 years of age
- Associated with morbidity due to postphlebitic limb
- Examples: deep vein thrombosis and pulmonary embolism.

Risk factors for VTE

- Immobility or paralysis
- Trauma or surgery in lower extremities, hips or abdomen
- History of VTE
- Obesity
- Increased progestogen levels (e.g. pregnancy, combined oral contraceptives, hormone replacement therapy)
- Inflammatory bowel disease
- Carcinoma
- Cardiac dysfunction
- Air travel (also referred to as 'economy class air travel syndrome')
- Thrombophilic states (e.g. anticardiolipin antibody syndrome).

Deep vein thrombosis

- Veins of lower limbs commonly affected
- Presentation: pain in calf, redness of skin, warmth in area, swelling of calf.

Aims of treatment in deep vein thrombosis

- To restore normal circulation
- To prevent damage to the valves and reduce risk of post-phlebitic limb.

Protocol of treatment in deep vein thrombosis

1. Initial heparin (heparin or LMWHs) treatment.
2. Warfarin for 3–6 months after the incident when there is a reversible cause or a precipitating factor, otherwise lifelong therapy.

Aim of treatment in pulmonary embolism

- When there is haemodynamic instability, removal of obstruction using thrombolytic drugs (see Chapter 21).

Thromboprophylaxis

- Without thromboprophylaxis, overall frequency of deep vein thrombosis after general surgery is about 25%. After 7–14 days, without thromboprophylaxis, frequency of deep vein thrombosis in total hip replacement, total knee surgery and hip fracture is about 50–60%.
- Low-dose heparin by subcutaneous injection is administered as prophylaxis in patients undergoing general surgery and major orthopaedic surgery to prevent post-operative deep vein thrombosis and pulmonary embolism.

Heparin (unfractionated heparin)

- Rapid anticoagulant effect
- Short duration of action
- Started as an intravenous loading dose and then continued as necessary with continuous intravenous infusion. May be administered subcutaneously; however, bioavailability following this route of administration is significantly decreased
- Monitoring: activated partial thromboplastin time (APTT), which reports clotting time in seconds. It reflects changes in the intrinsic pathway of the coagulation cascade. APTT prolongation may be due to heparin therapy, warfarin therapy (prothrombin time affected more and that is why prothrombin time is the test used to monitor warfarin therapy), liver dysfunction or vitamin K deficiency
- Example: heparin 25 000 units/mL.

Low-molecular-weight heparin (LMWHs)

These are derivatives of commercial heparin that have a mean molecular weight of 4000–5000 Da in contrast to the unfractionated heparin which has a mean molecular weight of 12 000–16 000 Da. Each is derived from natural heparins by various manufacturing methods. Examples are enoxaparin sodium, dalteparin sodium and tinzaparin sodium.

- Differences in pharmaceutical parameters between LMWHs exist.
- They have a longer duration of action than heparin.
- Once-daily subcutaneous administration. They exhibit improved bioavailability after subcutaneous injection compared with heparin.

LMWHs vs unfractionated heparin

- May be adopted as a prophylactic regimen
- More expensive
- Greater bioavailability
- Easier to administer by patients at home; increased patient compliance
- No need for monitoring of APTT – dose is calculated according to patient's body weight.

Advantages of low-molecular-weight heparins over unfractionated heparin

- Ease of administration
- Do not require routine daily monitoring.

Guidelines on LMWHs use

- Advantages of LMWH and comparable effectiveness indicate that they should replace unfractionated heparin in the prophylaxis of venous thromboembolism.
- In orthopaedic practice LMWHs are more effective than unfractionated heparin.
- May be used in the treatment of deep vein thrombosis, pulmonary embolism and unstable coronary artery disease (e.g. enoxaparin).

Contraindications to heparins

- Haemophilia
- Thrombocytopenia
- Peptic ulcer disease.

Side-effects

- Haemorrhage
- Heparin-induced thrombocytopenia
- Rebound hyperlipidaemia following withdrawal
- Hyperkalaemia
- Osteoporosis (risk lower for LMWH).

Heparin-induced thrombocytopenia

- It is immune-mediated and does not usually develop until after 5–10 days.
- Platelet count measured before initiation of therapy and monitored thereafter if treatment exceeds 4 days.
- Signs: 50% reduction of platelets, thrombosis, skin allergy.
- Stop heparin when condition occurs.
- Alternative anticoagulants such as hirudins (e.g. lepirudin, fondaparinux) may be considered.

Patient monitoring

- Occurrence of bleeding
- Occurrence of hyperkalaemia which:
  - occurs due to inhibition of aldosterone secretion by heparin
  - is associated with increased risk with longer duration of therapy, in diabeties, chronic renal failure and hyperkalaemia
  - suggests monitoring of plasma potassium concentration for patients at risk or where heparin therapy exceeds 7 days' duration.

Other parenteral anticoagulants: fondaparinux

This is used in the prophylaxis of venous thromboembolism in medical patients, patients undergoing major orthopaedic surgery of the legs or abdominal surgery, treatment of deep vein thrombosis and pulmonary embolism, treatment of unstable angina and myocardial infarction. It is available for once-daily administration as a subcutaneous injection.

Oral anticoagulants: warfarin

Warfarin (Figure 24.1) is a vitamin K antagonist which blocks the reduction of vitamin K epoxide that is necessary for its action as a cofactor in the synthesis of factors II, VII, IX and X in the coagulation cascade. It takes 48–72 hours for an effect because of the time needed for the degradation of factors that have already been formed.

- Contraindications: peptic ulcers, severe hypertension, renal impairment, pregnancy
- Initial dose: 10 mg daily for 2 days
- Maintenance dose: 3–9 mg daily at the same time of day
- Monitoring: international normalised ratio (INR) reports time taken to clot formation. It reflects changes in the extrinsic and common pathways

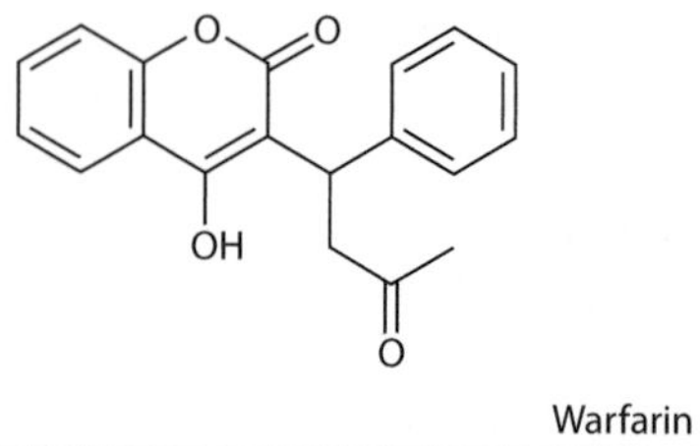

O O OH O Warfarin

Figure 24.1 Warfarin, a water-insoluble lactone that is weakly acidic due to hydroxy substitution, is a chiral compound where the *S*-enantiomer is more potent than the *R*-enantiomer.

of the coagulation cascade. Warfarin and heparin especially in high doses cause a prolongation of the prothrombin time (see also Chapter 11).

Clinically significant interactions

- Increased anticoagulant effect – pharmacodynamic effect (e.g. salicylates, gemfibrozil)
- Increased anticoagulant effect: inhibition of warfarin metabolism (e.g. cimetidine, erythromycin, mefenamic acid, metronidazole, ketoconazole, ciprofloxacin, sulphonamides)
- Reduced anticoagulant effect – pharmacodynamic effect (e.g. oral contraceptives, vitamin K).

Side-effects

- Haemorrhage: identify indicators of haemorrhage such as haematuria, skin petechia, oral bleeding. It may occur more commonly in trauma, infection, diabetics and the elderly.
- Long-term effects: rib fractures.

Cerebral thrombosis or peripheral arterial occlusion

Aspirin is more appropriate in reducing risk of transient ischaemic attacks than oral anticoagulants.

Thromboembolic disease in pregnancy

- Heparins are preferred because they do not cross the placenta; warfarin is associated with congenital malformations and fetal and neonatal haemorrhage. Warfarin should not be used during pregnancy.
- LMWHs have a lower risk of osteoporosis and of heparin-induced thrombocytopenia.
- Treatment should be stopped at onset of labour.

Arterial thromboembolism

This is associated with cerebral infarction (stroke) and transient ischaemic attacks. When transient ischaemic attacks occur, prophylaxis is required.

- In cerebral infarction anticoagulant treatment may increase risk of conversion of infarction of brain substance to haemorrhage. Control of hypertension is important.
- Use of antiplatelet drugs that inhibit thrombus formation on arterial side is indicated.

Antiplatelet drugs

Aspirin

- Blocks synthesis of thromboxane A_2 from arachidonic acid in platelets by acetylating and hence inhibiting enzyme cyclo-oxygenase.
- Prevents production of prostacyclin from endothelial cells; inhibits platelet aggregation.
- Dose: 75 mg daily for long-term use; a dose of 300 mg as soon as possible after ischaemic event is recommended.
- Gastrointestinal irritation and bleeding may occur, use of enteric-coated preparations may reduce damage due to direct contact in the gastric mucosa but will not exclude occurrence of this side-effect (see also Chapter 31).

Dipyridamole

- A platelet adhesion inhibitor
- An adjunct to oral anticoagulation for prophylaxis of thromboembolism associated with prosthetic heart valves. Modified-release formulations are used (usually in combination with aspirin) for secondary prevention of ischaemic stroke and transient ischaemic attacks
- 300–600 mg daily in three to four divided doses 30 minutes before food
- Side-effects: hypotension, nausea, headache, diarrhoea in the first weeks of treatment.

Clopidogrel

- Used in the prevention of atherosclerotic events in patients with a history of symptomatic atherosclerotic disease (ischaemic stroke, myocardial infarction)

- Cautions: haemorrhage; avoid for first few days after myocardial infarction and ischaemic stroke
- Side-effects: dyspepsia, abdominal pain, diarrhoea, bleeding disorders.

Practice summary

- User-friendly coagulometers using a fingerprick sample are available making it possible for pharmacists to participate in point-of-care prothrombin time monitoring in outpatient clinics and community pharmacies.
- Pharmacists should participate in providing patient counselling regarding drug therapy and side-effects to be expected.
- Interpretation of INR results:
  - INR maintained between 2 and 3.5 depending on condition being treated
  - INR over 7: serious threat of bleeding
  - if INR is low warfarin is increased
  - if INR is high warfarin is decreased.
- Warfarin is an oral anticoagulant drug that is prone to numerous interactions with other drugs. Patients should be advised to avoid taking other medicines unless recommended by a health professional who is aware that they are on warfarin therapy. Regular monitoring of the prothrombin time should be undertaken.

Questions

1 What patient monitoring is required in patients receiving warfarin? What advice should be given to the patients?

2 What are the signs of heparin-induced thrombocytopenia? Which parameters should be monitored?

Answers

1 Prothrombin time expressed as INR (international normalised ratio) should be monitored. Patients should be advised not to stop taking medication or start any other medication without pharmacist or doctor advice and to report any unexplained bleeding.

2 Heparin-induced thrombocytopenia is immune mediated and does not usually develop until after 5–10 days. Platelet count is measured before initiation of therapy and monitored thereafter if treatment exceeds 4 days. Signs include: 50% reduction of platelets, thrombosis, skin allergy. Heparin therapy should be withdrawn when condition occurs and alternative anticoagulants such as hirudins may be used. Parameters that should be monitored: platelet count, occurrence of bleeding.

Further reading

Anon (2008). Community pharmacy plays its part in making anticoagulation therapy safer. *Pharm J* 280: 78.

Coleman B, Patterson D, Long M and Farrell J (2003). Setting quality standards for a community pharmacist-led anticoagulant clinic. *Pharm J* 270: 308–311.

Rahman M H and Beattie J (2004). Drugs used to prevent surgical VTE. *Pharm J* 273: 717–719.

Sellier E, Labarere J, Bosson J L, Auvray M, Barrelier M T, Le Hello C *et al.* (2006). Effectiveness of a guideline for venous thromboembolism prophylaxis in elderly post-acute care patients. *Arch Intern Med* 166: 2065–2071.

Acknowledgements

Bernard Coleiro, Consultant Physician, Department of Medicine, Mater Dei Hospital, Malta.

25

Allergic rhinitis, asthma and chronic obstructive pulmonary disease

Learning objectives:

- To adopt a comparative approach towards antihistamine products
- To develop skills to identify appropriate use of drug therapy in allergic rhinitis
- To identify properties and characteristics of drugs used in asthma and chronic obstructive pulmonary disease.

Background

Cough is a common symptom which may indicate occurrence of infective conditions or allergy-related, chronic conditions. Histamine is a protein that is associated with the occurrence of allergic reactions.

Histamine

Histamine is an endocrine mediator that is found in many tissues and upon release its effects are mostly local. It is involved in allergic reactions and in the regulation of secretion of gastric acid.

Two main types of histamine receptors:

- H_1: in smooth muscle of intestine, bronchi, blood vessels
- H_2: in gastric parietal cells.

The histamine contents of human tissues are shown in Table 25.1.

Table 25.1 Histamine content of human tissues

Tissue	Histamine content (micrograms/g)
Lung	33 ± 10
Mucous membranes (nose)	15.6
Stomach	14 ± 4
Skin (face)	30.4
Skeletal muscle	0.97 ± 0.13

Pharmacological effects of histamine

- Circulatory effects: arteriolar dilatation, increased capillary permeability
- Smooth muscle: bronchi – bronchoconstriction
- Effects on secretions: stimulates gastric acid and pepsin secretion.

Antihistamines

These antagonise the effect of histamine.

- H_1-receptor antagonists are useful in the management of allergic reactions (hay fever, rhinitis, urticaria, food allergy). Reduce rhinorrhoea and sneezing, less effective against nasal congestion.
- May also exhibit effects at other receptors (cholinergic, dopaminergic and serotoninergic).
- Maximum effect occurs several hours after peak serum concentration has been obtained.

Uses of antihistamines are listed in Table 25.2.

> Chlorphenamine is used by slow intravenous administration as an adjunct to adrenaline in emergency treatment of anaphylaxis and angioedema.

Chemical classification

The antihistamines generally consist of two aromatic groups that are linked on the short chain to a tertiary aliphatic amine. The chemical classification of antihistamines is shown in Figure 25.1 and the characteristics of the five groups in Table 25.3.

Second-generation antihistamines

- Demonstrate selectivity to peripheral H_1 receptors
- Less anticholinergic effects than first-generation products
- Decreased affinity for adrenergic and serotoninergic receptors
- Amphoteric in nature, low penetration across blood–brain barrier resulting in a lower potential for sedation and psychomotor impairment.

Side-effects

- Cholinergic blockade
- Drying of secretions
- Dry mouth
- Urinary retention and constipation
- Visual disorders: blurred vision
- Central nervous system depression
- Sedation and dizziness
- Parodoxical treatment, insomnia and tremors

The sedative effects of selected first-generation antihistamine drugs are compared in Table 25.4.

Table 25.2 Uses of antihistamines

Common cold	For example, promethazine	Lessens rhinorrhoea, sedation
Allergies	For example, loratadine	Relieves sneezing, rhinorrhoea, itching of eyes, nose and throat, pruritus
Hypnotics	Doxylamine	See Chapter 29
Motion sickness	Dimenhydrinate	See Chapter 61

Table 25.3 Characteristics of antihistamines

Alkylamines	Very effective at low dosages, long duration of action, practical for daytime use due to low incidence of central sedative effects
Ethanolamines	High incidence of drowsiness and anticholinergic side-effects but a low occurrence of gastrointestinal side-effects, relatively short half-life
Phenothiazines	High incidence of drowsiness, suppress cough reflux, pronounced antiemetic and antimuscarinic effects, prolonged action
Piperazines	Moderate sedation, significant antiemetic effect leading to some products having a primary use in the treatment of motion sickness, vertigo, nausea and vomiting
Piperidines	Highly selective for H_1 receptors, moderate-to-low sedation

Alkylamines

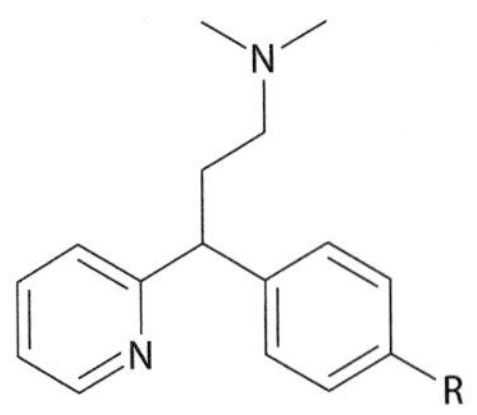

R=Br **brompheniramine**
R=Cl **chlorphenamine**

Ethanolamines

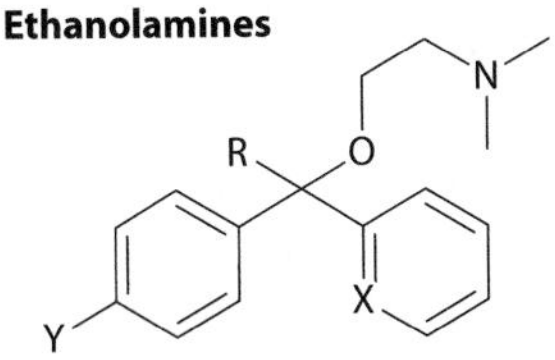

R=H; X=H; Y=H **diphenhydramine**
R=$-CH_3$; X=N; Y=H **doxylamine**
R=H; X=H; Y=Cl **carbinoxamine**

Phenothiazines

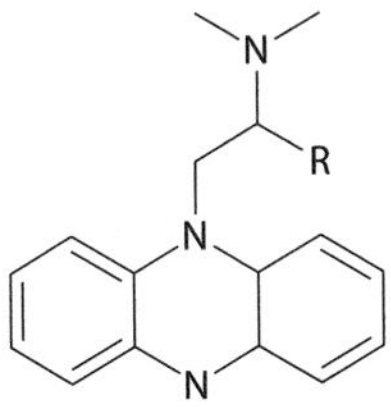

R=$-CH_3$ **promethazine**

Piperazines

R=Cl; R_1=$-CH_2CH_2-O-CH_2CH_2-OH$ **hydroxyzine**
R=H; R_1=$-CH_3$ **cyclizine**
R=Cl; R_1=$-CH_2-C_6H_5$ **meclizine**
R=H; R_1=$-CH_2CH_2-O-CH_2-COOH$ **cetirizine***

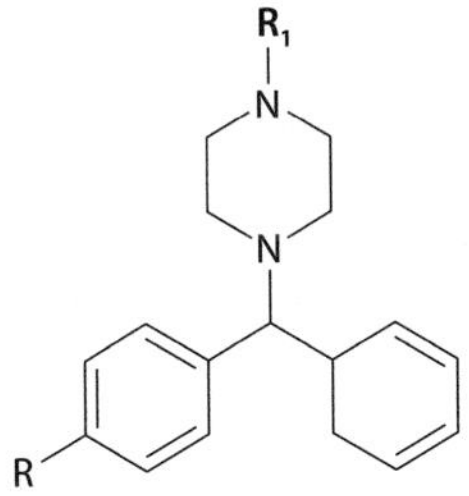

Piperidines

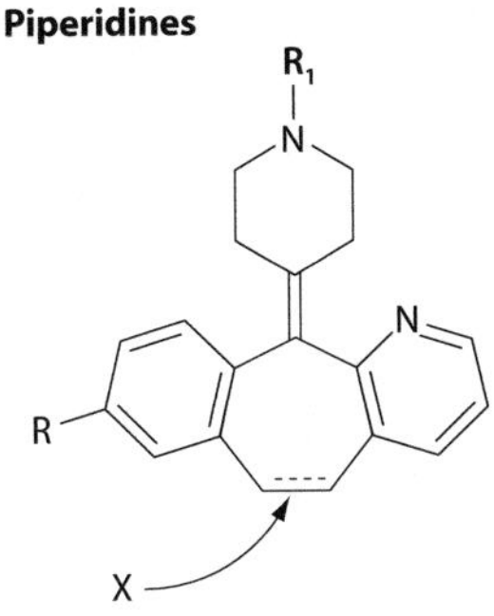

R=H; R_1=$-CH_3$; X=double bond **cyproheptadine**
R=$-Cl$; R_1=$-COO-C_2H_5$; X=single bond **loratadine***

Figure 25.1 Chemical structures of antihistamines. *Second-generation antihistamines.

Table 25.4 Comparison of sedative effects of selected first-generation antihistamine drugs

Drug	Degree of sedation
Diphenhydramine	+++
Promethazine	+++
Clemastine	++
Trimeprazine	++
Chlorphenamine	+
Mequitazine	+

- When choosing an antihistamine consider degree of drowsiness desired.
- Loratadine and fexofenadine have been shown to be associated with a lower incidence of sedation than acrivastine and cetirizine.
- Patients should still be advised to be careful when driving or operating machinery even when non-sedating antihistamines are used.
- Advise patient that consumption of alcohol with antihistamines increases risk of sedation.

Cautions/contraindications

- Elderly patients
- Neonates and children (particularly phenothiazines) due to higher susceptibility to antimuscarinic effects
- Cardiovascular disorders
- Benign prostatic hypertrophy
- Glaucoma
- Hepatic and renal disease
- Epilepsy.

Interactions

- Sedating antihistamines: alcohol, hypnotics, opioid analgesics, anxiolytics, antipsychotics
- Hazardous ventricular arrhythmias reported with non-sedating antihistamine products (astemizole and terfenadine).

Uses of antihistamines in paediatric patients are listed in Table 25.5.

- Antihistamines are rapidly absorbed from the gastrointestinal tract
- Tolerance may develop.

Other dosage form presentations of antihistamine

- Levocabastine, emedastine: nasal spray and eye drops
- Mepyramine: topical skin preparations; disadvantages: hypersensitivity and photosensitivity (see Chapter 47).

Other uses of antihistamines

- Migraine: doxylamine is used in compound analgesic preparations for migraine for its sedating properties and antiemetic effect
- Appetite stimulation: cyproheptadine, which is an antihistamine and serotonin antagonist, is used as an appetite stimulant, especially in anorexia nervosa. Side-effects include sedation and weight gain.

Table 25.5 Uses of antihistamines in paediatric patients

Drug	Recommended age	Availability of oral liqud dosage form
Cetirizine	Over 2 years	Yes
Desloratadine	Over 1 year	Yes
Fexofenadine	Over 6 years	No
Levocetirizine	Over 2 years	Yes
Loratadine	Over 2 years	Yes
Chlorphenamine	Over 1 year	Yes
Hydroxyzine	Over 6 months	Yes
Promethazine	Over 2 years	Yes

Allergic rhinitis

- Also referred to as hay fever
- Allergy to pollen grains
- Symptoms: sneezing, rhinorrhoea, nasal congestion, watery eyes, wheezing, coughing.

Description of presentation of allergic rhinitis

- Duration: intermittent or persistent
- Severity: mild or moderate–severe.

Treatment

- Non-sedating antihistamines vs sedating antihistamines: in patients with intermittent symptoms or mild symptoms of allergic rhinitis, antihistamines are recommended. The non-sedating antihistamines are preferred since they do not impact negatively on the patient's daily functioning.
- Steroid-containing nasally administered products (e.g. beclometasone, budesonide, fluticasone): used for persistent symptoms with nasal congestion.
- Cautions: untreated nasal infections, nasal surgery, pulmonary tuberculosis.
- Side-effects: dryness, irritation of nose and throat, epistaxis.
- Depot preparations are not recommended; they may cause local fat atrophy and local abscess formation.
- Decongestant-containing systemically administered products: these alleviate the symptoms of rhinorrhoea and nasal congestion.

Products for prophylaxis: sodium cromoglicate, ketotifen

- Used as prophylactic agents in mild-to-moderate symptoms

- May be used when symptoms are persistent
- Preferred in children to topical corticosteroids
- Side-effects: local irritation, transient bronchospasm.

Leukotriene receptor antagonists

- Montelukast and zafirlukast block the effects of cysteinyl leukotrienes in the airways. May be used in patients with concomitant asthma

Anticholinergic agents

- Products such as ipratropium bromide which have an anticholinergic effect may be administered topically to reduce watery, nasal secretions. However, their use is not clinically studied so much to date.

- Antihistamines should be used with caution in older patients and in paediatric patients
- In patients with allergy and a stuffy nose, combination products containing an antihistamine and a decongestant administered systemically may cause less drowsiness because the decongestant product which is a sympathomimetic agent will counteract the drowsiness brought about by the antihistamine.
- Patients using intranasal corticosteroids should be advised on proper administration technique so that the product is sprayed towards the nostril lining rather than on the septum. Repeated spraying of the corticosteroid on to the nasal septum may lead to damage.

Asthma and chronic obstructive pulmonary disease

Asthma

Asthma is a condition in which inflammation of small bronchi results in recurrent, reversible episodes of airway obstruction, causing dyspnoea, wheezing and cough.

Chronic obstructive pulmonary disease (COPD)

A progressive and irreversible condition characterised by diminished inspiratory and expiratory capacity of the lungs causing dyspnoea and chronic cough.

- Patients should be advised to stop smoking and to avoid smoking areas.
- Acute severe asthma attacks and deterioration of COPD may be exacerbated by upper respiratory tract infections.
- Hospitalisation may have to be considered in acute exacerbations of COPD and in acute severe asthma attacks.

Bronchodilators

These are useful in acute attacks and in maintenance therapy.

- Beta$_2$ agonists (e.g. salbutamol and terbutaline, which are short acting, and salmeterol, formoterol, which are long acting and should not be used for the management of an acute asthma attack) should be used with caution in hyperthyroidism, cardiovascular disease and hypertension
- Antimuscarinics (e.g. ipratropium, which is short acting, and tiotropium, which is long acting) should be used with caution in glaucoma (especially when administered by nebulisation), prostatic hyperplasia and bladder outflow obstruction.

- Salbutamol and terbutaline may be used for the relief of an asthma attack since they have a rapid onset of activity.
- Hypokalaemia may occur as a result of beta$_2$-agonist therapy, particularly when high doses are used or when administered

systemically. Care should be taken in patients receiving diuretics and corticosteroids.

Corticosteroids

These reduce bronchial inflammation. In asthma they are useful for the prevention of attacks and in COPD they reduce exacerbations.

- Administered on a regular basis to achieve the prophylactic effect
- Examples: beclometasone, budesonide, fluticasone
- May be used in combination with bronchodilators. Combination inhalers that present a corticosteroid and a long-acting beta$_2$ agonist are available.

Beclometasone and fluticasone are halogenated corticosteroids whereas budesonide is a non-halogenated corticosteroid (Figure 25.2). They are equally effective. The three of them exhibit a high relative lipophilicity. This characteristic may improve receptor affinity and increase retention of the drug in the nasal or lung tissues. This increased lipophilicity compared with oral steroids such as prednisolone and hydrocortisone (which are less effective if adopted for inhalation) results in a low oral bioavailability if administered orally.

- In acute severe asthma attacks, the administration of high-flow oxygen therapy (see Chapter 3) and a short-acting beta$_2$ agonist are first line of management.
- In COPD, mucolytics (Chapter 54) may be considered for the management of chronic productive cough.
- In severe COPD, long-term oxygen therapy may be considered.

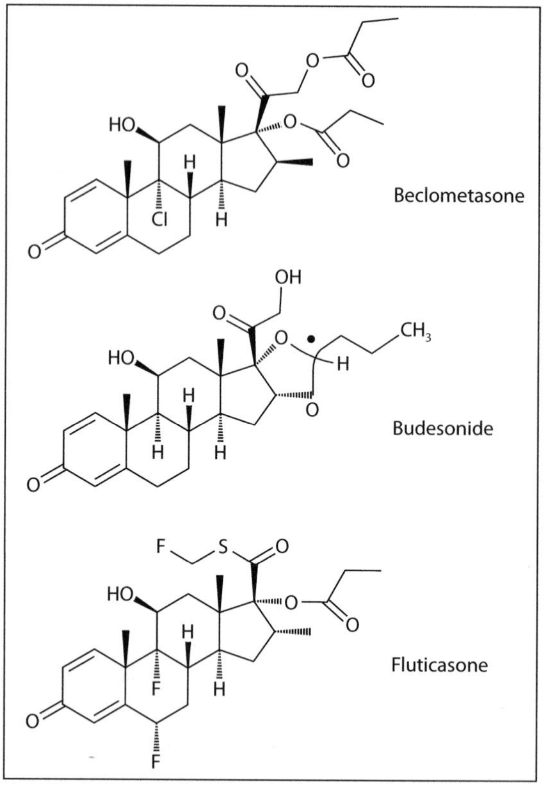

Figure 25.2 Chemical structures of beclometasone, budesonide and fluticasone.

Administration by inhalation

In asthma and COPD, drugs are preferably administered by inhalation since this route of administration delivers the drug directly to the respiratory system, minimising side-effects due to reduced systemic action.

- Pressurised metered-dose inhalers: require coordination between the act of actuation and inhaling for effective drug delivery
- Breath-actuated devices: drug delivery is activated by patient's inhalation
- Spacer device: used to improve drug delivery in patients who have difficulty in achieving the required coordination when using pressurised metered-dose inhalers (e.g. paediatric patients and the elderly) and to decrease local side-effects from inhaled corticosteroids
- Solutions for nebulisation: used in the management of severe asthma; require a nebuliser that is usually driven by oxygen.

- In severe cases or during severe acute attacks, oral or parenteral therapy with bronchodilators and corticosteroids may be required.
- When both bronchodilators and corticosteroids inhalers are prescribed, patients should be advised to first use the short-acting $beta_2$-agonist inhaler and then to use the corticosteroid inhaler.

Side-effects after inhalation therapy

- $Beta_2$ agonists: fine tremor, headache, palpitations, muscle cramps, nervous tension
- Corticosteroids: oral candidiasis; advise patient to rinse mouth after administration; the use of a spacer reduces incidence. After long-term inhalation of high doses, osteoporosis, glaucoma and in children growth retardation may occur.

Practice summary

- In allergic rhinitis, antihistamines are preferred in intermittent symptoms and mild symptoms. Cromoglicate is not as effective as intranasal corticosteroids and no more effective than antihistamines. Intranasal corticosteroids are more effective than antihistamines and are preferred in moderate-to-severe disease.
- In asthma and COPD, bronchodilators and corticosteroids are the mainstay of therapy. Combination therapy may be adopted.
- Inhalation therapy is the preferred route of drug administration. Patients need to receive advice on proper technique for drug administration.

Questions

1. Compare chlorphenamine and hydroxyzine.
2. Giving reasons for your answer, explain when bronchodilators are indicated.
3. What is a spacer device and when is it used?

Answers

1. Both are first-generation or sedating antihistamines. *Chlorphenamine* is an alkylamine. It is very effective at low dosages, has a long duration of action and is practical for daytime use due to low incidence of central sedative effects. Indications include symptomatic relief of an allergy such as hay fever, urticaria and emergency treatment of anaphylactic reactions. *Hydroxyzine* is a piperazine. It is associated with moderate sedation. Indications include pruritus and anxiety (short term). Chlorphenamine is recommended for children aged over 1 year and hydroxyzine for children over 6 months. Cautions, contraindications and side-effects are the same: elderly and paediatric patients, cardiovascular disorders, benign prostatic hypertrophy, glaucoma, hepatic and renal disease, epilepsy. Side-effects: sedation, dizziness, drying of secretions, dry mouth, urinary retention, constipation, blurred vision.
2. Bronchodilators are useful in acute attacks and maintenance therapy in asthma and COPD. They dilate the bronchi and the bronchioles, resulting in an increasing airflow.
3. A spacer is a device used by an asthmatic person to increase the effectiveness of an asthma inhaler. Spacers are specially designed plastic or metal tubes that fit an inhaler on one end, while the patient breathes normally on the other end. Their use eliminates the requirement to coordinate the actions of actuation and inhalation which is required with metered-dose inhalers.

Further reading

Anon (2003). International guideline on pharmacy management of hay fever. *Pharm J* 270: 428.

Mason P (2003). Management of hay fever in the pharmacy. *Pharm J* 270: 443–445.

Salib R and Howarth P (2002). Treating intermittent and persistent allergic rhinitis. *Prescriber* 5 May: 47–66.

26

Schizophrenia

Learning objectives:

- To describe characteristics of schizophrenia
- To understand use of antipsychotic medications
- To identify clinical issues associated with maintenance treatment for schizophrenia
- To develop skills to be able to participate in patient support and monitoring in the management of schizophrenia.

Background

Onset of schizophrenia commonly occurs in late adolescence or early adulthood. Increasing evidence supports a hypothesis that dopamine receptor defects exist in schizophrenia. This does not exclude other systems involving serotonin and noradrenaline. Clinical presentation can be extremely varied and the condition carries a high risk of suicide.

Definition

Schizophrenia is a *chronic* disorder of thought and affect, with the individual having a significant disturbance in interpersonal relationships and the ability to function in society on a daily basis.

Symptoms

- Positive (+) symptoms: hallucinations (visual or auditory), agitation, delusions (persecution, guilt)
- Negative (–) symptoms: loss of interest, loss of capabilities, lack of emotion, decreased initiation of goal-directed behaviour
- Cognitive symptoms: memory attention problems, inability to plan
- Affective symptoms: depression, increased risk of suicidal behaviour.

In the acute phase, the brain creates a false reality where the patient may report:

- audible thoughts
- hearing voices
- thought insertion
- thought broadcasting
- experiencing feelings not his or her own
- experiencing actions under control of external influence
- delusional perception.

Diagnostic criteria

The American Psychiatric Association[1] has developed diagnostic criteria that can be used in the diagnosis of schizophrenia:

A At least two of the following each present for a significant portion of time during a 1-month period:

1 delusions
2 hallucinations
3 disorganised speech (frequent derailment, incoherence)
4 grossly disorganised or catatonic behaviour
5 negative symptoms (affective flattening)

B Function in areas of work, social relations and self-care is low
C Continuous signs of illness for at least 6 months of which at least 1 month of symptoms from criterion A
D Not resulting from an organic mental disorder.

Assess occurrence of coexisting conditions, including other psychiatric disorders particularly depression and anxiety.

Financial impacts of schizophrenia

- Direct expenses of treatment and care including hospitalisation, professional services and clinic visits
- Lost production for patient and carer including economic burden to families and loss of productivity caused by illness and need for patient support.

Aims of treatment

- To reduce disruption of patient's and carers' lives as a consequence of inappropriate behaviour, anxiety, delusional thinking and hallucinations
- To reduce relapse: schizophrenia is associated with a relatively poor outcome with many patients experiencing exacerbation of symptoms that may require hospitalisation and suicide attempts.

Management options

A comprehensive management package that incorporates both pharmacotherapy as well as non-pharmacological interventions should be adopted. Non-pharmacological interventions include:

- social skills training
- occupational therapy
- behavioural therapy
- family therapy.

Antipsychotic drugs

- Phenothiazines (e.g. chlorpromazine)
- Thioxanthenes (e.g. flupentixol)
- Butyrophenones (e.g. haloperidol)
- Atypical (e.g. clozapine, olanzapine, risperidone).

Antipyschotics block dopamine receptors. First-generation (typical) antipsychotics have a high affinity towards dopamine D_2 receptors. The atypical antipsychotics (second and third generation) have a lower affinity for dopamine D_2 receptors but have significant affinity towards other receptors including serotonin and noradrenaline receptors. This difference in affinity to receptors is thought to be the cause of differences in the occurrence of side-effects.

The classification of neuroleptics based on potency is summarised in Table 26.1 and antipsychotic drugs are compared in Table 26.2.

The atypical antipsychotics pose a lower risk of extrapyramidal symptoms (EPS) but are associated with hypotension, weight gain and an increased risk of diabetes and hyperlipidaemia.

Table 26.1 Classification of neuroleptics based on potency

Potency	Drug	Potency (chlorpromazine = 1)
Weak	Perazine Thioridazine Promazine	0.5 0.5 0.5
Moderate	Chlorpromazine Clopenthixol	1 2–3
Strong	Trifluoperazine	10–20
Very strong	Fluphenazine Haloperidol	50 50

Table 26.2 Comparison of antipsychotic drugs

Antipsychotic	Risk of extrapyramidal symptoms	Risk of tardive dyskinesia	Effect on prolactin	Efficacy on symptoms
First generation (typical): haloperidol, chlorpromazine	High	High	Elevation	+
Second generation: risperidone	Dose variable	Possibly dose variable	Elevation	+, –
Third generation: olanzapine, quetiapine	Low	Low	Sparing	+, –, cognitive, mood

The occurrence of hyperprolactinaemia may lead to galactorrhoea, gynaecomastia, amenorrhoea, anovulation, decreased libido and decreased sexual arousal.

Extrapyramidal symptoms

- Parkinsonian symptoms:
  - onset is gradual
  - cease with drug withdrawal or administration of antimuscarinic agents
- Dystonia and dyskinesia:
  - abnormal face and body movements
  - occur after a few doses
- Akathisia:
  - restlessness
  - occurs after large initial doses
- Tardive dyskinesia:
  - involuntary movements of tongue, face, jaws
  - develops after long-term treatment
  - may persist after drug withdrawal.

Phenothiazines

Phenothiazines are tricyclic antipsychotic agents which consist of two benzene rings fused via a sulphur and a nitrogen atom. They are further classified according to the nature of the nitrogen-containing substituent on position 10 into aliphatics, piperazines and piperidines. An electronegative moiety at position 2 increases the antipsychotic activity as witnessed in chlorpromazine when compared with promazine (which effectively has the same chemical structure but lacks the chlorine moiety at position 2) (Figure 26.1).

The side-effects of phenothiazines are compared in Table 26.3.

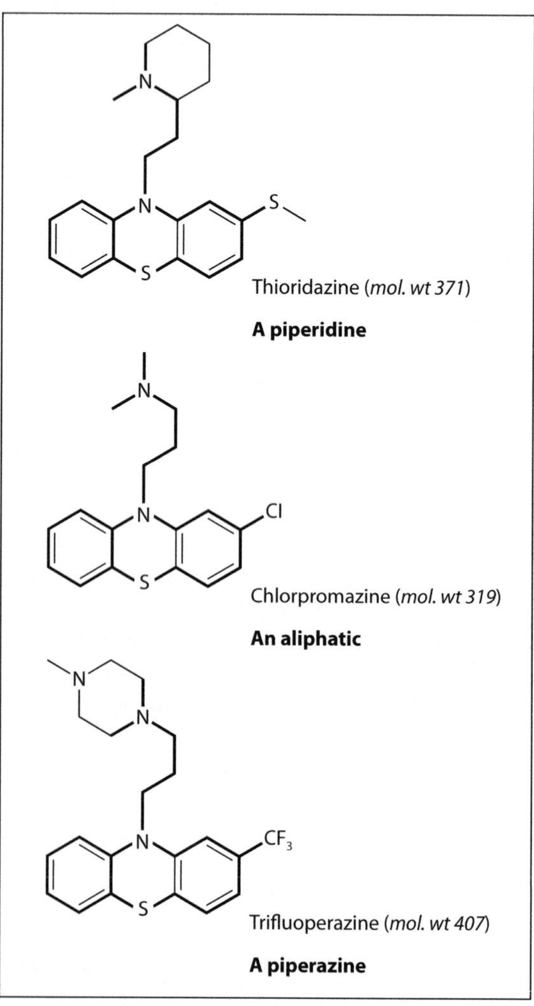

Figure 26.1 Examples of piperidine, aliphatic and piperazine structures.

Table 26.3 Comparison of side-effects of phenothiazines

Drug	Anticholinergic	Sedation	Hypotension	EPSs
Aliphatic Chlorpromazine	++++	+++++	+++++	++
Piperazine Trifluoperazine	++	+	++	++++
Piperidine Thioridazine	+++++	++++	+++++	+

EPSs, extrapyramidal symptoms.

Thioxanthenes and butyrophenones

Thioxanthenes (e.g. flupentixol; see Figure 26.2) are chemically related to phenothiazines. They consist of two benzene rings linked by a sulphur and a carbon atom.

Butyrophenones (e.g. haloperidol; see Figure 26.3) are heterocyclic compounds with a prolonged action. The presence of a tertiary amino group attached to the fourth carbon of the butyrophenone structure is required for neuroleptic activity. The presence of halogen atoms in haloperidol explains the relatively high potency of the drug.

The side-effects of antipsychotic drugs other than phenothiazines are compared in Table 26.4.

Common anticholinergic side-effects include dry mouth and throat (which could cause dental caries), constipation, urinary retention and dry eyes.

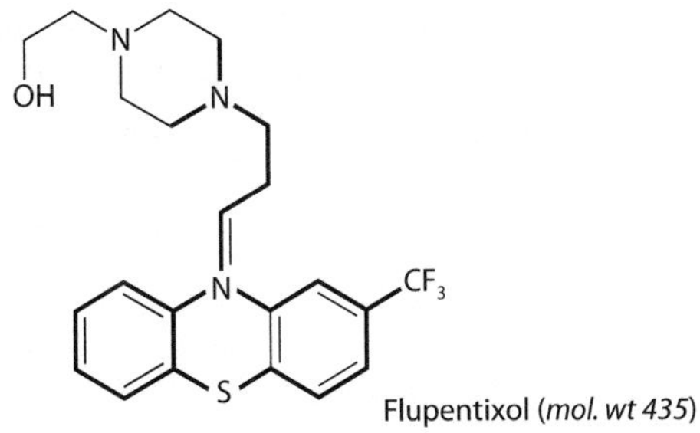

Flupentixol (*mol. wt 435*)

Figure 26.2 Chemical structure of flupentixol.

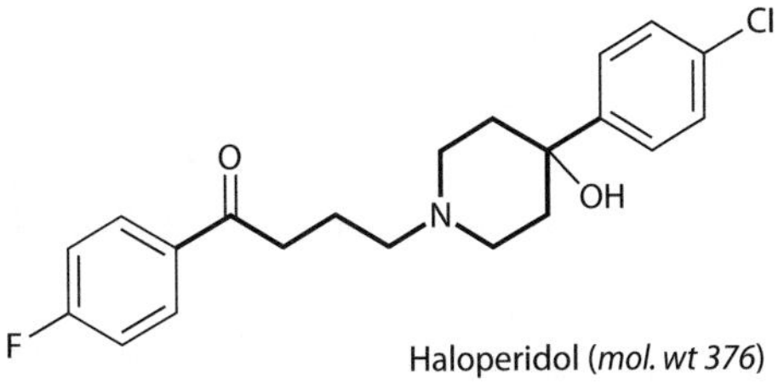

Haloperidol (*mol. wt 376*)

Figure 26.3 Chemical structure of haloperidol.

Table 26.4 Comparison of side-effects of other antipsychotic drugs

Drug	Anticholinergic	Sedation	Hypotension	EPSs
Thioxanthenes flupentixol	++	++	++	++++
Butyrophenones haloperidol	+	++	+	++++
Atypical clozapine	+++	+++	+++	

EPSs, extrapyramidal symptoms.

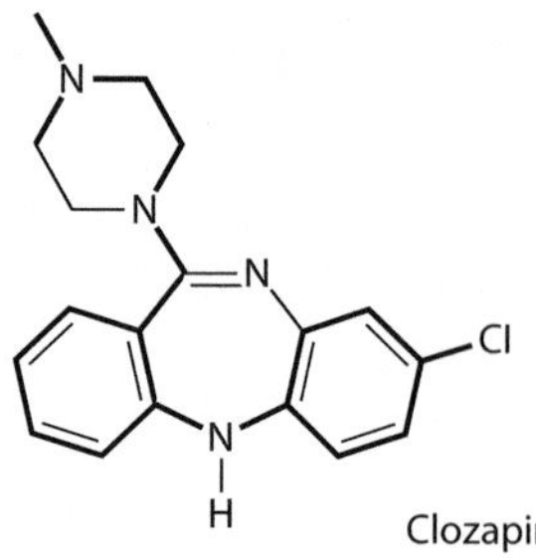

Figure 26.4 Chemical structure of clozapine.

Clozapine

Blood dyscrasias may occur with antipsychotic drugs. The use of clozapine (Figure 26.4) may lead to agranulocytosis in some patients. For this reason the use of clozapine is limited.

> Regular white blood counts should be carried out in patients receiving clozapine to reduce risk of agranuloctyosis. Patients should be advised to report immediately occurrence of fever, malaise or respiratory infections.

Risperidone

Risperidone (Figure 26.5) blocks D_2 and $5HT_2$ receptors. It is administered in a twice-daily regimen.

- A lower dose should be used in older patients and in patients with renal insufficiency.
- Potential interactions with anticholinergics may occur.
- It is associated with a low incidence of EPSs.
- Side-effects: insomnia, anxiety, agitation.

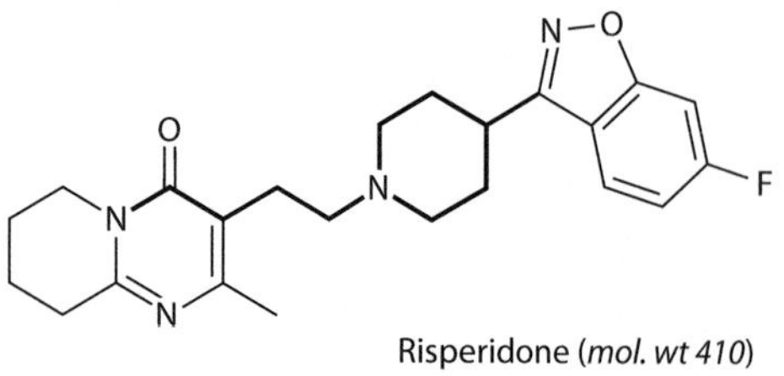

Figure 26.5 Chemical structure of risperidone.

Use of atypical antipsychotics

Atypical antipsychotics should be considered when:

- choosing first-line treatment in newly diagnosed cases
- unacceptable side-effects have occurred with conventional antipsychotic drugs
- outcomes of therapy with conventional antipsychotics are inadequate.

Initiation of pharmacotherapy

- Better response in the long term is expected when treatment is started early.
- New and acceptable medicines are available.
- Regular review of medicines by health professionals should be undertaken to identify drug-related problems and patient non-compliance.
- Continued treatment (maintenance therapy) is required in a number of cases and, to achieve this, the establishment of a therapeutic alliance with the patient and the carers is necessary.

Response to medication

The great majority of patients show substantial improvement with antipsychotic medicines. However, in some patients poor response may occur. In these patients, check compliance, assess dosing, monitor unacceptable stress levels and consider addition of mood stabilisers (see Chapter 27).

Patient counselling and monitoring

- At start-up: check for personal or family history of diabetes, dyslipidaemia, hypertension, cardiovascular disease, epilepsy.
- Patient advice: diet, exercise, weight control and information on how to take medication.
- Monitoring:
  - at baseline – blood glucose, lipid profile, blood pressure, ECG
  - check again after 3 months
  - assess clinical symptoms.

Special considerations in elderly patients (e.g. higher risk of occurrence of postural hypotension especially with blockers of alpha_1 receptors such as risperidone and olanzapine). Consider occurrence of comorbidities and use of other drugs.

Cautions when using antipsychotic agents

- Hepatic and renal impairment, cardiovascular disease, Parkinson's disease, epilepsy, depression, myasthenia gravis, prostatic hypertrophy, glaucoma, the elderly
- For the atypical: concomitant use with drugs that prolong QT interval, cardiovascular disease, epilepsy, the elderly.

Atypical antipsychotics and stroke

- Increased risk of stroke reported with olanzapine and risperidone in older people
- Risk factors for cerebrovascular disease and past history of stroke and transient ischaemic attacks increase risk.

Drug interactions

- Anti-arrhythmics – increased risk of arrhythmias:
  - clozapine with flecainide
  - haloperidol, phenothiazines, sertindole with amiodarone
- Antibacterial – increased risk of arrhythmias:
  - sertindole with macrolides
- Antibacterial – increased plasma concentration of antipsychotic:
  - olanzapine and ciprofloxacin.

Considerations in patient management

- Withdrawal of treatment requires close monitoring since it may result in a disastrous relapse. Occurrence of relapse may be delayed after cessation of treatment.
- Compliance: high rates of termination of antipsychotic treatment. Lieberman *et al.*[2] report that 74% of patients studied discontinued treatment before 18 months.

Long-acting depot injections

These are used when compliance with oral treatment presents a problem; however, once the drug is administered the dose is not reversible.

- May give rise to a higher frequency of EPSs
- Administered by deep intramuscular injection every few weeks
- Examples: haloperidol, risperidone, flupentixol.

Emergency administration of antipsychotics

- In acute attacks, antipsychotics may be used to control agitation and disturbed behaviour.
- They may be given by the intramuscular route (e.g. chlorpromazine, olanzapine).
- There is no first-pass effect with intramuscular route and so a lower dose can be used than for the oral route.

Practice summary

- All antipsychotics can reduce seizure threshold.
- Weight gain for atypical antipsychotics (check cardiovascular risk factor – could impact on patient adherence to treatment and in the long term on increased mortality): olanzapine > clozapine > risperidone > quetiapine > sertindole > zotepine.
- Atypical antipsychotics may alter glucose and lipid metabolism.

- Atypicals are associated with occurrence of sedation: clozapine > olanzapine > quetiapine.
- Care should be taken when using antipsychotics in patients with cardiovascular disorders.
- Clozapine should be introduced at the earliest opportunity in patients with treatment-resistant schizophrenia.

Question

1 Compare chlorpromazine, trifluoperazine and haloperidol.

Answer

1 All are first-generation neuroleptics indicated in schizophrenia. They are effective only for the positive symptoms of schizophrenia (hallucinations, agitation, delusions). The three preparations have a different chemical classification and potency resulting in differing side-effect profiles.

- Chlorpromazine is an aliphatic phenothiazine with moderate potency.
- Trifluoperazine is a piperazine phenothiazine with strong potency.
- Haloperidol is a butyrophenone (not a phenothiazine) which has a very strong potency.

Chlorpromazine causes anticholinergic side-effects, sedation and hypotension to a greater extent compared with trifluoperazine and haloperidol (haloperidol less than trifluoperazine). On the other hand, chlorpromazine poses the least risk for the occurrence of extrapyramidal symptoms (EPSs) whilst trifluoperazine and haloperidol cause EPSs to a greater extent. The extent of EPSs is related to potency. All may cause prolactin elevation.

Further reading

Guthrie S K (2002). Clinical issues associated with maintenance treatment of patients with schizophrenia. *Am J Health-Syst Pharm* 59(suppl 5): S19–S24.

Maguire G A (2002). Comprehensive understanding of schizophrenia and its treatment. *Am J Health-Syst Pharm* 59(suppl 5): S4–S11.

National Institute for Health and Clinical Excellence (2009). Schizophrenia: core interventions in the treatment and management of schizophrenia in primary and secondary care (update). http://www.nice.org.uk/guidance/index.jsp?action=byID&o=11786.

Taylor D M (2006). *Schizophrenia in Focus*. London: Pharmaceutical Press.

References

1 American Psychiatric Association (2000). *Diagnostic and Statistical Manual of Mental Disorders*, 4th edn. Washington: American Psychiatric Association.

2 Lieberman J A, Stroup T S, McEvoy J P, Swartz M S, Rosenheck R A, Perkins D A *et al.* Effectiveness of antipsychotic drugs in patients with chronic schizophrenia. *N Engl J Med* 2005; 353: 1209–1223.

27

Mood disorders

Learning objectives:

- To describe clinical signs and presentation of depression
- To identify characteristics of bipolar affective disorder and mania
- To understand pharmacotherapeutic options for affective disorders
- To develop skills to be able to assess the impact of psychotropic medications.

Background

- *Depression:* a medical condition that is characterised by a low mood and sleep disturbances that occur persistently.
- *Mania:* a medical condition that is characterised by an elevated, expansive or irritable mood that occurs persistently.
- *Bipolar disorder:* formerly known as manic depressive disease, refers to patients who present with mixed episodes of both mania and depression.

Depression

- Epidemiology: average age of onset – late 20s
- Aetiology: genetic predisposition, environmental factors (e.g. stressful events), biochemical factors, medication, other illness.

Pathophysiology of depression

Changes in brain monoamine neurotransmitters occur resulting in a reduction or functional deficiency of noradrenaline and serotonin.

Medications that may cause or exacerbate depression

- Cardiovascular agents: beta-adrenoceptor blockers, calcium channel blockers, clonidine, digoxin, methyldopa
- Central nervous system agents: alcohol, benzodiazepines, metoclopramide, zolpidem
- Hormonal agents: anabolic steroids, androgens, corticosteroids, gonadorelin analogues, oestrogens
- Others: H_2-receptor antagonists, isotretinoin, indometacin.

Physical illnesses that may precipitate mood disorders

- Addison's disease
- Carcinoma
- Neurological disorders
- Systemic lupus erythematosus
- Chronic inflammatory disease (e.g. rheumatoid arthritis)
- Thyroid disease
- Viral illness (e.g. AIDS).

Patient assessment tools

Patient assessment tools may be used by the clinical team to be able to identify mood disorders and assess patient progress. Examples include:

- Mental Status Exam (AMSIT): used to assess a patient's mental health
- rating scales such as Beck Depression Inventory (BDI), Hamilton Rating Scale for Depression (HAM-D) and Inventory for Depressive Symptoms (IDS). The BDI and IDS are brief scales that can be used in primary care settings to assess patient progress.

Diagnosis and classification

The American Psychiatric Association has described criteria for diagnosing depressive disorders.[1]

Criteria for diagnosing a major depressive episode

- Five or more of the following symptoms have been present during the same 2-week period and represent a change from the patient's previous functioning:
  - depressed mood (feels sad or empty, appears tearful)
  - markedly diminished interest or pleasure in daily activities
  - significant weight loss when not dieting, or weight gain
  - insomnia or hypersomnia nearly every day
  - psychomotor agitation or retardation
  - fatigue or loss of energy
  - feeling of worthlessness or inappropriate guilt
  - diminished ability to think or concentrate, indecisiveness
  - recurrent thoughts of death, recurrent suicidal ideation.
- Symptoms cause clinically significant distress or impairment in social and occupational areas.
- Symptoms are not due to medication or medical condition.
- Symptoms are not accounted for by bereavement.

Criteria for diagnosing a manic episode

- Three or more of the following symptoms have been present to a significant degree for at least 1 week:
  - inflated self-esteem and grandiosity
  - decreased need for sleep
  - more talkative than usual or pressure to keep talking
  - flight of ideas
  - distractibility
  - increase in goal-directed activity or psychomotor agitation
  - excessive involvement in pleasurable activities.
- Mood disturbance is sufficiently severe to cause marked impairment in occupational functioning or in social activities.
- Symptoms are not due to the direct physiological effects of a substance or a general medical condition.

Choices for the acute treatment of a major depressive disorder are summarised in Table 27.1.

Table 27.1 Choices in the acute treatment of a major depressive disorder

Medication	Formal psychotherapy	Medication and psychotherapy	Electroconvulsive therapy
Chronic case, recurrent, psychotic and melancholic	Less severe case, patient not psychotic	Used as a chronic treatment	Resorted to when patient is psychotic, severe
Past positive response	Past positive response	When there is a personality disorder	Failure to respond to medications
Failure to respond to psychotherapy	Medical contraindication to therapy		Require rapid response

Relapse risk factors

- Severity of illness: patients presenting with a major depressive disorder are more likely to experience multiple episodes in life.
- Social factors: peer pressure, environment, support from family and carers.
- Pharmaceutical issues: treatment terminated, low dose, occurrence of side-effects, non-compliance, failure to appreciate need to continue treatment.

Antidepressant drugs

Antidepressant drugs act by increasing the activity of monamines particularly dopamine, noradrenaline and serotonin.

Tricyclic antidepressants (TCAs)

These drugs have a three-ring structure in which two benzene rings are linked by a seven-membered central ring (Figure 27.1).

- Cautions: cardiac disease, history of epilepsy, the elderly, hepatic impairment, thyroid disease, history of mania, psychoses, glaucoma, history of urinary retention.

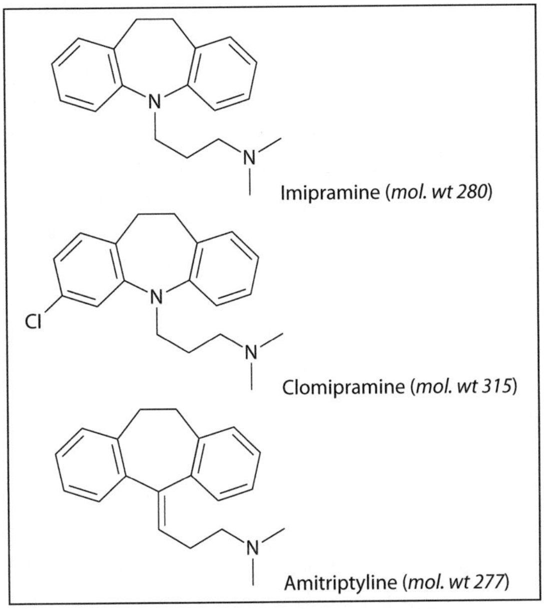

Imipramine (*mol. wt 280*)

Clomipramine (*mol. wt 315*)

Amitriptyline (*mol. wt 277*)

Figure 27.1 Chemical structures of some tricyclic antidepressants (TCAs).

Maprotiline

Maprotiline is structurally related to the tricyclic antidepressants. It consists of an additional ethylene bridge across the central six-carbon ring (Figure 27.2).

Selective serotonin re-uptake inhibitors (SSRIs)

Within the class of SSRIs, different drugs have differing chemical structure (Figure 27.3) but a similar side-effect profile. Their advantages over TCAs include a lower side-effect burden, safety in overdosage and once-daily administration. Pharmacoeconomic analyses have shown that despite the higher cost of SSRIs they are more cost-effective due to higher rates of medication adherence and decreased relapse (see also Chapter 28).

Fluoxetine: has a long half-life and an active metabolite that has a long half-life; this should be kept in mind when switching drugs.

- Cautions: epilepsy, history of mania, cardiac disease, diabetes, glaucoma, history of bleeding disorders, hepatic/renal disease, pregnancy and breast-feeding.

Safety issues and SSRIs

- Suicidal tendencies: use in patients under 18 years is not recommended.
- Gastrointestinal bleeding: SSRIs inhibit uptake and therefore storage of serotonin of platelets. This is significant because

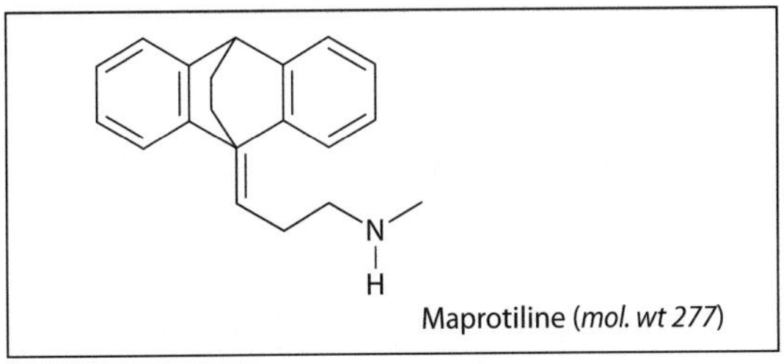

Maprotiline (*mol. wt 277*)

Figure 27.2 Chemical structure of maprotiline.

Citalopram (*mol. wt 324*)

Fluoxetine (*mol. wt 309*)

Fluvoxamine (*mol. wt 318*)

Paroxetine (*mol. wt 329*)

Sertraline (*mol. wt 306*)

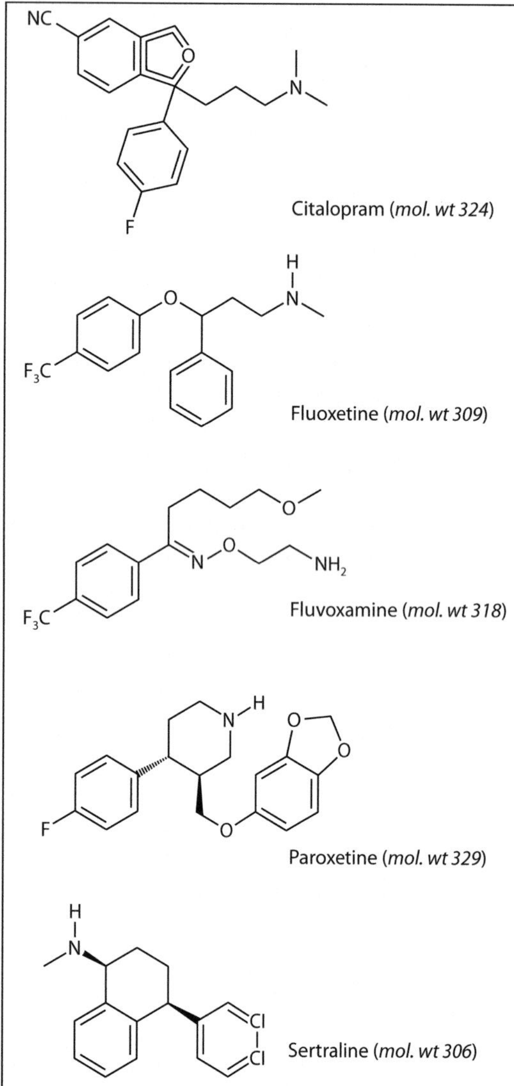

Figure 27.3 Chemical structures of some selective serotonin re-uptake inhibitors (SSRIs).

release of serotonin from platelets augments their aggregation.
- relative risk of gastrointestinal bleeding similar to use of NSAIDs
- avoid in elderly and in patients who are concurrently using NSAIDs
- consider use of a proton pump inhibitor in high-risk patients.

Venlafaxine

Venlafaxine (Figure 27.4) is a serotonin–noradrenaline re-uptake inhibitor (SNRI). Side-effects are very similar to those found with SSRIs. It also may present with side-effects due to increased noradrenaline activity such as hypertension. A risk of suicidal tendencies in children reported.

- Contraindications: heart disease, electrolyte imbalance, hypertension, severe renal and hepatic disease
- Cautions: ECG before treatment, monitor blood pressure, history of epilepsy and bleeding disorders, angle-closure glaucoma.

Tianeptine

- Similar to SSRIs in efficacy
- Has an anxiolytic effect
- Lacks anticholinergic side-effects.

Moclobemide (reversible monoamine oxidase inhibitor)

This is a reversible inhibitor of monoamine oxidase type A enzyme (RIMA). It is referred to as an monoamine oxidase inhibitor (MAOI) with RIMA activity. MAOIs interact with other drugs and tyramine-containing food (e.g. aged cheese, red wine, yeast extracts) leading to a potentiated pressor effect of tyramine and amine drugs. This may cause a dangerous rise in blood pressure. Moclobemide poses a lower risk for this interaction since it inhibits only the type A monoamine oxidase. However, patients should still be advised to avoid consuming large amounts of tyramine-rich food.

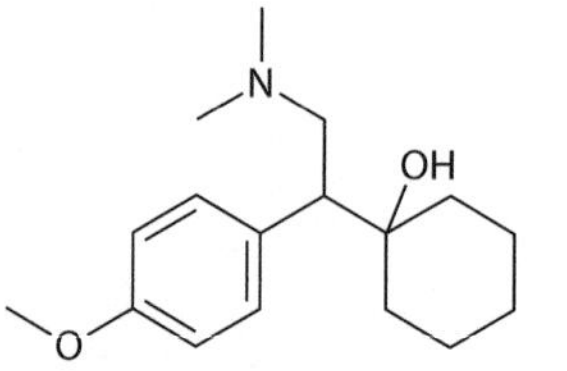

Venlafaxine (*mol. wt 329*)

Figure 27.4 Chemical structure of venlafaxine.

Other drugs

- Reboxetine: a selective inhibitor of noradrenaline re-uptake. May cause insomnia and postural hypotension
- Tryptophan: as a precursor of serotonin, it may be used as adjunctive therapy in patients who are refractory to treatment. Has been associated with eosinophilia–myalgia syndrome (EMS).

Doses and side-effects

Doses of antidepressant medications are summarised in Table 27.2 and potential side-effects are summarised in Table 27.3.

> TCAs are preferred where sedation is desired. However, they should be used with care or avoided in patients with cardiovascular disease.

Drug interactions

Examples of drug interactions are given in Table 27.4

Contraindications

- TCAs: recent myocardial infarction, arrhythmias, severe liver disease, manic phase
- SSRIs: manic phase.

Table 27.2 Doses of antidepressant medications

Medication	Usual adult daily dosage range for depression (mg)	Relative cost
TCAs:		
Amitriptyline	75–200	£
Clomipramine	10–250	£
Imipramine	75–200	£
Heterocyclic:		
Maprotiline	75–225	£
SSRIs:		
Fluoxetine	20–60	££
Paroxetine	20–50	££
SNRI:		
Venlafaxine	75–375	££

SNRI, serotonin–noradrenaline re-uptake inhibitor; SSRIs, selective serotonin re-uptake inhibitors; TCAs, tricyclic antidepressants.

Discontinuation syndrome

Discontinuation syndrome is an adverse reaction that occurs following withdrawal of antidepressants. SSRIs are associated with a higher risk of discontinuation syndrome than TCAs.

- Occurrence may be mistaken for recurrence of an acute depressive effect.

Table 27.3 Potential side-effects of antidepressants

Drug	Anticholinergic effects	Drowsiness	Orthostatic hypotension	Cardiac arrhythmias	GI distress	Weight gain
Amitriptyline	4+	4+	4+	3+	0	4+
Clomipramine	4+	4+	2+	3+	1+	4+
Imipramine	3+	3+	4+	3+	1+	4+
Maprotiline	2+	3+	2+	2+	0	2+
Fluoxetine	0	0	0	0	3+	0
Paroxetine	1+	1+	0	0	3+	1+
Venlafaxine	1+	2+	0	1+	3+	1+

GI, gastrointestinal.

Table 27.4 Examples of interactions (excluding between antidepressant classes)

Class	Drug	Rationale
TCAs, SSRIs	Antiepileptics	Antagonism to anticonvulsant effect
TCAs, SSRIs	Sibutramine	Increased risk of CNS toxicity
TCAs, SSRIs	Warfarin	Increased/decreased anticoagulant effect Increased anticoagulant effect
TCAs	Alcohol	Increased sedative effect
TCAs	Moxifloxacin	Increased risk of ventricular arrhythmias
SSRIs	NSAIDs	Increased risk of bleeding
SSRIs	Lithium	Increased risk of CNS effects

CNS, central nervous system; NSAIDs, non-steroidal anti-inflammatory drugs; SSRIs, selective serotonin re-uptake inhibitors; TCAs, tricyclic antidepressants.

- Its occurrence may indicate that the patient has stopped treatment or is not taking the drug regularly, leading to the onset of discontinuation syndrome.
- When drug is being discontinued consider tapering off drug therapy or for SSRIs switching to fluoxetine which is less likely to cause this effect due to a long half-life.

The symptoms of discontinuation syndrome are listed in Table 27.5.

Since fluoxetine has a long half-life and is metabolised into an active metabolite, it appears to be much less likely to be associated with discontinuation symptoms reported with other SSRIs (e.g. paroxetine, citalopram, sertraline).

Hyponatraemia and antidepressants

This association occurs especially in elderly patients due to inappropriate secretion of antidiuretic hormone. It is more frequently reported with SSRIs.

Table 27.5 Symptoms of discontinuation syndrome

Symptom group	Common symptoms	SSRIs	TCA
Dysequilibrium	Light-headedness, vertigo	+	
Sensory symptoms	Paraesthesia, numbness	+	
General somatic symptoms	Lethargy, headache, tremor, sweating	+	+
Sleep disturbance	Insomnia, nightmares	+	+
Gastrointestinal symptoms	Nausea, vomiting, diarrhoea	+	+
Affective symptoms	Irritability, anxiety, low mood	+	+

SSRIs, selective serotonin re-uptake inhibitors; TCAs, tricyclic antidepressants.

- Signs: drowsiness, confusion, convulsions
- Risk factors: older age, female, diuretic therapy, low body weight, low baseline serum sodium concentration.

Herbal medicine: St John's wort

St John's wort is a herbal preparation that is used in mild depression. It is a drug metabolism enzyme inducer, leading to significant drug interactions when administered with other drugs such as:

- anticoagulants – reduced effect of warfarin
- SSRIs – increased serotonergic effects
- antiepileptics – reduced plasma concentration of carbamazepine and phenytoin
- cardiac glycosides – reduced plasma concentration of digoxin
- oral contraceptives – reduced contraceptive effect.

> Patients who are started on SSRIs should be advised against the concomitant use of St John's wort.

Treatment of mania

In the acute management of mania, mood stabilisers such as lithium and anticonvulsant therapy such as valproate and carbamazepine are recommended as monotherapy. The use of atypical antipsychotic drugs (aripiprazole, olanzapine, quetiapine, risperidone, ziprasidone) (see Chapter 26) as monotherapy or in combination with lithium or anticonvulsants may be considered. The atypical antipsychotics are used to manage acute agitation and aggression. Benzodiazepines (see Chapter 28) may be used as adjunctive treatment to treat agitation and hyperactivity and to produce sedation and reduce anxiety.

Lithium

- Has a narrow therapeutic index
- Is excreted renally
- Hyponatraemia and dehydration (which may be due to diuretics) lead to increased renal reabsorption which may result in lithium toxicity
- May worsen severe cardiac disease, induce hypothyroidism and weight gain, and complicate the presentation of diabetes mellitus
- Baseline lithium work-up: creatinine and electrolytes, thyroid function tests, urinalysis, ECG.

Routine therapeutic monitoring

- Serum lithium concentrations: every 3–6 months for six months; every 6–12 months thereafter
- Creatinine, electrolytes: every 3–6 months; every 6–12 months thereafter
- Thyroid function tests: every 3–6 months; every 6–12 months thereafter
- Urinalysis: every 12 months.

Side-effects

See Table 27.6 for the side-effects of lithium.

> Since bioavailability varies from one preparation to another, care should be taken if changing preparation.

Treatment of bipolar disorder

Antidepressants including TCAs, the heterocyclics, MAOIs and SSRIs pose the risk of switching a depressed patient to a manic phase within a few weeks after initiation of therapy. SSRIs and venlafaxine seem to be less likely to induce this switch. For this reason it is recommended that, for maintenance therapy in bipolar disorder, mood stabilisers including antipsychotics (see Chapter 26), lithium or anticonvulsants are considered as first line of therapy. Antidepressants, preferably SSRIs or venlafaxine, may be considered as adjunct therapy.

Practice summary

- Efficacy of antidepressants is similar; choice depends on side-effects to be avoided.

Table 27.6 Side-effects of lithium

Side-effects	Management strategies
Tremors	Reduce dose, give once daily at bedtime, use slow-release preparations, add propranolol
Polydipsia or polyuria	Reduce dose, give once daily at bedtime, use slow-release preparations, add amiloride
Nausea, diarrhoea	Take with food, reduce dose, give once daily at bedtime, use slow-release preparations
Weight gain	Restrict diet, switch to carbamazepine
Hypothyroidism	Use levothyroxine
Mental dulling	Give once daily at bedtime, use slow-release preparations, switch to valproic acid or carbamazepine

- Outcome can be improved by applying non-pharmacological factors in addition to pharmacotherapy.
- Preference of SSRIs as first-line therapy due to better patient acceptability.
- Lag period of 1–4 weeks which may be longer in elderly patients before positive outcomes of therapy are experienced.
- Compliance is a problem in patients with mood disorders, resulting from ambivalence to take antidepressants or mood stablisers due to social stigma, side-effects, periodic lack of insight into need for medication (non-compliance range 10–60% reported in most studies).

Question

1 Describe the discontinuation syndrome associated with selective serotonin re-uptake inhibitors.

Answer

1 Gastrointestinal disturbances, headache, anxiety, dizziness, paraesthesia, sleep disturbances, fatigue, influenza-like symptoms and sweating are the most common features which result if an SSRI is stopped abruptly after regular administration for 8 weeks or more or a marked reduction of the dose. The dose should preferably be reduced gradually over a period of about 4 weeks, or longer if withdrawal symptoms emerge (6 months in patients who have been on long-term maintenance treatment).

Fluoxetine has a long half-life and is metabolised into an active metabolite. It appears to be much less likely associated with discontinuation symptoms reported with other SSRIs. Patient may be switched to fluoxetine and weaned off slowly.

Further reading

Akerblad A, Bengtsson F, Ekselius L and Knorring V L (2003). Effects of an educational compliance enhancement programme and therapeutic drug monitoring on treatment adherence in depressed patients managed by general practitioners. *Int Clin Psychopharmacol* 18: 347–354.

Bleakley S (2009). The management of depression. *Pharm J* 282: 285–288.

Jacob S and Spinler Sa A (2006). Hyponatraemia associated with selective serotonin-re-uptake inhibitors in older adults *Ann Pharmacother* 40: 1618–1622.

National Institute for Health and Clinical Excellence (2006). Bipolar disorder: the management of bipolar disorder in adults, children and adoloscents in primary and secondary care. http://guidance.nice.org.uk/CG38.

National Institute for Health and Clinical Excellence (2004). Depression: management of depression in primary and secondary care. http://www.nice.org.uk/CG023.

Spigset O and Martensson B (1999). Drug treatment of depression. *BMJ* 318: 1188–1191.

Vieta E, Fresno D and Amann B (2006). Atypical antipsychotics in bipolar disorders. *Hosp Pharm Eur* May/June: 53–56.

Reference

1 American Psychiatric Association (2000). *Diagnostic and Statistical Manual of Mental Disorders*, 4th edn revised. Washington DC: American Psychiatric Association.

28

Anxiety disorders

Learning objectives:

- To differentiate between the characteristics of the various anxiety disorders
- To understand management of anxiety
- To appreciate the use of antidepressants and antipyschotics in the treatment of anxiety disorders.

Background

Although anxiety is a universal feeling, anxiety disorders are among the most frequently diagnosed psychiatric disorders. Patients with anxiety disorders tend to be high users of healthcare facilities for non-psychiatric reasons.

Characteristics

- Disproportionate response to fear triggers such as flying or to social situations
- Significant impact on quality of life and personal achievement
- Aetiology: hereditary component, personality traits, childhood experiences
- Pathology: disrupted serotoninergic, glutamatergic, GABA-ergic, noradrenergic systems and involvement of the corticotrophin-releasing factor.

Examples of psychiatric disorders associated with anxiety

- Depression
- Dementia
- Eating disorders
- Mood disorders
- Schizophrenia
- Substance use.

Examples of drugs associated with anxiety symptoms

- CNS depressant withdrawal: benzodiazepines
- CNS stimulants: caffeine, ephedrine, phenylephrine, pseudoephedrine, salbutamol
- Others: fluoroquinolones, levodopa, sibutramine, thyroid hormone, statins, triptans
- Psychotropics: antipsychotics, bupropion, SSRIs, TCAs, venlafaxine.

Examples of common medical disorders associated with anxiety symptoms

- Cardiovascular system: angina, arrhythmias, hypertension
- Endocrine system: hyperthyroidism, hypoglycaemia, premenstrual syndrome
- Gastrointestinal system: colitis, irritable bowel syndrome, peptic ulcer
- Neurological system: epilepsy, migraine, pain
- Respiratory system: asthma, COPD, pulmonary oedema.

Symptoms of anxiety

- Feeling of apprehension
- Somatic symptoms: palpitations, chest pain, shortness of breath, dizziness, dysphagia, gastrointestinal disturbance, headache and tremor.

Classification of anxiety disorders

A Phobic disorders: social phobia, simple phobia
B Panic disorder: with or without agoraphobia
C Agoraphobia without a history of panic disorder
D Generalised anxiety disorder (GAD)
E Obsessive–compulsive disorder (OCD)
F Post-traumatic stress disorder
G Atypical anxiety disorder.

Non-pharmacological measures

- Relaxation therapy
- Cognitive therapy

Lifestyle measures to counteract stress

1. Recognise activities and factors that induce stress
2. Assess what adjustments to lifestyle are possible
3. Do not try to be 'superhuman'
4. Practise relaxation and cognitive therapies for 10 minutes a day
5. Adopt healthy eating habits and reduce alcohol consumption
6. Take up daily regular exercise
7. Maintain hobbies, friends and social time.

- Psychotherapy
- Behavioural therapy.

Drug treatment in anxiety

Some drugs used in the treatment of anxiety are listed in Table 28.1.

Generalised anxiety disorder

This is a persistent condition characterised by excessive anxiety and worry about two or more life circumstances without panic or phobic symptoms. It is not usually due to situation-specific triggers. The patient feels on edge, has difficulty in concentrating, feels muscle tension and is irritable.

Benzodiazepines are the drugs of choice in an acute attack and, for long-term management, SSRIs or TCAs are preferred.

Table 28.1 Drug treatment in anxiety

Drug	Efficacy	Onset of action	Risk of withdrawal symptoms	Administration
Benzodiazepines	++	Immediate	+++	For acute attack
Buspirone	+	Delayed	–	Short term (4 weeks)
Beta-blockers	+	Immediate	+	Medium term for symptom control
TCAs	++	Delayed	+	Medium–long term for GAD, panic disorder
SSRIs	++	Delayed	++	OCD, post-traumatic stress disorder, social phobia

GAD, generalised anxiety disorder; OCD, obsessive–compulsive disorder; SSRIs, selective serotonin re-uptake inhibitors; TCAs, tricyclic antidepressants.

Benzodiazepines

- Potent anxiolytic effect exerted at lower doses than those required for a hypnotic effect (see also Chapter 29)
- Rapid onset of effect makes them useful in acute attacks
- Side-effects: tolerance (develops to a lesser extent for anxiolytic effect than psychomotor effects), psychomotor impairment (memory loss), affective reactions (aggravate depression, suicidal tendencies), dependence
- Abuse and withdrawal syndrome limit use in chronic conditions
- Effectiveness is similar for different benzodiazepines; choice is influenced by pharmacokinetic parameters and incidence of side-effects.

The half-lives of some benzodiazepines are listed in Table 28.2.

Buspirone

Compared with benzodiazepines, buspirone lacks anticonvulsant, muscle-relaxant, hypnotic and dependence properties.

- Probably acts as a serotonin partial agonist, enhances dopaminergic neurotransmission and facilitates noradrenergic activity
- Side-effects: dizziness, nausea, gynaecomastia, extrapyramidal symptoms
- No potential for dependence.

Beta-blockers (adrenergic blocking agents)

- Example: propranolol
- Used in patients with prominent cardiovascular symptoms of anxiety such as palpitations and tremors
- Used when anxiety is related to performance and stress.

Antihistamines

- Example: hydroxyzine
- Little evidence to support effectiveness but sedative properties may be useful
- Can be used on an as-necessary basis
- Side-effects: anticholinergic effects.

TCAs, SSRIs and SNRIs (see also Chapter 27)

- Preferred for medium- to long-term treatment
- Due to side-effect profile and safety profile in overdosage, SSRIs and SNRIs are preferred to TCAs.

The characteristics of non-benzodiazepine anxiolytic drugs are summarised in Table 28.3

Time required after initiating antidepressants for patients with anxiety disorders to experience positive outcomes with therapy may be longer than time required when antidepressants are used in the management of depression. Risk of withdrawal syndrome has to be kept in mind when withdrawing therapy.

Table 28.2 Half-life of benzodiazepines

Anxiolytics	Half-life (hours)	Active metabolites
Chlordiazepoxide	3–30	+ long half-life
Diazepam	20–50	+ long half-life
Lorazepam	10–20	–
Temazepam	10–20	Insignificant
Triazolam	1.5–5	Insignificant

Panic disorder

This disorder is characterised by recurrent and unexpected panic attacks. The patient may show hyperventilation prior to attack. Symptoms may be misinterpreted as being caused by physical illness, commonly heart disease.

An attack involves an intense period of fear with four or more of the following symptoms developing abruptly and reaching a peak within 10 minutes:

Table 28.3 Characteristics of non-benzodiazepine anxiolytic drugs

Drug	Half-life (hours) (active metabolite half-life)	Dose
Buspirone	2–4 (reports up to 11)	5 mg two to three times daily
Propranolol	2–4	40 mg twice daily
Amitriptyline	10–25 (13–93)	75–150 mg daily
Clomipramine	16–20	10–100 mg daily
Imipramine	4–18 (12–61)	50–100 mg daily
Fluoxetine	2–3 days (7–15 days)	20 mg daily
Citalopram	33	10–20 mg daily
Fluvoxamine	15	100 mg daily
Paroxetine	20	20 mg daily
Sertraline	26 (36)	50 mg daily
Venlafaxine	5 (11)	75 mg daily

- Palpitations ± tachycardia
- Sweating
- Tremor
- Shortness of breath
- Choking feeling
- Chest pain or discomfort
- Nausea/abdominal symptoms
- Dizzy or faint feeling
- Depersonalisation/unreality
- Fear of losing control
- Fear of dying
- Paraesthesia
- Chills or hot flushes.

Management

The drugs used to treat panic disorders are summarised in Table 28.4.

Obsessive–compulsive disorder

Obsession

- Recurrent and persistent ideas, thoughts or images that are experienced as intrusive and senseless
- Person attempts to ignore or suppress such thoughts or to neutralise them
- Person recognises that the obsessions are the product of his or her mind.

Compulsion

- Repetitive, purposeful and intentional behaviours that are performed in response to an obsession.
- Behaviour is designed to neutralise or to prevent discomfort or some dreaded event or situation.
- Person recognises that the behaviour is excessive or unreasonable.

Management

- Drugs that inhibit re-uptake of serotonin (e.g. clomipramine, fluoxetine, fluvoxamine, sertraline)
- Treatment should be continued for several months (12) in patients who respond to therapy

Table 28.4 Drugs used to treat panic disorders

Classification	Drug	Comments
Benzodiazepine	Alprazolam, diazepam	Effective Problems: side-effects, withdrawal
SSRIs	Paroxetine, escitalopram, citalopram	Effective Problems: lag time, initial worsening of panic disorders
TCAs	Imipramine	Effective Problems: lag time, initial worsening of panic disorders, side-effects

SSRIs, selective serotonin re-uptake inhibitors; TCAs, tricyclic antidepressants.

- Consider use of an antipsychotic as an adjunct in patients who do not respond to therapy.

Social phobia

This is marked, persistent fear of social situations where individual worries about exposure to society. Symptoms include blushing and diarrhoea. It occurs in young adults.

Management

- SSRIs (e.g. paroxetine, escitalopram) are considered drugs of choice
- Beta-blockers could be used in performance-related anxiety.

Post-traumatic stress disorder

This is a reaction to a traumatic event which carries the threat of death or serious injury to the patient or significant others. It involves continued experience in dreams and flashbacks.

Symptoms that were not present prior to event and, occur with a duration of at least 1 month include:

- Insomnia
- Irritability or outbursts of anger
- Poor concentration
- Exaggerated response to non-threatening stimuli.

Management

- SSRIs are the drugs of choice (e.g. paroxetine, sertraline)
- TCAs (e.g. amitriptyline); SNRIs may be considered as second-line therapy
- The use of antispychotics could be considered where paranoia or flashbacks are prominent.

Practice summary

- Symptomatic treatment is adopted to achieve rapid resolution of symptoms:
  - benzodiazepines when symptoms are severe and disabling
  - beta-blockers when there are significant autonomic symptoms.
- Long-term pharmacological intervention:
  - SSRIs: chronic symptoms of more than 4 weeks or underlying depression
  - lag time of 2–4 weeks: in panic disorders and OCD symptoms may persist up to 4–10 weeks after treatment is started
  - antidepressants (e.g. SSRIs and venlafaxine) are associated with initial worsening of panic symptoms; consider co-prescribing benzodiazepines in the short term.
- Use of antipsychotics:
  - have a tranquillising effect without impairing consciousness and without causing paradoxical excitement
  - to alleviate severe anxiety as a short-term measure
  - examples: phenothiazines (chlorpromazine, prochlorperazine, trifluoperazine); butyrophenone (haloperidol).

Question

1 Describe the use of benzodiazepines in anxiety disorders.

Answer

1 Benzodiazepines can be effective in alleviating anxiety states and are indicated for the short-term relief of severe anxiety. Diazepam, alprazolam and chlordiazepoxide have a sustained action. Shorter-acting compounds such as lorazepam may be preferred in patients with hepatic impairment and the elderly, but they carry a greater risk of withdrawal symptoms. Unwanted effects include: tolerance which would require higher doses to achieve same desired effect, aggravation of depression, and increased

suicidal tendencies and dependence. Occurrence of dependence and risk of withdrawal syndrome limit use in chronic conditions. Effectiveness is similar for different benzodiazepines and choice is influenced by pharmacokinetic parameters and incidence of side-effects.

Further reading

Bleakley S (2008). An overview of anxiety disorders. *Pharm J* 281: 511–514.

National Institute for Health and Clinical Excellence (2004). Anxiety: management of anxiety (panic disorder with or without agoraphobia, and generalised anxiety disorder) in adults in primary, secondary and community care. http://www.nice.org.uk/CG22.

29

Sleep disorders

Learning objectives:

- To understand normal sleep physiology
- To classify insomnia
- To appreciate conditions that may disturb sleep
- To understand management of insomnia.

Background

Sleep disorders impact on both physical and mental well-being, resulting in decreased productivity, a reduction in overall feeling of well-being and in quality of life.

Diagnosis of insomnia

- Taking more than 30 minutes to fall asleep
- Difficulty maintaining sleep – waking up for more than 30 minutes and having a sleep efficiency ratio of less than 85%
- Sleep disturbed for more than three nights a week
- Significant impairment of daytime functioning.

Classification of insomnia

- Transient: lasts for 2–3 days and is due to external factors such as jet lag, noise. Occurs in individuals who normally do not complain of insomnia.
- Short-term: lasts up to 3 weeks and is usually associated with physical or emotional trauma.
- Chronic: insomnia on most nights lasting for 3 weeks or more. Psychiatric disorders and alcohol consumption are common factors leading to chronic insomnia. Treatment should address the underlying condition selecting drug therapy that also alleviates insomnia.

Sleep cycle

- Controlled by the reticular-activating system in the brain
- Consists of two states: *rapid eye movement* (REM) cycles alternating with cycles of *non-rapid eye movement* (NREM)
- Quality of sleep depends on the ratio between the REM and NREM cycles
- Sleep may be studied through the use of electroencephalogram to monitor electrical brain activity
- Disturbance could occur as wakefulness, early waking, difficulty in falling asleep.

Types of sleep

- During NREM sleep, repair of bodily tissues takes place. This phase is further subdivided into four stages. The activating neurotransmitter is serotonin.

- REM sleep is associated with the restoration of memory function, along with repair of brain tissue and laying down of memories. During this phase the eyes may move with the eyelids closed. Blood pressure, heart rate and breathing rate may vary. Dreams are associated with this phase. Catecholamines are involved.
- If the ratio between NREM and REM sleep is disrupted, the sleep efficiency ratio is very low, meaning that the patient will report a feeling of tiredness despite having slept an appropriate amount of hours. In adults NREM sleep constitutes 75–80% and REM sleep 20–25% of the sleep duration.

Effect of drugs

Some drugs have an effect on the percentage of REM sleep (Table 29.1).

Drugs that can disrupt sleep include:

- antiepileptics: gabapentin, phenytoin, lamotrigine, topiramate
- antidepressants: SSRIs
- beta-blockers
- calcium channel blockers
- NSAIDs
- levothyroxine
- proton pump inhibitors.

Table 29.1 Effect of drugs on the amount of REM sleep

	REM suppression with administration	REM rebound following withdrawal
Amphetamine	Yes	Yes
Nitrazepam	Yes	Yes
Amitriptyline	Yes	Small/nil

REM, rapid eye movement.

Sleep management

Goal 1: Understanding sleep

- What is sleep?
- What is a 'good night's sleep'? Nocturnal sleep requirements decrease with age and there is great inter-individual variation. So when a patient complains of insomnia the patient's perspective of a good night's sleep has to be established.
- Understanding sleeplessness: is the patient experiencing difficulty falling asleep, early morning wakefulness or difficulty maintaining sleep?

Goal 2: Identify factors that are disturbing sleep

- Combat sleeplessness naturally: use herbal teas (e.g. chamomille and valerian)
- Provide sleep hygiene advice
- Ask the patient to complete a sleep diary to understand sleep patterns, patient's lifestyle and symptoms.

Sleep hygiene

- Establish a routine
- Exercise early
- Say no to naps
- Comfort comes first
- Cut out late cravings
- Relax before retiring
- Use bedroom for sleep and relaxation
- Deal with frustration or thoughts before going to bed
- Unwind the mind.

Factors affecting the ability to relax and sleep are summarised in Table 29.2.

Goal 3: Identify suitable medical treatments and address underlying conditions

There is not, as yet, an ideal hypnotic available. The effectiveness of currently available hypnotics in stimulating deep and satisfying sleep is limited. The sleep efficiency ratio achieved is low indicating, that the

Table 29.2 Factors affecting the ability to relax and sleep	
Physical	Pain, gastrointestinal upset, night cramps, nocturia, sleep apnoea, itch
Psychological	Stress, tension, bereavement
Psychiatric	Anxiety, depression, mania, eating disorders
Physiological	Jet lag, late night eating, late night exercise, environmental factors
Pharmacological	Caffeine, alcohol, nicotine, drugs

hypnotics induce sleep but do not achieve a physiologically normal sleep cycle.

Hypnotic drugs

The choice of hypnotic drug is influenced by:

- age
- concomitant disease states
- duration of action
- type of insomnia
- onset of action required
- risk of adverse effects
- cost.

The main hypnotic drugs available are benzodiazepines (e.g. nitrazepam, diazepam, lorazepam), non-benzodiazepines (e.g. zaleplon, zolpidem, zopiclone), sedative antihistamines (e.g. promethazine) and chlomethiazole (used for elderly patients, also used in alcohol withdrawal symptoms).

Benzodiazepines

Benzodiazepines are relatively safe when compared with phenobarbital and morphine since the lethal dose is over 1000 times greater than the typical therapeutic dose. They enhance the binding of gamma-aminobutyric acid (GABA) to the receptor. This results in a greater entry of chloride ions, which hyperpolarises the cell making it difficult to depolarise, and therefore reduces its neural excitability. This action leads to a lower output of excitatory neurotransmitters such as noradrenaline, serotonin and dopamine.

Benzodiazepines increase total sleep. However, they cause a mild suppression of REM sleep.

Half-lives of benzodiazepines

- Nitrazepam: 20+ hours
- Flurazepam: 2–4 hours (produces active metabolite with a very long half-life)
- Lormetazepam: 11 hours.

Structure–activity relationship

The structure of benzodiazepines (Figure 29.1) is based on 5-phenyl-1,4-benzodiazepine-2-one. Halogen substitution on ring A at position 7 increases functional hypnotic and anxiolytic effects. A 3-hydroxy moiety on ring B as in lorazepam increases excretion rate. Annelation of the 1,2-bond on ring B with S-triazole, as in triazolam, maintains clinical effectiveness since it promotes ligand binding.

Cautions and contraindications

- Benzodiazepines should not be used in patients with sleep apnoea, respiratory depression and conditions that predispose to respiratory weakness including myasthenia gravis and acute pulmonary insufficiency.
- Benzodiazepines should be used with caution in patients with a history of respiratory disease, muscle weakness or myasthenia gravis, in patients with a history of drug or alcohol dependence, in pregnancy and breast-feeding, and in hepatic and renal impairment.

Side-effects

- Dependence (physical and psychological): treatment with benzodiazepines should be short term (2–4 weeks)

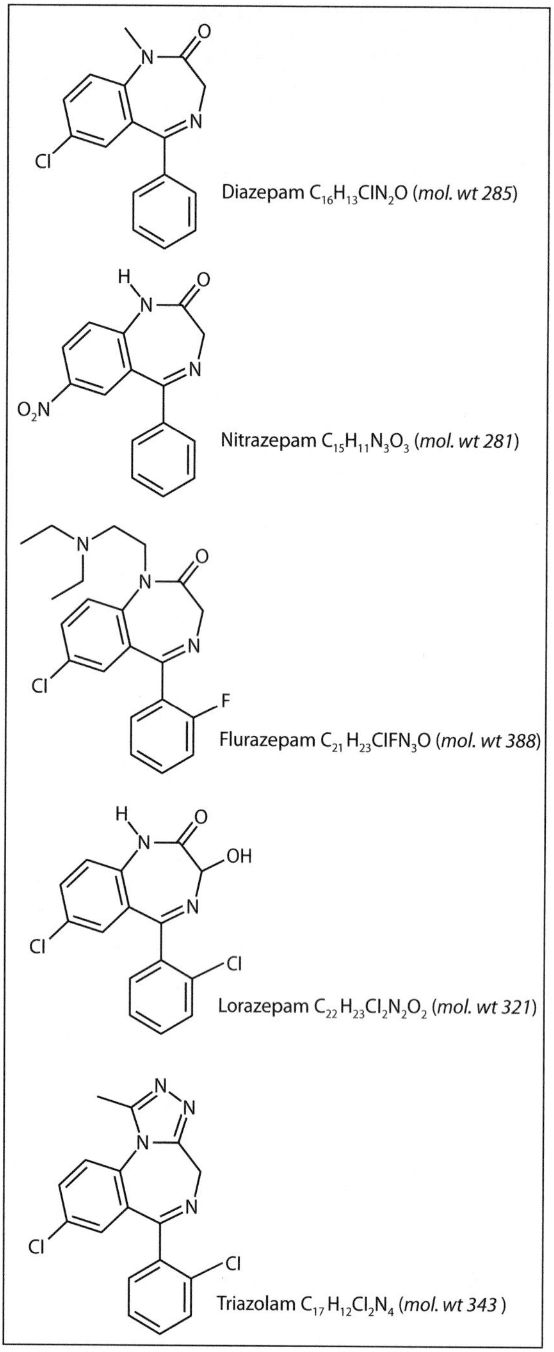

Diazepam $C_{16}H_{13}ClN_2O$ (*mol. wt 285*)

Nitrazepam $C_{15}H_{11}N_3O_3$ (*mol. wt 281*)

Flurazepam $C_{21}H_{23}ClFN_3O$ (*mol. wt 388*)

Lorazepam $C_{22}H_{23}Cl_2N_2O_2$ (*mol. wt 321*)

Triazolam $C_{17}H_{12}Cl_2N_4$ (*mol. wt 343*)

Figure 29.1 Chemical structures of some benzodiazepines.

- Tolerance: particularly to the hypnotic effect
- Hangover effects: drowsiness and light-headedness the day after drug administration, confusion and ataxia, less common with short-acting benzodiazepines
- Withdrawal syndrome: abrupt withdrawal should be avoided.

> Benzodiazepines, particularly triazolam and lorazepam, are associated with memory impairment. This is a dose-dependent effect and, if it is reported by patient, dose should be lowered.

Benzodiazepine withdrawal syndrome

Due to the occurrence of dependence, abrupt withdrawal of a benzodiazepine may lead to anxiety, headaches, increased pulse rate, increased blood pressure, increased body temperature, tremor, rebound insomnia, confusion, toxic psychosis and convulsions. The withdrawal syndrome may occur immediately upon stopping the drug (for short-acting products) or take up to 3 weeks to develop.

Drugs that are more potent and rapidly eliminated (e.g. lorazepam, triazolam) have more frequent and severe withdrawal problems. Gradual withdrawal should be effected. The prescriber may consider changing to a long-acting benzodiazepine such as diazepam before considering withdrawal.

Less potent and more slowly eliminated drugs (e.g. flurazepam) continue to improve sleep even after discontinuation, and are therefore associated with less severe withdrawal problems.

Other hypnotics

Zaleplon, zolpidem, zopiclone

These drugs act at the benzodiazepine receptor and have a rapid onset of action and a short duration of action. They are useful in patients who have difficulty in falling asleep. They are associated with dependence to a lesser extent when compared with benzodiazepines. Cautions and contraindications to the use of these drugs are similar to those noted for benzodiazepines.

In the USA, eszopiclone, the *S*-isomer of zopiclone is used.

Antihistamines

Antihistamines such as promethazine are useful for their sedative effect. The sedative effect of antihistamines may decrease rapidly with continued treatment. See also Chapter 25.

Half-lives of non-benzodiazepine hypnotics

- Zaleplon: 1 hour
- Zolpidem: 2 hours
- Zopiclone: 5 hours
- Promethazine: 17–34 hours.

Use of hypnotics

- Hypnotics increase sleeping time but may produce a hangover effect in the morning.
- Hypnotics produce a reduction in the occurrence and duration of REM sleep, resulting in patients feeling irritable and unrested the day after.
- Patients who have used benzodiazepine hypnotics for long periods can be gradually weaned using non-benzodiazepine hypnotics as doses of the benzodiazepine are gradully lowered.
- Hypnotics should be considered only when the insomnia is severe and disabling.

Drug treatment in insomnia

Drug treatment schedules for insomnia are summarised in Table 29.3.

Geriatric patients

- In older patients hypnotics are potentially hazardous and should be avoided.
- A reduction in urinary clearance and accumulation of drug in adipose tissue may result in a prolonged half-life, leading to confusion and ataxia that increase risk of falls and injury.
- Clomethiazole may be considered for short-term use in severe insomnia in older patients or in restlessness and agitation because of its lower risk of hangover effects. However it may cause dependence and common side-effects include nasal congestion and irritation, conjunctival irritation and headache.

Table 29.3 Drug treatment in insomnia

Type of insomnia	Choice of drugs	Administration
Transient insomnia	Benzodiazepine	Stat
Short-term insomnia	Benzodiazepine	For 1–2 weeks
Chronic insomnia	Treat cause, using antidepressants, antipsychotics benzodiazepine/ non-benzodiazepine intermittently	Use lowest effective dose

Paediatric patients

- Children are more susceptible to the central nervous system depressant effects of benzodiazepines. Hypnotics are not recommended for children. Sedating antihistamines are preferred.

Natural products that can be used in sleep disturbance

Melatonin

This is produced by the pineal gland when exposed to darkness; bright light and physical activity result in decreased secretion. It regulates sleep by affecting the circadian rhythm and increases total sleep time and causes a faster onset of sleep. It is useful in patients suffering from jet lag and in patients suffering from insomnia due to night shift work.

Ramelteon, a melatonin receptor agonist, is available in the USA.

Valerian

This contains valerenic acid which inhibits GABA metabolism.

Passionflower

This contains maltol and ethylmaltol.

Snoring

Snoring occurs when air does not flow smoothly through the nasal and throat pathways. Predisposing factors are obesity, alcohol intake, drugs (hypnotics, antidepressants, antipsychotics), age, gender and sleep apnoea.

Anti-snoring aids include:

- nasal strips – when snoring is due to small or collapsing nostrils
- mandibular devices – when snoring is due to tongue displacement.

Sleep apnoea

This is a neurological disorder characterised by repetitive periods during sleep with breathing cessation for at least 10 seconds. It results in impacting negatively on quality of sleep.

Obstructive sleep apnoea is the most common type. During sleep the throat is closed and breathing stops temporarily, resulting in patient gasping for air and falling back to sleep. Snoring is a presenting complaint.

Diagnosis carried out by polysomnography.

Sleep apnoea is associated with obesity, smoking and alcohol. There is increased risk in patients with hypertension, coronary artery disease and cerebrovascular disease, and a relationship with metabolic syndrome is being examined. Patients with sleep apnoea tend to be high users of healthcare services due to increased risk of cardiovascular morbidity and use of psychoactive medicines, especially if obstructive sleep apnoea is undiagnosed.

In obstructive sleep apnoea, anatomic devices such as a mandibular splint are used. In central sleep apnoea a continuous positive airway pressure machine (CPAP) is indicated. The CPAP machine provides a constant flow of air through a mask that is worn by the patient during sleep, thus preventing breathing cessation. CPAP is a symptomatic management since once it is stopped apnoea episodes re-occur.

The use of hypnotics in sleep apnoea is not indicated since they may interfere with the stimulation of breathing once this has stopped.

Restless leg syndrome

This is a neurological condition characterised by uncomfortable sensations in the legs that demand movement when at rest and at night. The condition contributes to insomnia and patients complain of impaired daytime functioning due to disturbed sleep.

The condition is common in: geriatric patients, Parkinson's disease, hypothyroidism, kidney disorders, rheumatoid arthritis, neuropathy, chronic venous insufficiency and iron-deficiency anaemia.

Investigation to assess whether restless leg syndrome occurs as a secondary condition should be undertaken. Most commonly it may present as a sign of undiagnosed anaemia. The underlying condition should be treated.

Non-pharmacological management includes sleep hygiene, reducing caffeine and alcohol intake, regular exercise, smoking cessation.

Treatment for idiopathic restless leg syndrome

Choice depends on severity of symptoms and concomitant disease states. Dopamine agonists (see Chapter 33) such as pramipexole and ropinirole are used, but they may induce insomnia. The use of opioids may be considered to induce an analgesic effect, but their use is limited due to side-effect profile and dependence. Anticonvulsants such as carbamazepine and gabapentin and magnesium supplementation may be considered. For patients with iron-deficiency anaemia, iron supplementation is required.

Practice summary

- In the management of insomnia, behavioural interventions should be considered since these are free from any side-effects and have a sustained effect.
- Duration of use of hypnotics should be minimal and preferably of less than 4 weeks' duration.
- When hypnotics are used, exit strategies should be planned when treatment is started, and patient information on the duration of treatment and advice on the effects of the drugs explained (e.g. care when driving or operating machinery).
- Snoring could be a sign of sleep apnoea. Occurrence of sleep apnoea may go undiagnosed but may impact on daytime activities, cardiovascular morbidity and overuse of psychoactive medications.
- The occurrence of restless leg syndrome requires investigations to identify the possible occurrence of underlying pathology.

Question

1 Give an example of a benzodiazepine that has a short duration of activity. Explain the clinical implications of this characteristic.

Answer

1 Benzodiazepines with a short half-life include lorazepam and triazolam. The duration of action is implicated in the frequency of rebound insomnia resulting from discontinuation of benzodiazepine therapy. The drugs that are more potent and rapidly eliminated have more frequent and severe withdrawal problems, and a higher risk of rebound insomnia when compared with the more slowly eliminated drugs such as diazepam. Rebound insomnia results in a worsening presentation of the original symptoms of difficulty in falling asleep or in maintaining sleep.

Further reading

Allen S (2005). Insomnia and its management. *Pharm J* 274: 243–246.

Allen S (2005). Sleep and sleeping disorders. *Pharm J* 274: 187–190.

Holmes J, Millard J, Greer D and Silcock J (2003). Trends in psychotropic drug use in older patients in general hospitals. *Pharm J* 271: 584–586.

Lam J and Ip M (2007). An update on obstructive sleep apnea and the metabolic syndrome. *Curr Opin Pulm Med* 13: 484–489.

Morin A K, Jarvis C I and Lynch A M (2007). Therapeutic options for sleep-maintenance and sleep-onset insomnia. *Pharmacotherapy* 27: 89–110.

Nathan A (2005). Snoring and the evidence behind the various treatments available. *Pharm J* 274: 309–312.

Reese J P, Stiasny-Kolster K, Oertel W H and Dodel R C (2007). Health-related quality of life and economic burden in patients with restless legs syndrome. *Exp Rev Pharmacoeconomics Outcomes Res* 7: 503–521.

Tarasiuk A, Greenberg-Dotan S, Simon-Tuval T, Oksenberg A and Reuveni H (2008). The effect of obstructive sleep apnoea on morbidity and health care utilization of middle-aged and older adults. *J Am Geriatr Soc* 56: 247–254.

30

Eating disorders

Learning objectives:

- To identify characteristics of eating disorders
- To identify use of therapeutic agents
- To develop skills to be able to promote lifestyle changes to address obesity and eating disorders.

Background

The term 'eating disorders' generally refers to anorexia nervosa and bulimia nervosa which are two conditions that commonly coexist with other psychiatric conditions including depression and anxiety (obsessive–compulsive disorder, post-traumatic stress disorder) and with substance abuse. In this chapter the term 'eating disorders' is applied in a broader sense to include obesity and lack of appetite.

Poor appetite

Complaints of poor appetite are commonly associated with:

- paediatric patients
- illnesses: cancer, Parkinson's disease
- elderly patients
- postoperative patients.

Strategies to increase appetite

- Eat frequent small meals instead of three large meals
- Provide a pleasant atmosphere at meal times
- Garnish meals with fresh fruit, vegetables, parsley, herbs
- Vary smells and textures of foods at meals
- Vary food selections
- Get lots of fresh air.

Agents that increase appetite

- Metopine
- Carnitine
- Lysine
- Vitamin B complex
- Energy- and nutrient-providing drinks.

In palliative care, corticosteroids (e.g. prednisolone and dexamethasone) are used to improve appetite and maintain a state of well-being.

Asthenia

This term is used to describe chronic fatigue due to sleep disorders, stress or chronic disease.

- Symptoms: headache, malaise, anorexia, xerostomia, diaphoresis, pallor, heartburn, abdominal pain, flatulence.
- Treatment is sulbutiamine: precursor to thiamine (vitamin B_1), improves memory and intellectual tiredness, and reduces fatigue.

Obesity

Obesity is a disorder that is becoming increasingly predominant among Western societies. It occurs as a result of an abnormal energy balance, usually resulting from excessive caloric intake and inadequate caloric loss. This reflects excess energy being stored as body fat.

Causes of obesity

- Physiological factors: disturbances in the hunger and satiety centres in the hypothalamus, effects on neurotransmitters, neuropeptides and hormones that regulate food intake
- Genetic factors: genetic predisposition together with environmental factors tend to result in occurrence of obesity
- Metabolic abnormalities: hypothyroidism, diabetes, psychiatric disorders, pregnancy, congestive heart failure
- Lifestyle factors: sedentary lifestyle, food intake patterns
- Psychological factors: cultural and socio-economic influences
- Medications.

Drugs that may cause weight gain

- Antidepressants (e.g. TCAs, SSRIs)
- Antiepileptics (e.g. carbamazepine, gabapentin, valproate)
- Antipsychotics (e.g. olanzapine)
- Beta-blockers
- Corticosteroids
- Oral hypoglycaemics: sulphonylureas
- Insulin
- Mood stabilisers (e.g. lithium).

Disorders associated with obesity

- Hypertension
- Congestive heart failure
- Diabetes
- Hyperlipidaemia
- Cerebrovascular disease
- Gallbladder disease
- Obstetric complications
- Osteoarthritis
- Varicose veins
- Flat feet
- Hiatus hernia.

Critical periods in life for obesity development

Obesity in children has been rising. Obesity that starts during critical periods in life appears to increase risk of persistent obesity and of related complications. Critical periods include gestation and early infancy, age between 5 and 7 years, and adolescence.

Childhood obesity should be given priority and management should emphasise behavioural changes necessary to achieve a reduction in weight gain.

Obesity management plan

- Diagnosis: body mass index (BMI) – obesity >30 kg/m^2, overweight 25–29.9 kg/m^2; waist circumference men >102 cm, women >88 cm
- Investigations: blood pressure, blood tests (blood glucose, lipid profile, thyroid function tests). Hypothyroidism is a potential cause for weight gain
- Smoking cessation for smokers
- Lifestyle and behavioural recommendations.

Lifestyle and behavioural recommendations

- Reduction of caloric intake: a weight reduction programme should include educating the patient on evaluation of caloric content of food items. Patients should receive information on reducing fat and how to avoid rapid reduction in body weight. Crash diets and starvation diets are to be avoided since they result in a rapid weight reduction. However, patients do not learn to modify and adjust food intake patterns, so weight regain will occur once dieting is stopped.

- Behavioural modification: patients should learn how to limit eating in between meals and snacking on high-fat food items. Keeping a diary of food intake patterns could help individuals to recognise over-indulgence in food. Individuals may find encouragement and support from attending weight reduction groups.
- Exercise.

Exercise recommendations

- At least three times a week
- For 25–30 minutes
- Schedule exercise sessions when they best fit into your lifestyle
- Develop a realistic schedule.

Natural products

- Methylcellulose: increases bulk and produces a feeling of satiety
- Chitosan: derived from polysaccharide chitin, it attaches to lipids or fats in the stomach to prevent their absorption.

Pharmacotherapy and obesity

Pharmacotherapy may be considered when:

- reducing diet has been established and an unsatisfactory response observed
- a plateau is reached after initial success with dieting alone
- relapse is encountered after prolonged periods of progress.

An anti-obesity drug should be considered only for those with a body mass index of 30 kg/m² or greater in whom at least 3 months of managed care involving supervised diet, exercise and behaviour modification fails to achieve a realistic reduction in weight.

In the presence of risk factors (such as diabetes, coronary heart disease, hypertension and obstructive sleep apnoea) it may be appropriate to prescribe a drug to individuals with a BMI of 27 kg/m² or greater, provided that such use is permitted by the drug's marketing authorisation. Drugs should never be used as the sole element of treatment.[1]

Pharmacotherapy available today includes drugs that act on the gastrointestinal tract (orlistat) or centrally acting appetite suppressants (sibutramine).

Development of appetite suppressants

In the 1950s and 1960s the effect of amphetamines as appetite suppressants led to amphetamines being used in the management of obesity. However, they have addictive and euphoric properties. Later, other appetite suppressants that had a centrally acting effect such as phentermine and diethylpropion were developed. Compared with the amphetamines these had a lower occurrence of addiction and unwanted effects. Their use is still restricted in many countries.

In the 1990s fenfluramine and dexfenfluramine provided an alternative to amphetamines and sympathomimetic products. Fenfluramine and dexfenfluramine stimulate serotonin release. They resulted in a lower occurrence of addiction and a few cardiac and CNS side-effects. They were withdrawn from the market in the mid-1990s, however, because of an association with valvular heart disease and primary pulmonary hypertension.

Lipase inhibitor – orlistat

Orlistat is a reversible inhibitor of lipases, which interferes with hydrolysis of dietary fat. It has a topical action resulting in decreased absorption of ingested fat and is suitable for patients who have a high intake of fat in their diet.

- Capsules are taken with meals or up to 1 hour after and should be omitted if meals contain no fat.
- If patient takes a multivitamin preparation, this should be taken 2 hours after the orlistat dose.

- Effects are seen within 24–48 hours after dose.
- Side-effects: interference with absorption of fat-soluble vitamins, oily spotting in faeces, flatus and faecal urgency.
- Low-dose orlistat has been granted centralised over-the-counter status by the European Medicines Agency.

Guidance on use of orlistat

- Used for patients aged between 18 and 75 years who have lost at least 2.5 kg body weight by lifestyle modifications
- Treatment should continue beyond 3 months if weight loss is greater than 5%, beyond 6 months if loss is greater than 10%
- Treatment should not usually continue beyond 1 year and never beyond 2 years.

Sibutramine

This drug inhibits re-uptake of serotonin and noradrenaline. It acts centrally, resulting in increased adrenergic and serotonin activity leading to down-regulation of alpha- and beta- adrenergic receptors and serotonin receptors. This causes a sensation of satiety.

- May be used as an adjunctive management of obesity in patients with other risk factors such as type 2 diabetes and dyslipidaemia
- After initiating treatment, weight loss occurs slowly
- Patient advice: dose to be taken in the morning, check before using other medications concurrently (e.g. avoid nasal decongestants due to sympathomimetic effect, antidepressants and antipsychotics due to increased risk of CNS toxicity)
- Monitoring: blood pressure, pulse rate
- Contraindications: psychiatric illness, history of cardiovascular disease, uncontrolled hypertension, hyperthyroidism, prostatic hypertrophy
- Cautions: epilepsy, glaucoma, predisposition to bleeding, family history of motor or vocal tics, history of depression, ocular hypertension
- Side-effects: headache, dizziness, depression, anxiety, insomnia, hypertension, constipation, dry mouth, nausea.

Guidance on use of sibutramine

- Treatment should not be continued for more than 1 year
- Treatment should be discontinued if weight loss after 3 months is less than 5%, when weight loss stabilises at less than 5% and in individuals who regain 3 kg or more after previous weight loss.

Anorexia nervosa

This is a syndrome characterised by self-starvation, extreme weight loss, body image disturbance and an intense fear of becoming obese. A BMI index $<17.5\ kg/m^2$ is used to describe anorexia nervosa. Weight loss, refusal to maintain normal BMI, irrational fear of becoming overweight and amenorrhoea are classic symptoms.

Bulimia nervosa

This is a condition characterised by binge eating usually followed by some form of purging. Individuals experience a sense of lack of control over volume of food intake or food intake within short time frames which is followed by inappropriate behaviour to prevent weight gain such as self-induced vomiting, misuse of laxatives and diuretics, or excessive exercise.

Table 30.1 summarises the complications of anorexia nervosa and bulimia.

Binge eating disorder

This is a newly delineated disorder characterised by bingeing not followed by purging. It results in excessive caloric eating and occurs commonly in obese individuals and in the older age group. It is related to negative emotional stress.

Table 30.1 Complications of anorexia nervosa and bulimia

Manifestation	Anorexia nervosa	Bulimia
Endocrine/metabolic	Amenorrhoea, osteoporosis, abnormal temperature regulation	Menstrual irregularities, metabolic alkalosis
Cardiovascular	Bradycardia, hypotension, arrhythmias	
Renal	Oedema	Hypokalaemia
Gastrointestinal	Decreased gastric emptying	Constipation/diarrhoea oesophagitis, dental erosion
Haematological	Anaemia	

Recognising patients with eating disorders

- Girls in early to late teens who exhibit weight loss (anorexia) or significant weight fluctuations (bulimia)
- Young women repeatedly purchasing laxatives, appetite suppressants and diuretics
- Complaints of irregular period or amenorrhoea
- History of depression or drug abuse
- Young men and boys may also present with eating disorders.

Causes of eating disorders

- Personality: low self-esteem, fear of becoming fat, sensitivity to rejection, perfectionism
- Genetic and environmental factors
- Biochemistry: serotonin and noradrenaline activity lower in patients with eating disorders.

Pharmaceutical care plan

Aims

- To improve overall nutritional status
- To restore weight
- To establish normal eating patterns
- To restore gonadal function
- To correct any secondary conditions e.g. anaemia

Management

- Restore body weight through weight restoration programmes
- Rehydrate
- Behavioural therapy

Monitoring

- Full blood count (to evaluate for anaemia)
- Renal and liver function tests
- Electrolytes
- ECG
- Bone density assessment
- Body weight.

Pharmacotherapy of anorexia nervosa, bulimia nervosa and binge eating disorder

SSRIs are more effective in bulimia nervosa and in binge eating disorder than in anorexia nervosa, probably because in anorexia nervosa there is reduced dietary tryptophan.

SSRIs may be considered in anorexia nervosa in patients with prominent depressive or obsessive–compulsive symptoms which continue after normal body weight has been achieved. They reduce binge eating and vomiting in patients with binge eating disorder and in bulimia nervosa. Duration of treatment for at least 6 months is recommended for a better long-term outcome compared with shorter duration of therapy.

Practice summary

- Eating disorders are conditions in which relapse could occur.
- Ideal body weight is commonly assessed according to the body mass index (weight in kilograms/square of height in metres).
- A comprehensive management approach is required in the management of eating disorders which includes behavioural modification, patient support and education on food patterns.
- In obesity, pharmacotherapy should be considered as an adjunct to exercise, diet and behavioural modification in patients without risk factors with a BMI index of 30 kg/m^2 or greater or in patients with an obesity-related risk factor and a BMI index of 27 kg/m^2 or greater.

Question

1 Compare sibutramine and orlistat.

Answer

1 Orlistat is a reversible inhibitor of lipases interfering with hydrolysation of dietary fat. It has a topical action. Side-effects include interference with absorption of fat-soluble vitamins, oily spotting, flatus and faecal urgency. Orlistat can be used by patients aged between 18 and 75 years. Treatment with orlistat should continue beyond 3 months if weight loss is greater than 5%, beyond 6 months if loss is greater than 10%. Treatment should not usually continue beyond 1 year and never beyond 2 years. Sibutramine inhibits re-uptake of serotonin and noradrenaline. It acts centrally and causes a sensation of satiety. Patients should be advised to take the dose in the morning and not to use other drugs before seeking advice from a health professional. Blood pressure and pulse rate should be monitored. Sibutramine is contraindicated in psychiatric illness, glaucoma, history of cardiovascular disease and side-effects include dry mouth, headache and constipation.

Further reading

Ali O (2002). Getting to grips with obesity: incidence and associated risks. *Pharm J* 268: 616–618.

Ali O (2002). Getting to grips with obesity: non-drug strategies. *Pharm J* 268: 652–654.

Ali O (2002). Getting to grips with obesity: pharmacotherapy. *Pharm J* 268: 687–689.

Ali O (2002). Getting to grips with obesity: how pharmacists can contribute to obesity management. *Pharm J* 268: 720–722.

Anon (2006). Sibutramine – four years experience. *Aust Adverse Drug React Bull* 25: 11.

Eissa M A H and Gunner K B (2004). Evaluation and management of obesity in children and adolescents. *J Pediatr Heatlh Care* 18: 35–38.

Riedl A, Becker J, Rauchfuss M and Klapp B R (2008). Psychopharmacotherapy in eating disorders: a systematic analysis. *Psychopharmacol Bull* 41: 1–22.

Sonnenberg G E, Matfin G and Reinhardt R R (2007). Drug treatment for obesity: where are we heading and how do we get there? *Br J Diabetes Vasc Dis* 7: 111–118.

Reference

1 Martin J (ed.). *British National Formulary*, 57th edn. London: Pharmaceutical Press, 2009, p. 218.

Acknowledgements

Claire Sillato-Copperstone, assistant lecturer, Institute of Health Care, University of Malta, Malta.

31

Pain management and fever

Learning objectives:

- To recognise sources of pain, categories of pain and therapeutic response required
- To understand pyrexia and drugs used as antipyretic agents
- To identify properties and characteristics of opioid and non-opioid drugs
- To appreciate use of analgesics in pain management
- To develop skills required in the use of opioid analgesics and patient monitoring required
- To review occurrence and management of headache.

Background

Pain is an uncomfortable experience that occurs as a result of tissue damage and which has an emotional dimension in addition to the physical damage. The extent to which the same level of pain interferes with the emotional dimension and with a patient's lifestyle varies from one individual to another due to variation in the pain threshold.

Examples of painful conditions

- Gingival pain
- Headache: tension headache, migraine, sinus headache
- All pains of rheumatological conditions, sciatica
- Myalgia, arthralgia
- Menstrual and post-partum pains
- Traumatic pain
- Cancer pain.

The categories of pain are summarised in Table 31.1.

Types of pain

- Nociceptive pain: arising from pain receptors (e.g. twisted ankle)
- Neuropathic pain: arising from nervous system (e.g. trigeminal neuralgia, shingles)
- Pain with no apparent cause.

Factors affecting the pain threshold are listed in Table 31.2.

Pain is an uncomfortable sensation and individuals may react differently.

The pain pathway is illustrated in Figure 31.1.

The endogenous analgesia system

Endogenous peptide agonists, such as enkephalins and endomorphins, act on opioid receptors which present as:

Table 31.1 Categories of pain

	Acute	Chronic non-malignant pain	Chronic malignant pain
Duration	Hours to days	Months to years	Unpredictable
Associated pathology	Present	Often none	Usually present
Prognosis	Predictable	Unpredictable	Increasing pain
Associated problems	Uncommon	Depression, anxiety	Numerous (e.g. fear of loss of control)
Social effects	Minimal	Profound	Variable depending on patient characteristics, patient support
Treatment	Primarily analgesics	Multimodal, drugs play a minor role	Multimodal, drugs play a major role

Table 31.2 Factors affecting pain threshold

Lowering	Raising
Insomnia, fatigue	Sleep, rest
Discomfort, pain	Relief of symptoms
Anxiety, depression	Sympathy, anxiolytics, antidepressants
Fear, anger, isolation	Companionship, understanding
Boredom	Activity

- μ receptor: agonist effect causes analgesia at supraspinal level, euphoria, respiratory depression, dependence
- κ receptor: analgesia at spinal level, miosis, sedation
- δ receptor: dysphoria, hallucination.

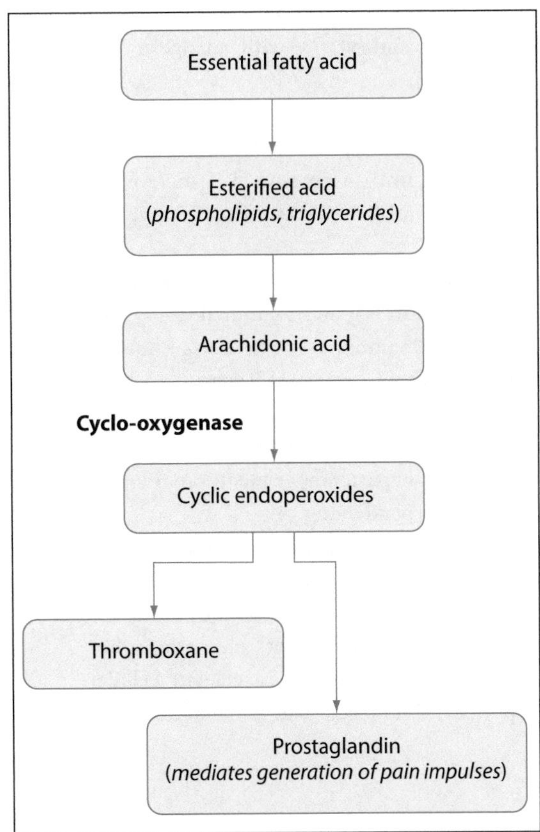

Figure 31.1 Pain pathway.

Assessment of pain

- Psychosocial assessment: impact of pain on psychological well-being and social activities
- Medication history: analgesics used and outcome
- Assessment of previous pain problems: history of pain problems
- Factors that influence pain: activities that increase or decrease occurrence of pain
- Qualitative analysis using visual analogue: patient can describe quantitatively the impact of pain
- Measurement instruments: to evaluate impact of pain on patient's physical and psychological well-being
- Diaries: to identify activities that may relate to the occurrence or deterioration of the condition.

Pain management

- Analgesics
- Acupuncture and massage
- Neurosurgery or neurolytic nerve block
- Physical therapy
- Psychological techniques.

Analgesic drugs

Opioid and non-opioid analgesic drugs are commonly used (Figure 31.2).

Paracetamol

This is an antipyretic with analgesic properties (Figure 31.3).

- Dosage forms: tablets (500 mg), soluble tablets (500 mg), oral suspension (125 mg/5 mL, 250 mg/5 mL), suppositories (125 mg, 250 mg, 500 mg)
- Dosage: adults: 0.5–1 g every 4–6 hours to a maximum of 4 g daily; children: every 4–6 hours up to a maximum of 4 doses in 24 hours:
  - 3 months–1 year 60–120 mg
  - 1–5 years 120–250 mg
  - 6–12 years 250–500 mg
- Cautions: hepatic impairment, renal impairment, alcohol dependence
- Overdosage: hepatotoxicity. Paracetamol is metabolised to a quinone imine which is extremely toxic. This metabolite is normally eliminated in the liver by a reaction with gluthatione. In overdosage, the quinone reacts with cellular proteins and nucleic acid in the liver.

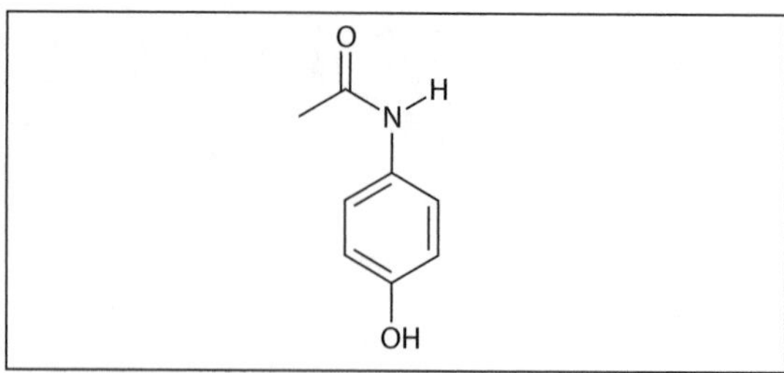

Figure 31.3 Chemical structure of paracetamol.

Compound analgesics

These contain a non-opioid drug with an opioid component (e.g. co-codamol is paracetamol and codeine).

A number of cold preparations contain paracetamol. Advise patients using cold preparations that contain paracetamol against the concomitant use of paracetamol to avoid overdosage.

Non-steroidal anti-inflammatory agents

Aspirin

Aspirin (Figure 31.4) has analgesic, antipyretic and anti-inflammatory actions; the anti-inflammatory action is experienced at high doses when side-effects are more common. It inhibits cyclo-oxygenase, resulting in decreased release of prostaglandins, and has an antiplatelet effect, irreversibly inhibiting cyclo-oxygenase in platelets and preventing formation of thromboxane A_2 (platelet aggregation agent).

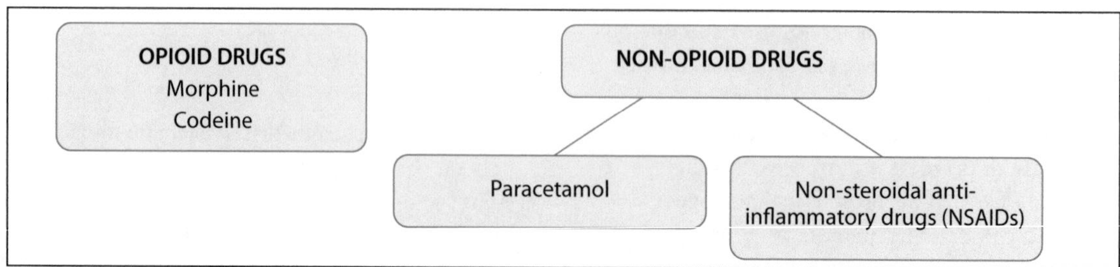

Figure 31.2 Analgesic drugs.

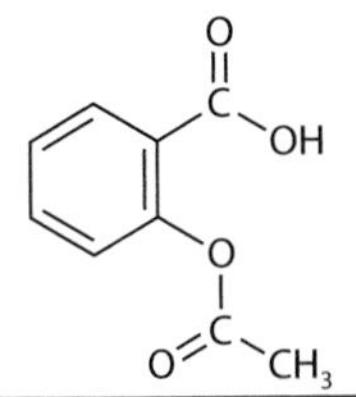

Figure 31.4 Chemical structure of aspirin.

- Dosage forms: tablets, dispersible tablets (300 mg), low-dose aspirin tablets (75 mg)
- Indications: headache, transient musculoskeletal pain, dysmenorrhoea, pyrexia; low-dose: prophylaxis of cerebrovascular disease and myocardial infarction
- Dosage regimen: maximum adult daily dose 4 g daily (300–900 mg every 4–6 hours)
- Side-effects: gastrointestinal disturbances (irritation, blood loss, peptic ulceration), increased bleeding time, bronchospasm
- Cautionary labels: take after food, use enteric-coated tablets to decrease physical damage during drug administration
- Contraindications: children (occurrence of Reye's syndrome – fatty liver degeneration accompanied by encephalopathy), haemophilia and bleeding disorders, acute or history of peptic ulcers
- Cautions: asthma, allergic disease, the elderly, hepatic and renal impairment, pregnancy
- Pregnancy: during the third trimester use of aspirin may present potential bleeding disorders in mother and fetus, delayed onset and increased duration of labour with increased blood loss
- Drug interactions: enhanced anticoagulant effect of warfarin
- See also Chapter 44.

Some examples of NSAIDs are shown in Figure 31.5.

NSAIDs – selective inhibitors of cyclo-oxygenase 2

- Improve gastrointestinal tolerance
- Indicated for symptomatic relief in osteoarthritis and rheumatoid arthritis in patients at high risk of developing a gastroduodenal ulcer
- Not to be used as routine treatment

Patients at risk of NSAID-associated damage to the gastric mucosa

- >60 years of age
- Previous history of peptic ulcer disease
- Administration of high doses of NSAIDs or more than one NSAID
- Smokers
- Heavy alcohol drinkers
- Patients with *Helicobacter pylori*
- Other drugs causing gastric damage
- Anticoagulants.

- Contraindications/cautions: in congestive heart failure, hypertension, oedema
- Example: celecoxib.

Opioid analgesics

- Morphine (Figure 31.6): the standard drug against which other opioids are compared
- Diamorphine (heroin): more potent
- Codeine (Figure 31.7): higher bioavailability than morphine but less potent
- Tramadol: presents fewer of the typical opioid side-effects.

What is inflammation?

- An event that occurs in response to a disease state or pathogen
- Immunological reaction involving:
  - cells: white blood cells, tissue cells (mast cells, macrophages)
  - mediators: eicosanoids, cytokines, bradykinin, histamine, neuropeptides.

Principal anti-inflammatory agents

- Glucocorticoids (e.g. hydrocortisone, betamethasone, dexamethasone)
- Non-steroidal anti-inflammatory drugs (e.g. aspirin, ibuprofen, diclofenac, mefenamic acid, celecoxib, meloxicam).

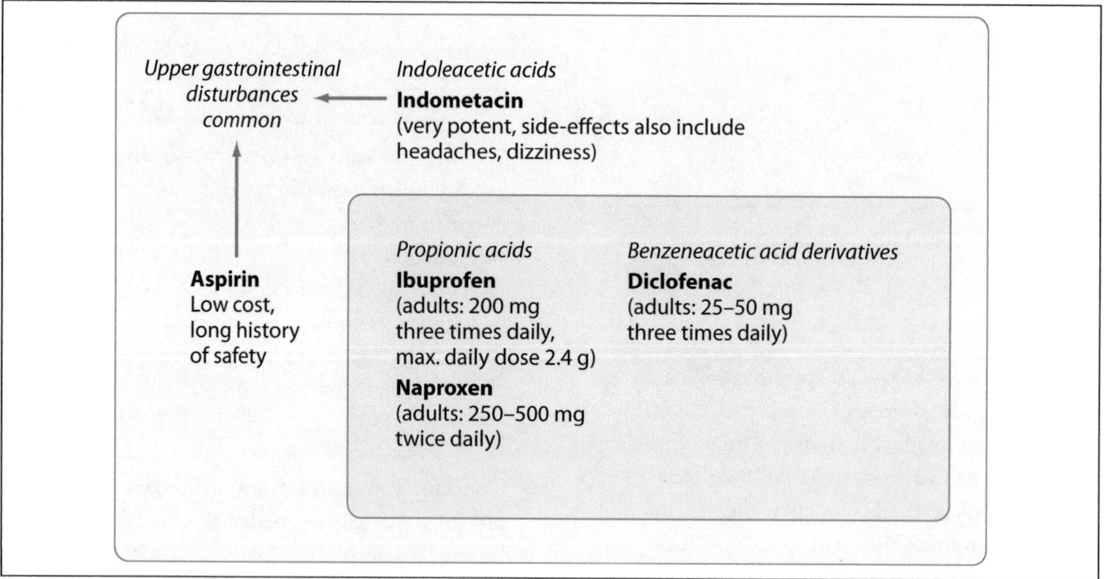

Figure 31.5 Non-steroidal anti-inflammatory drugs.

Effects

- Analgesia (elevate pain threshold, alter reaction to pain)
- Euphoria (relieve anxiety and fright)
- Sedation (induce sleep)
- Reduce gut motility (control diarrhoea; see Chapter 15)
- Control cough (cough suppression; see Chapter 54).

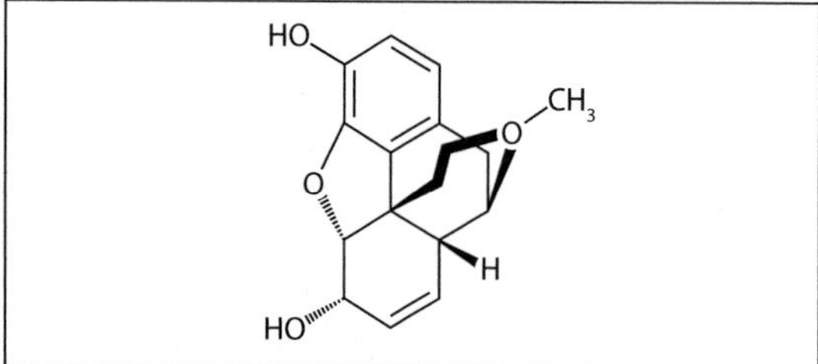

Figure 31.6 Chemical structure of morphine.

Figure 31.7 Chemical structure of codeine.

Side-effects

- Psychological and physical dependence
- Respiratory depression
- Nausea and vomiting
- Constipation.

Contraindications: respiratory disease, head injury, raised intracranial pressure.

> Opioids can cause respiratory depression. They should be avoided in patients with acute respiratory insufficiency, sputum retention, bronchiectasis and chronic bronchitis.

Morphine

- Used in chronic, severe pain in advanced cancer and in post-operative pain
- Has a central analgesic action, produces euphoria and a sense of detachment, all of which could be useful in advanced cancer and in palliative care
- Duration of action is of about 7 hours
- May cause drowsiness, aggravation of gastrointestinal pain
- Administration:

- normal release morphine elixir: effect within 20 minutes, peak 60 minutes
- modified-release tablets: peak 4–8 hours
- injections: considered when patient presents with persistent nausea and vomiting, difficulty in swallowing and when patient is not cooperative.

Diamorphine

- More soluble than morphine allowing effective doses to be injected in smaller volumes
- May cause less nausea and hypotension than morphine. This characteristic is particularly useful in patients in cardiac and emergency units.

Pethidine

- Used peri-operatively and in obstetrics
- Causes less euphoria and sedation than morphine
- Has a rapid onset of action and a short duration of action (2 hours)
- Metabolised to norpethidine which can cause seizures in renal impairment due to accumulation.

Fentanyl

- Used for intra-operative analgesia but is not suitable for post-operative analgesia since the duration of action is short
- For long-term analgesia, transdermal patches may be preferred
- Remifentanil: has a rapid onset of action (2 minutes) and a short duration of action.

In patients receiving opioid analgesics, prophylaxis for nausea and vomiting should be considered using antiemetics and when opioid is being used long term consider a laxative such as lactulose due to incidence of constipation as a side-effect. Opioids can cause confusion, especially in older patients.

Guidelines for analgesia

- Nociceptor-generated pain: follow the analgesic ladder (Table 31.3)
- Neuropathic pain: include use of adjuvant analgesics such as anticonvulsants (e.g. carbamezepine), antidepressants (e.g. imipramine) and others (e.g. baclofen)
- Unknown cause: opioids with adjuvant analgesics such as anticonvulsants, antidepressants.

Table 31.4 shows adjuvant drugs used in the treatment of pain.

- Mild pain: paracetamol, NSAIDs
- Moderate pain: paracetamol, NSAIDs, codeine
- Severe pain: strong opioid drugs (e.g. morphine).

Table 31.3 The analgesic ladder

Class	Drug	Relative potency	Duration of action (hours)
Stage 1 non-opioid	Paracetamol NSAIDs		
Stage 2 weak opioids	Codeine Dextropropoxyphene	0.08 0.16	4 8
Stage 3 strong opioids	Morphine Fentanyl	1 50	4 1

NSAIDs, non-steroidal anti-inflammatory drugs.

Table 31.4 Adjuvant drugs used in the treatment of pain

Drug class	Type of pain	Example
Anticonvulsants	Neuropathic pain	Carbamazepine Phenytoin
Antidepressants	Neuropathic pain, burning pain	Amitriptyline
Muscle relaxants	Muscle spasm	Baclofen
Steroids	Nerve compression	Dexamethasone Prednisolone
Bisphosphonates	Bone pain	Pamidronate
Antispasmodics	Smooth muscle spasm	Hyoscine

Special techniques

Neural blockade

This involves the injection of local anaesthetic close to the sensory area where the pain is occurring so as to block conduction of pain impulses. The use of adrenaline in combination with the local anaesthetic is considered to increase duration of action of the anaesthetic due to the vasoconstriction that occurs.

Patient-controlled analgesia (PCA)

An opioid drug is delivered in a pump system which delivers a pre-set dose on activation. A safety feature (lock-out time) ensures that the patient does not re-activate and get release of drug immediately after an activation. The pump delivers the drug by subcutaneous injection. It gives the patient a feeling of control over pain management and results in individual dosing.

Local anaesthetics

The durations of action of some common local anaesthetics are compared in Table 31.5.

Concomitant administration of a vasoconstrictor (e.g. adrenaline) to increase duration of action may be considered. Such practice is contraindicated if the anaesthetic is being used near extremities, due to ensuing vasoconstriction.

Table 31.5 Durations of action of local anaesthetics

Drug	Duration of action
Benzocaine	+
Lidocaine	++
Bupivacaine	+++

Reasons for analgesic treatment failure include inadequate management (dose, frequency, drug selection), occurrence of side-effects, fear of addiction and patient misunderstanding.

Classification of headache

- Primary headache disorders (e.g. muscle contraction headache, vascular headache)
- Psychogenic disorders
- Secondary headache disorders (e.g. sinus headache).

Sinus headache

- Presentation: localised to the periorbital area or forehead; blowing the nose intensifies pain

Assessing headache attacks

- Time of day when attacks occur
- Duration of attack
- Intensity of pain
- Location of pain
- Precipitating factors (e.g. food, activities)
- Factors that relieve or improve headache
- Concomitant phenomena
- Significance to patient – impact on lifestyle.

- Possible cause: infection or blockage of the paranasal sinuses
- Duration: several days or more
- Onset: gradual
- Management: analgesics and nasal decongestants
- See Chapters 25 and 54.

Muscle contraction (tension) headache

- Presentation: bilateral, diffuse pain often over the top of the head
- Possible cause: tight muscles in the upper back, neck
- Duration: up to several days
- Onset: gradual
- Management: acute: analgesics; chronic: relaxation, short-term benzodiazepines, antidepressants.

Vascular headache (migraine)

- Presentation: recurrent hemicranial, throbbing headache, nausea, vomiting
- Possible cause: distension or dilatation of intracranial arteries or traction or displacement of large intracranial veins
- Duration: aura 30 minutes before onset of attack; several days
- Onset: acute
- Management: NSAIDs, compound analgesics, $5HT_1$ agonists.

$5HT_1$ agonists

- Examples: sumatriptan, zolmitriptan
- Considerable value in acute migraine attack in patients who fail to respond to conventional analgesics
- Caution: pre-existing cardiac disease (angina, hypertension, transient ischaemic attacks, stroke) since they cause vasoconstriction, hepatic impairment
- Side-effects: tingling sensations, numbness, dizziness, vertigo
- Patient education: report occurrence of severe tightness.

Triptans should be started as soon as symptoms of migraine occur.

Migraine-precipitating factors

- Psychological factors: stress, personality
- Environmental factors: noise, light, disturbed sleep patterns
- Physiological factors: epilepsy, allergy, hypoglycaemia
- Dietary factors: cheese, alcohol, caffeine withdrawal or excessive caffeine intake
- Iatrogenic factors
- Drugs: ethinylestradiol, indometacin, H_2-receptor antagonists.

Management of migraine

- Acute treatment: analgesics or $5HT_1$ agonist ± metoclopramide (if accompanied by nausea)
- Prophylaxis: beta-blockers (e.g. propranolol), calcium channel blockers, tricyclic antidepressants (e.g. amitriptyline), pizotifen, anticonvulsants (e.g. valproate, topiramate).

Headache in childhood

- Occurs commonly: by age 7 years 40% of children experienced headaches and by age 15 years 75% of individuals would have experienced headaches

- Before adoloscence headache is mainly migraine and with adoloscence pattern changes to muscle contraction headache.

Medication overuse headache (MOH)

- Rebound patterns of headache from repeated use of symptomatic headache medications (analgesics, ergot alkaloids, triptans)
- Most frequent secondary cause of chronic daily headache (headache for >4 hours on >15 days/month)
- Diagnosis: detailed patient drug history and medication use
- Withdrawal of MOH-inducing medication
- High occurrence with combination analgesics containing caffeine and with triptans.

Management of selected pain syndromes

- Dysmenorrhoea: use of oral contraceptive agents when menstrual cycle disorders are associated with clinical dysmenorrhoea (see Chapter 40)
- Trigeminal neuralgia: characterised by abrupt, intense bursts of pain along one side of the face. Carbamazepine and phenytoin may be considered during the acute phase
- Herpetic and postherpetic neuralgia: post-herpetic neuralgia may persist for a number of months. Antiviral agents are used during the herpetic phase and amitriptyline and gabapentin may be considered in the postherpetic phase
- Post-amputation and phantom limb pain: antidepressants are considered.

Transcutaneous electrical nerve stimulation (TENS)

- Used for chronic pain
- Consists of a small, battery-operated instrument that delivers rapid pulses of a small electric current to electrodes applied to the skin
- Provides relief and is indicated within a pain management programme.

Pyrexia

Pyrexia or fever occurs when the body temperature is higher than the normal core temperature of 37°C. Body temperature is controlled in the hypothalamic heat-regulating centre. Fever occurs when interleukin 1 generates prostaglandins which disturb the heat-regulating centre. Complications of fever include febrile convulsions and status epilepticus.

Measurement of fever

- Oral temperature: normal 37.8°C
- Rectal temperature: normal 38.8°C
- Axillary temperature: normal 37.2°C.

Medical devices for measurement of fever

The advantages and disadvantages of mercury-in-glass and electronic thermometers are summarised in Table 31.6.

Management of pyrexia

- Use of antipyretic agent
- Light clothing
- Maintain good airflow
- Sufficient fluid intake
- Sponging with tepid water.

Antipyretics

- Act on hypothalamic heat-regulating centre in the central nervous system
- Paracetamol and NSAIDs (e.g. ibuprofen)
- Febrile convulsions should be avoided. If they, occur patient is treated with intravenous or rectal administration in solution of diazepam.

Practice summary

- Adopt oral administration wherever possible.

Table 31.6 Comparison of mercury-in-glass and electronic thermometers

	Mercury in glass	Electronic
Advantages	Patient familiarity Low cost Compact size	Safer to use in children Register quickly
Disadvantages	Can break easily	Cost

- Treatment goals have to be realistic.
- The three principal compounds – aspirin, ibuprofen and paracetamol – are all effective for mild-to-moderate pain; the first two are indicated more where pain is due to inflammation such as musculoskeletal, dental and dysmenorrhoea.
- Aspirin and ibuprofen have similar indications but ibuprofen appears to be more effective with a lower profile of adverse effects.
- Paracetamol is preferred in children under 16 years, and patients with a history of asthma or gastrointestinal problems.
- Aspirin and NSAIDs interact with warfarin.
- Soluble preparations have a faster onset of action and for NSAIDs produce less gastric irritation.
- Review treatment regularly; if one type of analgesic fails, move up the ladder.
- Avoid recurrence of pain; drugs with a short duration of action are not suitable in the management of sustained severe pain.
- Consider adjuvant drugs, social and psychological support in addition to analgesics.
- In chronic pain adopt patient self-report measures which assess occurrence of pain, for example at rest, during movement or during sleep.

Questions

1. What are the advantages of bupivacaine over benzocaine?
2. Describe the mode of action of ibuprofen and list indications for use.
3. List common adverse reactions that could be expected with NSAIDs.
4. What are the distinguishing characteristics between indoleacetic acid NSAIDs and propionic acid NSAIDs?
5. What is pyrexia and what devices can be used to monitor the condition?
6. What is adjuvant analgesia?

Answers

1. Bupivacaine has a longer duration of action.
2. *Mode of action:* ibuprofen inhibits the cyclo-oxygenase 1 (COX-1) enzyme, resulting in a decrease in inflammatory mediators such as prostaglandins and leukotrienes. It, however, also inhibits the COX-2 enzyme which results in a decrease in the protective prostaglandins in the stomach and the kidney, hence causing side-effects such as gastrointestinal irritation and renal impairment. *Indications:* headache, transient musculoskeletal pain, dysmenorrhoea, pyrexia.
3. Gastrointestinal disturbances (irritation, blood loss, peptic ulceration), increased bleeding time, bronchospasm.
4. Indoleacetic acids (e.g. indometacin) are very potent with many side-effects including gastrointestinal disturbances, headaches and dizziness. Propionic acid derivatives (e.g. ibuprofen, naproxen and diclofenac) are less potent with fewer side-effects. This distinction is attributed to a difference in structure.
5. Pyrexia is body temperature that is higher than the normal core temperature of 37°C. Body temperature is controlled in the hypothalamic heat-regulating centre. Fever occurs when interleukin 1 (IL-1)-generated prostaglandins disturb the heat-regulating centre. Medical devices used to measure pyrexia include mercury-in-glass and electronic thermometers.
6. In adjuvant analgesia, products with a primary indication other than for pain are used in combination with analgesics, for example tricyclic antidepressants such as amitriptyline which is used in neuropathic pain.

Further reading

Aronoff G (2006). The use of opioids in chronic pain management. *Hosp Pharm Eur* January/February: 67–71.

Dickman A (2007). Opioid analgesics in palliative care. *Pharm J* 278: 745–748.

Hankin C S, Schein J, Clark J A and Panchal S (2007). Adverse events involving intravenous patient-controlled analgesia. *Am J Health-Syst Pharm* 64: 1492–1499.

Helme R D (2006). Drug treatment of neuropathic pain. *Aust Prescrib* 29: 72–75.

Pizzuto M, Wirth F, Azzopardi L M, Zarb-Adami M and Serracino-Inglott A (2009). Palliative care in cancer patients. *Hosp Pharm Eur* 42: 66–69.

32

Dementia and Alzheimer's disease

Learning objectives:

- To appreciate the use of pharmacotherapy in dementia
- To develop skills to support patient and caregivers to cope with condition and benefit from drug therapy prescribed
- To identify use of adjunctive therapy in the management of dementia.

Background

Dementia is a syndrome of acquired abnormality in cognitive functions (including memory, language, judgement), behaviour and participation in social life. Dementia leads to a deterioration in emotional control (patients may at times become aggressive), a change in social behaviour patterns and motivation.

Alzheimer's disease is a common example of dementia. Alzheimer's disease is a systemic neuro-degenerative disease that causes slow and gradual progressive dementia.

Aetiology

- Loss of neurons in cerebral cortex and hippocampus
- Deficiency of neurotransmitters, particularly acetylcholine, due to decreased occurrence of acetyltransferase
- May be as a result of various pathophysiological pathways and may depend on multiple factors
- Possibility that NSAIDs, oestrogen therapy, antioxidants (vitamin E) and higher education decrease likelihood of disease.

Presentation

- Average age of onset is 75 years (range 52–89 years)
- Span 2–20 years, average 8 years' duration
- Insidious onset
- Short-term memory lapse developing into deterioration of cognitive function, urinary incontinence, depression and hallucinations
- Scales such as the Global Deterioration Scale may be used to describe the extent of cognitive decline, which ranges from very mild decline (forgetfulness) to very severe decline (loss of psychomotor and verbal skills and incontinence). Cognitive decline impacts negatively on work and social life and leads to agitation and aggression.

Diagnostic criteria

- Establishment of dementia by clinical examination and using scales such as the Mini-Mental State Examination (MMSE)
- Occurrence of deficits in two or more areas of cognition: language, memory, perception

- Progressive worsening of memory and other cognitive functions, impairment in daily living and altered behavioural patterns
- Dementia is not associated with disturbance of consciousness
- Absence of other systemic disorder or brain disease that may account for deficits in memory and cognition
- Review drug therapy to identify use of medications that may have a negative impact on cognitive function (e.g. benzodiazepines).

Aims and objectives of disease management

Aims

- To modify and slow disease progression
- To optimise cognitive and functional states
- To support caregiver.

Objectives

- To achieve healthy diet and maintain weight control
- To induce patient to keep active and take up exercise and suggest participation in patient support groups
- To avoid polypharmacy to reduce tablet-taking burden on patient and carers
- To monitor use of medications that may have an effect on the central nervous system.

Pharmacotherapy

- Acetylcholinesterase inhibitors (e.g. donepezil, galantamine, rivastigmine, which is also licensed for dementia associated with Parkinson's disease) are used in mild-to-moderate disease.
- NMDA (*N*-methyl-D-aspartate) antagonists (e.g. memantine) are used in moderate-to-severe disease.

> Pharmacotherapy alleviates the symptoms but the condition will gradually deteriorate to an extent where the patient becomes unable to communicate and to cope independently.

Acetylcholinesterase inhibitors

These slow the rate of cognitive and non-cognitive deterioration. In addition to activity on acetylcholinesterase, galantamine stimulates nicotinic receptors and rivastigmine inhibits butyrylcholinesterase activity, which is another pathway for acetylcholine metabolism. They are associated with a lag time of 3 months.

- Efficacy is judged on assessment of cognition, behaviour and daily activities.
- Side-effect profile is low; gastrointestinal cholinergic side-effects may occur.
- Cautions: cardiac disease, asthma, COPD, pregnancy, breast-feeding, and hepatic and renal impairment.

> Acetylcholinesterase inhibitors are better tolerated if taken with or after food.

NMDA antagonists

These have a neuroprotective effect since in Alzheimer's disease there is probably an age-related change in NMDA receptors. They are indicated for moderate-to-severe disease and may be used in patients who cannot tolerate cholinesterase inhibitors.

- Side-effect profile is low: constipation, hypertension, headache, dizziness and drowsiness
- Cautions: history of convulsions, renal impairment and pregnancy.

Other possible therapies

Other possible therapies that are currently being evaluated include: MAOIs, antioxidants and *Gingko biloba*.

Pharmacoeconomics and Alzheimer's disease

- Enormous direct and indirect cost burden
- Use of cholinesterase inhibitors in mild-to-moderate disease may allow patients to stay longer at home rather than being institutionalised
- Treatment postpones disease onset but decision has to be taken when treatment should be withdrawn (end-point of treatment) if patients are not responding or tolerating the drugs
- Assessment of outcome of therapy using quality-of-life scores; functional and behavioural assessment should be carried out within 3 months of initiating therapy.

Drugs that should be avoided

Drugs that can cause confusion as a side-effect should be used with caution in patients with dementia or Alzheimer's disease:

- anticholinergics – antidepressants
- benzodiazepines, particularly long-acting
- opioid analgesics
- long-acting sulphonylureas.

Care and social support

Directed towards the patient

- Optimise patient's sensory input (good lighting, hearing aids)
- Follow structural routine
- Offer reassurance
- Adopt clear and simple communication
- Avoid confrontation
- Provide frequent reorientation with home environment.

Directed towards the caregiver

- Ensure safety at home
- Get help and use day-care facilities
- Take up legal and financial planning
- Educate on how to manage stress levels
- Reassure and counsel to avoid guilty feelings as a result of reactions by patients.

Achieving compliance in patients with dementia is very difficult. Pharmacists should establish contact with carers to explain use of medication, to offer patient and carer support and to provide signposting services.

Management of mood disorders

Behavioural and psychological symptoms present in patients with dementia and Alzheimer's disease. The following suggested therapies are available:

- depression: SSRIs
- anxiety: buspirone, propranolol, SSRIs
- insomnia: zolpidem
- delirium: haloperidol
- psychosis, aggression: risperidone, atypical antipyschotics.

Antipsychotic therapy should be considered for non-cognitive symptoms that are interfering with patient's lifestyle and where carers report negative aspects of patient's behaviour.

The use of atypical antipsychotic drugs is uncertain since concerns about the safety have emerged. The disadvantages of the atypical antipsychotics include weight gain, diabetes mellitus, cardiac conduction abnormalities, cerebrovascular events and extrapyramidal symptoms. Patients with dementia may be at a higher risk of developing stroke associated with use of antipsychotics (see also Chapter 26).

Before starting an atypical antipsychotic in patients with dementia, who are in most cases elderly, baseline assessment of cardiac function and occurrence of extrapyramidal symptoms should be undertaken and concurrent medication reviewed.

In the management of insomnia and anxiety, benzodiazepines should be avoided due to their negative effect on cognitive function.

Practice summary

- Compliance may be an issue – treatment is not effective with intermittent administration, patient may have cognitive impairment which will impact negatively on compliance, and family supervision needs to be recruited.
- Patient, family and carers need social support.
- Titration of dose: start at low dose and titrate up.
- Patient monitoring: assess cognitive and non-cognitive deterioration.

Question

1 When is memantine used in Alzheimer's disease? List common side-effects that may occur with its use.

Answer

1 Memantine is an *N*-methyl-D-aspartate (NMDA) antagonist with a neuroprotective effect indicated for moderate-to-severe Alzheimer's disease. The rationale for its use is that in Alzheimer's disease there is probably an age-related change in NMDA receptors. Memantine may be used in patients who cannot tolerate cholinesterase inhibitors. The side-effect profile includes constipation, hypertension, headache, dizziness and drowsiness, and less commonly vomiting, thrombosis, confusion, fatigue, hallucinations and abnormal gait. Very rarely seizures, pancreatitis, psychosis, depression and suicidal ideation may occur.

Further reading

Bullock R (2003). Guide to identifying and treating dementia. *Prescriber* 19 October: 34–44.

Douglas I J and Smeeth L (2008). Exposure to antipsychotics and risk of stroke: self-controlled case series study. *BMJ* 337: a1227.

Herrmann N and Lanctot K L (2006). Atypical antipsychotics for neuropsychiatric symptosm of dementia: malignant or maligned? *Drug Safety* 29: 833–843.

Husband A and Worsley A (2006). Different types of dementia. *Pharm J* 277: 579–582.

Jones R (2000). Alzheimer's disease. *Pharm J* 264: 846–850.

National Institute for Health and Clinical Excellence (2006). Dementia: Supporting people with dementia and their carers in health and social care. http://www.nice.org.uk/guidance/cg42 (updated September 2007).

Schneider L S, Tariot P N, Dagerman K S, Davis S, Hsiao J K, Ismail S *et al.* (2006). Effectiveness of atypical antipsychotic drugs in patients with Alzheimer's disease. *N Engl J Med* 355: 1525–1538.

Thompson F C, Fraser K, Kelly J, Martin M and Lyons D (2001). Drug treatment of dementia. *Hosp Pharm* 8: 41–49.

Yaari R and Corey-Bloom J (2007). Alzheimer's disease. *Semin Neurol* 27: 32–41.

33

Parkinson's disease

Learning objectives:

- To appreciate principles in pharmacotherapy of parkinsonism
- To develop skills to identify concerns of the patient with anti-parkinsonian drugs and develop an individualised drug therapy programme.

Background

This condition was described in 1817 by Dr James Parkinson as 'the shaky palsy'. It is a progressive neurological disorder characterised by impaired voluntary movements.

Aetiology

- Idiopathic
- Environmental toxin: MPTP
- Cerebral damage
- Viral encephalitis
- Drugs.

Drug-induced parkinsonism

Parkinsonism may be induced by:

- phenothiazines (e.g. trifluoperazine, chlorpromazine)
- tricyclic antidepressants (e.g. amitriptyline)
- butyrophenones (e.g. haloperidol)
- metoclopramide.

Symptoms may disappear with treatment withdrawal or may persist after discontinuation of treatment.

Pathology

- Reduced concentration of dopaminergic neurons in corpus striatum and substantia nigra
- Striatal cholinergic hyperactivity
- Symptoms: bradykinesia, tremor at rest, muscle rigidity, abnormal posture
- Signs: shuffling gait, blank facial expression, speech impairment, inability to perform skilled tasks
- Secondary manifestations:
  - psychiatric: sleep disorders, depression, anxiety
  - gastrointestinal related: constipation, dysphagia
  - skin: seborrhoeic dermatitis
  - visual deficits
  - urinary dysfunction.

Depression is a common condition related to parkinsonism. Signs need to be taken into account when reviewing patient. Antidepressant drug therapy, when required, should be identified after considering current drug therapy and disease state.

Staging Parkinson's disease

A common scale that is used to assess disease progression is the Hoehn and Yahr scale.[1]

- Stage I: unilateral involvement only
- Stage II: bilateral or midline involvement
- Stage III: bilateral involvement, first sign of impaired righting reflexes
- Stage IV: fully developed, severely disabling disease
- Stage V: confined to bed or chair unless aided.

Pharmacotherapy

- Drugs that increase dopamine level: levodopacarbidopa
- Drugs that stimulate dopamine receptors: dopamine agonists
- Drugs that inhibit dopamine metabolism: monoamine oxidase-type inhibitor, catechol-O-methyltransferase inhibitors
- *Others*: amantadine, anticholinergic agents.

Patients and their carers should be advised about the drug therapy and expected side-effects and limitations of current pharmacotherapy in parkinsonism. Therapy with more than one product may be required to control the symptoms while avoiding as much as possible the occurrence of side-effects. Patients should be advised against abrupt withdrawal of anti-parkinsonian drugs since this may induce neuroleptic malignant syndrome.

Levodopa

Levodopa is a precursor of dopamine and is the mainstay treatment. It is given in combination (co-careldopa) with carbidopa, a dopa-decarboxylase inhibitor, to reduce the peripheral conversion of levodopa to dopamine, allowing for administration of lower doses of levodopa and resulting in decreased occurrence of side-effects.

It is mostly effective against bradykinesia and rigidity with minimal effect on tremor.

- Cautions: pre-existing cardiovascular disease since it may cause arrhythmias, peptic ulceration, pulmonary disease, history of convulsions and skin melanoma, psychiatric illness or dementia, endocrine disease such as diabetes, hyperthyroidism, osteomalacia, phaeochromocytoma, hepatic or renal impairment, glaucoma.
- Side-effects: nausea and vomiting, dry mouth, anorexia, postural hypotension, cardiac arrhythmias, involuntary movements, behavioural changes including depression, anxiety, psychoses and dementia (higher risk in the elderly, and patients with dementia or psychiatric illness) and drowsiness.
- Disadvantages: involuntary movements that may occur as side-effects of treatment due to motor complications, and end-of-dose deterioration which leads to decreased benefit with time with same amount of drug administration. This is due to dopaminergic neuron loss with time.
- Drug interactions: phenothiazines, butyrophenones, tricyclic antidepressants, phenytoin, metoclopramide, benzodiazepines, anticholinergics since they decrease effect of levodopa.
- The modified-release oral formulations are used to decrease fluctuations in blood levels of levodopa and decrease occurrence of response fluctuations. Also, the number of doses per day are reduced, ensuring better patient acceptability and compliance. A disadvantage to modified-release oral formulations is that they may present with a delayed onset of action in the morning to counteract immobility when the patient needs to get out of bed. In such cases either the modified-release formulation is administered about 1 hour before rising or else immediate-release formulation is used in the morning.
- Drug holidays: this describes the practice of withdrawal of levodopa therapy for a brief period. This may improve therapeutic outcome when therapy is re-instated possibly because levodopa causes downregulation of dopamine receptors. Disadvantages of drug holidays are

that patient may experience immobility which will impact negatively on the physical and psychological well-being of the patient. Patient needs to be monitored closely.

Dopamine agonists

These are bromocriptine and the newer dopamine agonists cabergoline, pergolide, pramipexole, ropinirole and rotigotine. They have a levodopa-sparing effect since they are used early in treatment, delaying the use of levodopa to later stages of the disease. May be used in combination with levodopa.

- Less effective than levodopa in improving overall motor performance. An advantage over levodopa is that they have a longer half-life and therefore require less frequent dosing.
- Caution in cardiovascular disease since they may cause arrhythmias, in psychiatric disease or in dementia.
- Side-effects: nausea, constipation, drowsiness, postural hypotension, confusion especially in the elderly, involuntary movements, behavioural changes.
- Drug interactions: neuroleptic drugs decrease effect of dopamine agonists.

Bromocriptine

This has an effect on prolactin release from the pituitary gland. It is used in hyperprolactinaemia.

Ergot-derived dopamine agonists

Examples include bromocriptine, cabergoline and pergolide.

- May cause fibrotic reactions (pulmonary, retroperitoneal, pericardial). This requires measurement of renal function, ESR and serum creatinine, and a chest X-ray before initiating therapy and on a yearly basis thereafter.
- Patient monitoring for occurrence of signs of fibrotic reactions namely dyspnoea, persistent cough, chest pain, cardiac failure, abdominal pain and tenderness.
- Non-ergot-derived dopamine agonists (pramipexole, ropinirole, rotigotine) are preferred.

- Co-careldopa and dopamine receptor agonists may cause excessive daytime sleepiness or sudden onset of sleep. Patients should be advised about this in order to be careful when driving and operating machinery especially during initiation of therapy until occurrence of side-effects is understood.
- Domperidone may be used as an antiemetic to counteract the nausea caused by levodopa or dopamine agonists or both when used in combination. Patient is advised to take antiparkinsonian agents with meals.

Catechol-*O*-methyltransferase inhibitors

Catechol-O-methyltransferase (COMT) inhibitors such as entacapone and tolcapone increase the elimination half-life of levodopa, thus prolonging the activity of levodopa in the brain. Lower doses of levodopa may be used and there is an increased amount of time when levodopa therapy has a positive impact on the disease. They do not have antiparkinsonian activity and are used as an adjunct to co-careldopa.

- Side-effects: nausea, diarrhoea or constipation, abdominal pain, urine discoloration, dry mouth
- Tolcapone may cause hepatotoxicity. Patients should be advised to report any signs of liver disease such as anorexia, fatigue, abdominal pain, dark urine or pruritus. Liver function tests should be carried out regularly.

Monoamine oxidase B inhibitors

Inhibitors of monoamine oxidase type B, such as rasagiline and selegiline, enhance central dopamine effects and delay the need for and allow for reduction in doses of levodopa.

- Sudden withdrawal may exacerbate the condition.
- Side-effects: gastrointestinal disturbances.

Amantadine

This is a synthetic antiviral agent. It improves bradykinesia, tremor and rigidity, and probably potentiates dopamine activity by causing release of dopamine from storage vesicles in neurons.

- Administered in early disease so as to delay use of levodopa
- Withdrawal may exacerbate symptoms
- Dose-limiting side-effects: cognitive impairment, orthostatic hypotension, nausea, hallucinations.

Anticholinergic drugs

Examples include benztropine, orphenadrine, procyclidine and trihexyphenidyl. They are used when tremor is a characteristic symptom and in drug-induced parkinsonism.

- Cautions: cardiovascular disease, hypertension, psychotic disorders, prostatic hypertrophy, pyrexia, the elderly, glaucoma
- Side-effects: blurred vision, dry mouth, constipation, urinary retention, mental confusions, delusions, hallucinations, impaired memory.

Management of symptoms

- Constipation: high fibre, increase fluid intake, stool softeners, osmotic laxatives
- Blurred vision: artificial tears eye drops
- Insomnia: use of sedating antihistamines
- Diet: soft food.

Drugs used in tremor and tics

- Haloperidol: used in motor tics and symptoms of Gilles de la Tourette's syndrome and related choreas
- Propranolol or other beta-blockers: to treat tremor including postural tremor in parkinsonism which is not controlled by antiparkinsonian agents
- Primidone: an antiepileptic drug which may be used in tremor
- Trihexyphenidyl: used to improve tremor
- Piracetam: used as an adjunct treatment in myoclonus of cortical origin.

Practice summary

- Treatment is symptomatic and there is treatment failure after some years due to end-of-dose deterioration; patients may suffer from on–off effects where they abruptly experience treatment failure lasting for a few minutes to hours.
- There is controversy over when to commence therapy since current treatment reaches end-of-dose effect.
- Quality-of-life assessment using tools to measure mobility or potential for falls and assessment of occurrence of complicating factors (e.g. neuropsychiatric disease, autonomic dysfunction, falls and sleep disorders).
- Coordinate with other health professionals, namely psychotherapists, physiotherapists and speech and language therapists, and provide emotional support and address social needs.
- Ensure patient compliance with treatment since treatment failure may be attributed to loss of activity of drug therapy when patient is in actual fact not compliant with treatment.

Questions

1. Mention the unwanted effects of levodopa. Mention four conditions when levodopa should be used with caution.
2. Giving examples, discuss therapeutic alternatives to levodopa in the management of parkinsonism.

Answers

1. Common unwanted effects of levodopa include nausea and vomiting, sedation, hypotension, cardiac arrhythmias and involuntary movements. Levodopa should be used with caution in pre-existing cardiovascular disease,

peptic ulcer, pulmonary disease, psychiatric illness.

2 Dopamine agonists such as cabergoline, pergolide, pramipexole, ropinirole, rotigotine as well as amantadine and monoamine oxidase B inhibitors may be considered in the initial stages of the disease. They are less effective than levodopa but they have a levodopa-sparing effect and levodopa may be used at a later stage in the disease. Anticholinergic drugs such as benztropine, orphenadrine, procyclidine and trihexyphenidyl are more effective in drug-induced parkinsonism.

Further reading

Lim S-Y and Fox S H (2008). An update on the management of parkinson's disease. *Geriatrics Aging* 11: 215–222.

National Institute for Health and Clinical Excellence (2006). Parkinson's disease: Diagnosis and management in primary and secondary care. http://www.nice.org.uk/CG035.

Reference

1 Hoehn M and Yahr M. Parkinsonism: onset, progression and mortality 1967. *Neurology* 2001; 57(10 suppl 13): S11–26.

34

Anti-infective agents

Learning objectives:

- To appreciate principles of drug selection in anti-infective therapy
- To review classification of anti-infective agents
- To identify characteristics of different classes of anti-infective agents
- To develop skills required to manage clinical use of anti-infective agents
- To review anti-infective prophylaxis in surgery.

Definitions

- Anti-infective agents: products used in the management or prophylaxis of infective conditions caused by bacteria, mycobacteria, fungi, protozoa or viruses
- Antibacterial agents: used in the management or prophylaxis of infections caused by bacteria
- Antibiotics: agents derived from natural source
- Antimicrobials: agents produced synthetically.

Background

- Generations of drugs: within the same class of anti-infective agents the products can be classified according to characteristics in their structural development leading to different generations within a class of drugs.
- Spectrum of activity: antibacterials such as aminopenicillins have the potential to affect a wide range of bacterial species; these are referred to as broad-spectrum antibacterials. Other products, such as clindamycin, affect only a few bacterial species and are termed narrow-spectrum antibacterials.
- Antimicrobial prophylaxis: examples include contacts of patients with meningococcal meningitis, and use of antibacterials before and after dental procedures in patients at risk of endocarditis.
- Nosocomial infections: infection caused by exposure to treatment in a hospital or a healthcare institution.
- Exogenous infection: infection caused from organisms that the body is exposed to.
- Endogenous infection: infection caused from organisms that were within the body.
- Acute sepsis: infection that leads to the formation of pus or to the multiplication of bacteria in the blood.

Patients at risk of developing nosocomial infections

- Immunocompromised patients
- Patients in intensive and critical care

- Malnourished patients
- Cancer patients
- Patients with diabetes
- Geriatric and paediatric patients.

Signs and symptoms of a bacterial infection

- Body temperature: >38°C or <36°C
- Tachycardia: heart rate >90 bpm
- Tachypnoea
- Increase in white blood cells.

Mode of action of antibacterial drugs

Antibacterials that cause killing of bacteria at clinical doses are referred to as bactericidal. Drugs that interfere with bacterial multiplication at clinical doses are referred to as bacteriostatic. Some bactericidal and bacteriostatic drugs are listed in Table 34.1.

Sites of action of antibacterial drugs

- Peptidoglycan cell wall: penicillins, cephalosporins
- Protein synthesis: aminoglycosides, chloramphenicol, fusidic acid, macrolides, tetracyclines
- Nucleic acids: quinolones
- Folic acid synthesis: sulphonamides, trimethoprim.

Table 34.1 Bactericidal (killing of the bacteria) vs bacteriostatic (growth retardation)

Bactericidal	Bacteriostatic
Penicillins	Macrolides
Cephalosporins	Tetracyclines
Quinolones	Sulphonamides
Aminoglycosides	Trimethoprim

Complications of antibacterial therapy

- Hypersensitivity:
  - immediate: urticaria, wheezing, anaphylactic response
  - delayed: rashes, rarely haemolytic anaemia, interstitial nephritis, leukopenia
  - cross-sensitivity: e.g. penicillins with cephalosporins, about 10% of patients who are penicillin sensitive are also sensitive to cephalosporins
- Direct toxicity: gastrointestinal side-effects (e.g. diarrhoea)
- Superinfections: especially with broad-spectrum antibiotics, risk of superinfections with *Candida albicans* causing oral or vaginal thrush.

Concerns about overuse of antibacterial agents

- Some patients demand antibacterials every time that there is illness.
- Overuse of antibacterial agents may result in the suppression or destruction of weak organisms, leaving the very virulent pathogens in the clinical scenario.
- Overuse of antibacterial agents may lead to the development of resistance of microorganisms against anti-infective agents.
- Economic considerations: the use of anti-infective agents without clinical evidence for the need of treatment or prophylaxis using an anti-infective agents is going to increase cost of treatment without a valid rationale.

Choice and use of systemic antibacterial drugs

Causative organism

- Assess severity of infection and withhold systemic drugs in trivial infections
- Obtain specimens for culture before starting anti-infective treatment so as to identify organisms before any bacteriostatic or

bactericidal effect has kicked in (e.g. urine sample for urinary tract infections).

Drug characteristics

- Site of infection: drug should attain adequate concentrations at the location of infection (e.g. otitis media, toenail infection)
- Toxicity: adverse effect profile
- Single or combination therapy (e.g. use of combination therapy in bacterial meningitis)
- Drug interactions with medications that the patient is already taking or medications that are required (e.g. antihistamines and macrolides)
- Cost.

Patient characteristics

- Age: e.g. tetracyclines are avoided in children due to risk of teeth staining and dental hypoplasia in growing teeth
- Comorbidities: e.g. renal disease – dose reduction for cefaclor, ciprofloxacin, macrolides; liver disease – dose reduction for ofloxacin, erythromycin
- Allergy: avoid penicillins and cephalosporins in penicillin-sensitive individuals
- Pregnancy: avoid aminoglycosides (risk of auditory or vestibular nerve damage), tetracyclines (risk of dental discoloration in neonate, maternal hepatotoxicity with large parenteral doses).

Choice within a class of drug

- Degree of antibacterial activity: e.g. cloxacillin (narrow spectrum) vs amoxicillin (broad spectrum)
- Efficiency of absorption: e.g. ampicillin vs amoxicillin (better absorption)
- Convenience of administration: e.g. clarithromycin (lower dosage frequency) vs erythromycin
- Incidence of adverse effects
- Relative cost.

> The antibacterial drug used should reach the site of infection in an effective concentration, and should cause no toxicity and no clinically significant interactions with other drugs being taken by the patient.

Selection of antibacterial therapy is illustrated in Figure 34.1.

> - Intravenous administration of anti-infective agents is considered in the event of a serious infection, when the drug has poor oral bioavailability and when patient is unable to take drugs orally (peri-operative, unconscious).
> - Combination anti-infective therapy is considered when a broad spectrum of activity is required, in mixed infections, for a synergistic effect and to decrease drug resistance.

Comorbidities and antibacterial prescribing

Conditions in which certain antibacterial drugs are best avoided are summarised in Table 34.2.

Some examples of drug interactions with antibacterials are listed in Table 34.3.

Patient monitoring during antibacterial treatment

- Monitor white blood cell count
- Clinical signs of infection (e.g. pyrexia, pulse and respiratory rate, occurrence of urinary urgency when urinary tract infection is suspected)
- Occurrence of side-effects (e.g. gastrointestinal effects or signs of sensitivity reactions).

Penicillins

Penicillins are beta-lactam antibacterial agents in which a cyclic amide ring consisting of four atoms is fused to a substituted five-membered thiazolidine

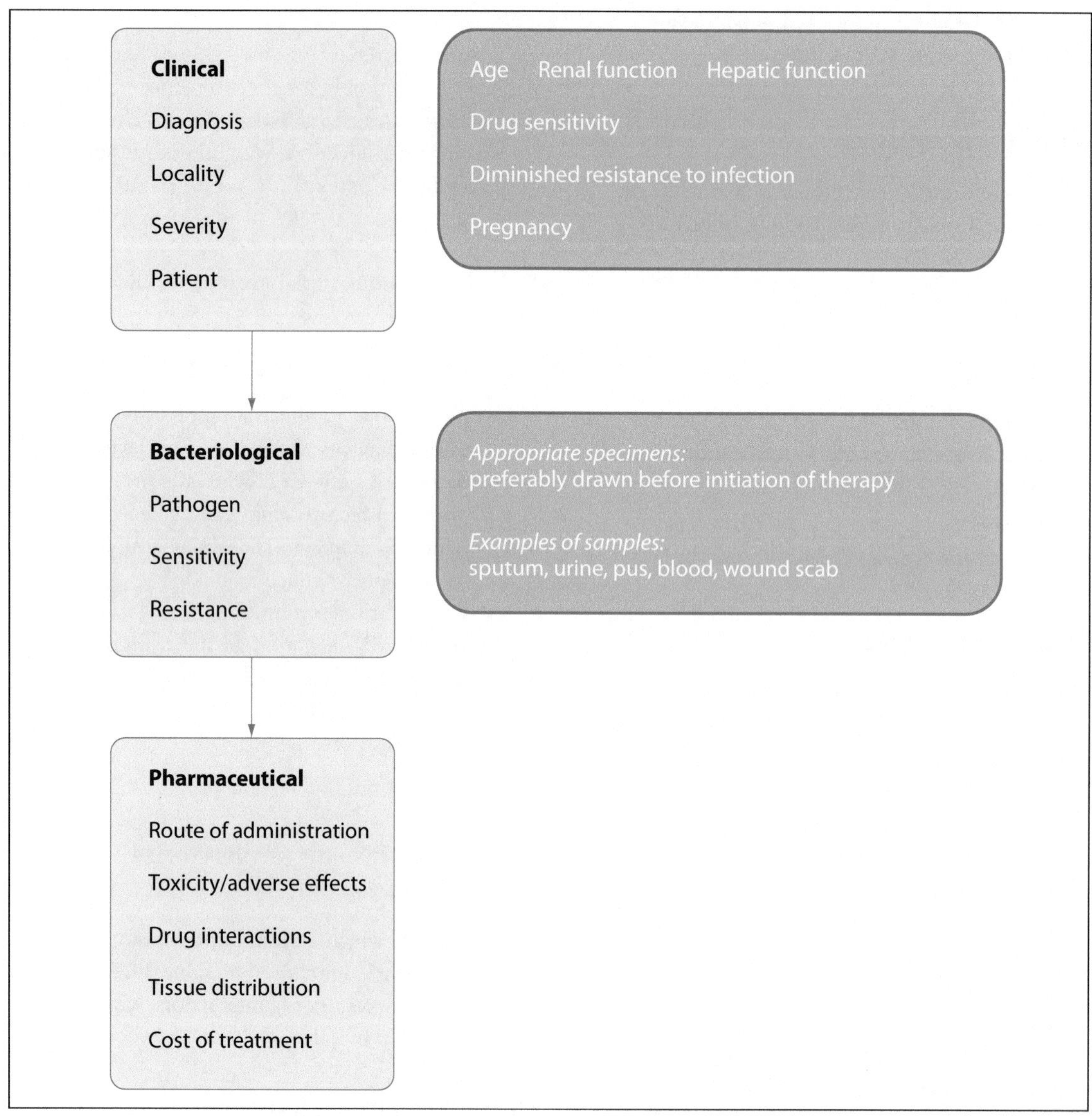

Figure 34.1 Selection of antibacterial therapy.

Table 34.2 Comorbidities and antibacterial prescribing

Condition	Drug to avoid/caution	Comments
Arrhythmias	Macrolides	Prolongation of QT interval
Penicillin allergy	Penicillins and cephalosporins	Hypersensitivity reactions
Epilepsy	Quinolones	May induce convulsions
Psychiatric disorders	Quinolones	May increase risk of seizures
Myasthenia gravis	Aminoglycosides Tetracyclines	May cause muscle weakness

Table 34.3 Examples of drug interactions with antibacterials

Broad-spectrum antibacterials and oral contraceptives	Contraceptive effect of oestrogens possibly reduced
Quinolones with NSAIDs	Increased risk of convulsions
Quinolones, tetracyclines, macrolides with warfarin	Possibly enhance anticoagulant effect
Macrolides with antipyschotics	Increased risk of arrhythmias

NSAIDs, non-steroidal anti-inflammatory drugs.

ring. Due to this configuration the beta-lactam is sensitive to hydrolysis.

Benzylpenicillin

Benzylpenicillin or Penicillin G (Figure 34.2) is acid labile and requires parenteral administration. It is beta-lactamase sensitive, with a narrow spectrum of activity, mainly against Gram-positive cocci.

Phenoxymethylpencillin penicillin

In phenoxymethylpenicillin or penicillin V (Figure 34.3) the addition of a phenoxymethyl moiety on the amide side chain inhibits hydrolysis of the beta-lactam ring and provides the product with acid stability. The drug can be administered orally. It has a spectrum similar to benzylpenicillin.

Aminopenicillins

In ampicillin and amoxicillin (Figure 34.4) the addition of a primary amino group on the side chain results in aminopenicillins where acid stability is retained but the spectrum is shifted to include Gram-negative bacteria. These products are therefore described as broad-spectrum antibacterials. The addition of a hydroxyl group in amoxicillin leads to better absorption profiles compared with ampicillin. The products are penicillinase labile.

The addition of clavulanic acid (co-amoxiclav contains amoxicillin with the beta-lactamase inhibitor clavulanic acid) counteracts the tendency of the penicillinases to destroy the antibacterial agent. Clavulanic acid has minimal antibacterial effects.

Penicillinase-resistant agents

The beta-lactamase enzymes (penicillinases) destroy the antibacterial agents. By having steric hindrance near the side-chain amide bond, penicillinase-resistant agents such as flucloxacillin (Figure 34.5) are resistant to them. They are acid stable and are

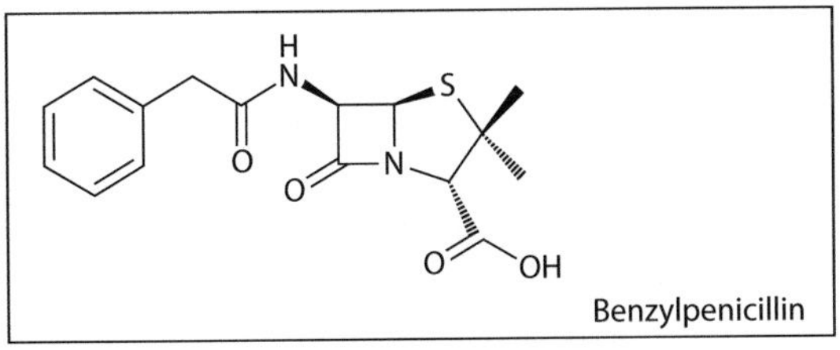

Benzylpenicillin

Figure 34.2 Chemical structure of benzylpenicillin.

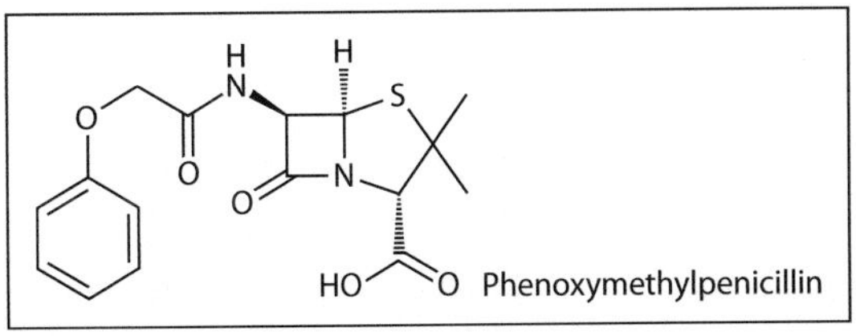

Phenoxymethylpenicillin

Figure 34.3 Chemical structure of phenoxymethylpenicillin

Amoxicillin

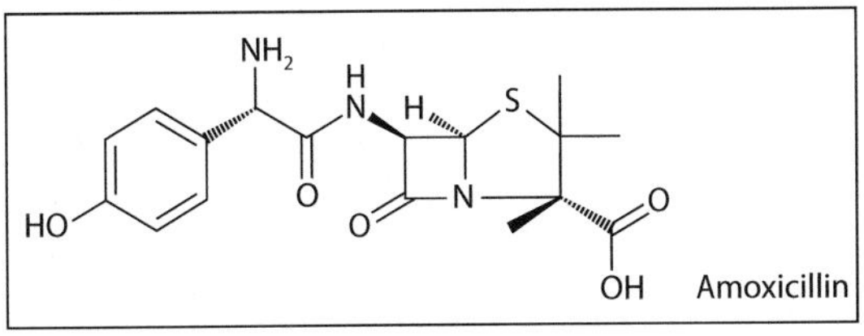

Figure 34.4 Chemical structure of amoxicillin.

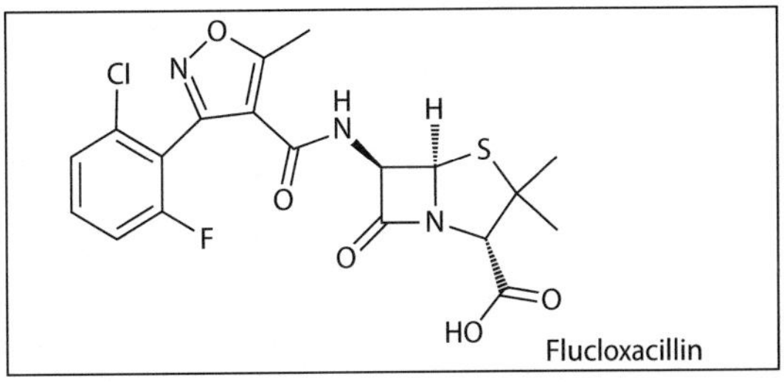

Flucloxacillin

Figure 34.5 Chemical structure of flucloxacillin.

mostly active against Gram-positive cocci, particularly *Staphylococcus aureus*.

Antipseudomonal penicillins

In the antipseudomonal penicillins ticarcillin and piperacillin (Figure 34.6) the amino group in the side chain has been converted to a variety of ureas. These are broad-spectrum products but have greater activity than the aminopenicillins against Gram-negative bacteria; some are active against *Pseudomonas* species. They are available for parenteral administration and are penicillinase sensitive.

General properties of penicillins

- Have good penetration to most tissues but poor entry to cerebrospinal fluid since they are poorly lipid soluble. Meningeal inflammation increases cerebrospinal fluid penetration and in fact may be used in meningitis.
- May be used in combination with aminoglycosides; there is a synergistic effect.

Cephalosporins

Cephalosporins feature a beta-lactam ring that is annealed to a six-membered dihyrothiazine ring. The cephalosporins are described in three generations:

- First generation: e.g. cefalexin, cefadroxil, cefradine (Figure 34.7). Active against Gram-positive cocci. Cefalexin and cefadroxil reflect ampicillin and amoxicillin structures respectively.
- Second generation: e.g. cefuroxime, cefaclor (Figure 34.8). Active against Gram-positive cocci and some activity against Gram-negative bacteria. The addition of a chlorine atom in cefaclor gives it greater activity against Gram-negative bacteria than cefuroxime.
- Third generation: e.g. cefotaxime, ceftriaxone, ceftazidime (Figure 34.9). Active against Gram-negative bacteria; less active against Gram-positive cocci.

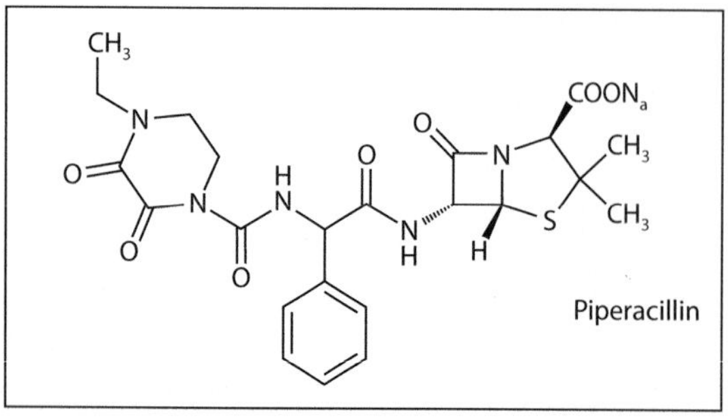

Figure 34.6 Chemical structure of piperacillin.

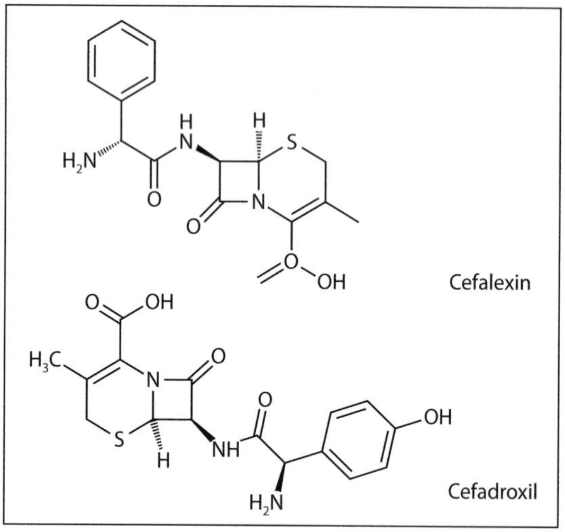

Figure 34.7 Chemical structures of cefalexin and cefadroxil.

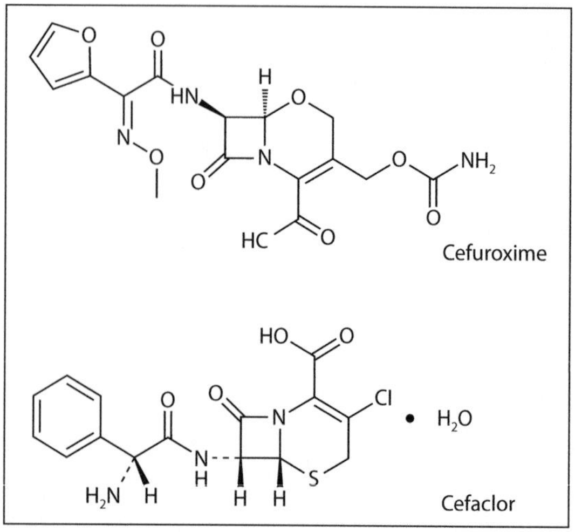

Figure 34.8 Chemical structures of cefuroxime and cefaclor.

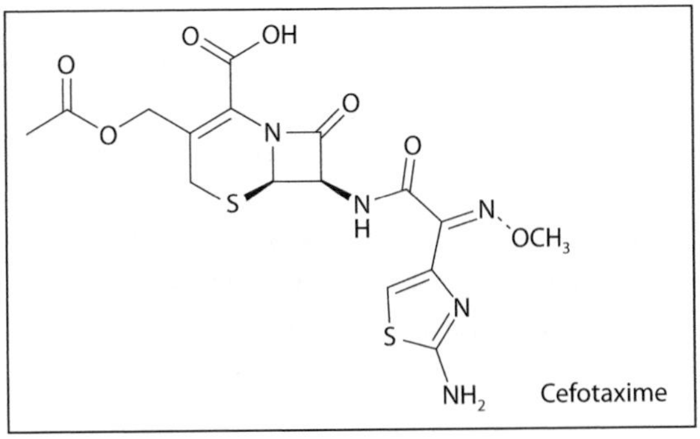

Figure 34.9 Chemical structure of cefotaxime.

Macrolides

These are broad-spectrum drugs, active against Gram-positive bacteria (including some penicillinase-producing strains), *Haemophilus influenzae* (activity greater for azithromycin), Chlamydia, Mycoplasma and *Legionella* species. Examples are erythromycin (Figure 34.10), clarithromycin and azithromycin (long half-life).

- Considered in penicillin-hypersensitive patients
- Side-effects: gastric pain, nausea and vomiting which are less prominent with clarithromycin and azithromycin
- Cautions: hepatic and renal impairment, predisposition to QT interval prolongation

Chemical structure

Macrolides have a large lactone (cyclic ester) ring. The structure for erythromycin is shown in Figure 34.10. Clarithromycin (Figure 34.11) has enhanced lipophilicity and a methyl ether introduced on the C-6 hydroxyl group,

In azithromycin, an azalide antibiotic, an *N*-methyl group is included and the carbonyl moiety is removed.

The chemical amendments of clarithromycin and azithromycin result in inhibition of the formation of the cyclic internal ketal responsible for the gastro-intestinal cramps that are associated with erythromycin.

Telithromycin

This is a ketolide, a derivative of erythromycin. It has a spectrum similar to that of macrolides. It should be used only to treat beta-haemolytic streptococcal pharyngitis and tonsillitis, sinusitis and community-acquired pneumonia when conventional treatment is contraindicated.

- Disadvantages: may precipitate hepatic disorders, visual disturbances or transient loss of consciousness.

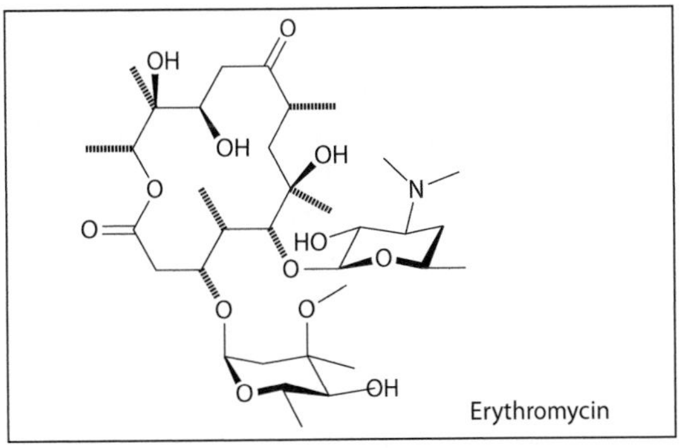

Figure 34.10 Chemical structure of erythromycin.

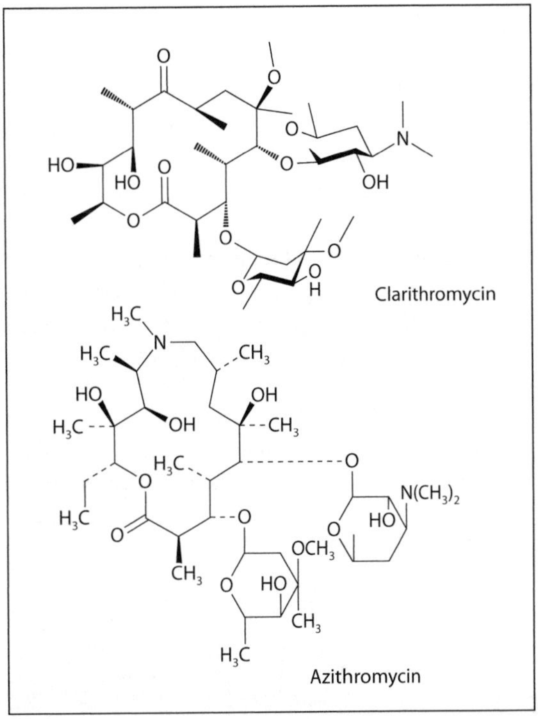

Figure 34.11 Chemical structure of clarithromycin and azithromycin.

Tetracyclines

These include tetracycline (Figure 34.12), doxycycline (long half-life) and minocycline (has a broader spectrum and is active against *Neisseria meningitidis*). They are broad-spectrum antibiotics that are active also against *Chlamydia*, *Rickettsia*, *Mycoplasma* and *Brucella* species.

- Widely distributed after administration
- Use in acne treatment as systemic or topical treatment
- Absorption affected by concomitant use of antacids and milk (except for minocycline)
- Contraindications in children, pregnancy: they bind to calcium in bones and teeth causing impaired bone growth and dental discoloration during active mineralisation
- Cautions: myasthenia gravis, systemic lupus erythematosus, hepatic failure
- Contraindications: renal disease (except doxycycline and minocycline)
- Chemical structure: partially reduced naphthacene ring system, amphoteric substances.

Quinolones

Nalidixic acid (Figure 34.13) was the first quinolone developed. It is used for uncomplicated urinary tract infection. Fluoroquinolones are broad-spectrum products that are active against Gram-positive and Gram-negative bacteria, particularly against Gram-negative bacteria such as *Pseudomonas*, *Neisseria* and *Shigella* species. Examples are ciprofloxacin (Figure 34.14), levofloxacin and moxifloxacin (have greater activity against pneumococci than ciprofloxacin).

- Good tissue distribution
- Block GABA neurotransmitter causing a lowering of the seizure threshold and confusion
- Caution in children, pregnancy: arthropathy in weight-bearing joints; epilepsy, myasthenia gravis, renal and hepatic impairment
- Care: photosensitivity may occur, convulsions may be a side-effect and risk is greater in patients taking NSAIDs, risk of crystalluria (ensure adequate fluid intake), risk of tendon damage (including rupture) increased in elderly patients or those receiving corticosteroids
- Side-effects: nausea, vomiting, dyspepsia, abdominal pain, diarrhoea, headache, dizziness, sleep disorders, rash and pruritus.

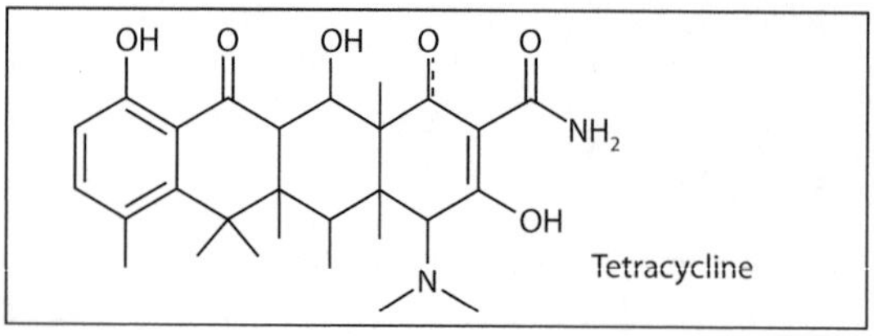

Sulphonamides and trimethoprim

- Co-trimoxazole has synergistic activity between sulfamethoxazole and trimethoprim
- Broad-spectrum of activity
- Good tissue distribution
- Use decreased due to side-effects: blood dyscrasias (bone marrow suppression and agranulocytosis), erythema multiforme (including Stevens–Johnson syndrome), renal failure due to sulphonamide
- Cautions: hepatic and renal impairment, may cause crystalluria (adequate fluid intake recommended), existing haematological conditions, elderly patients

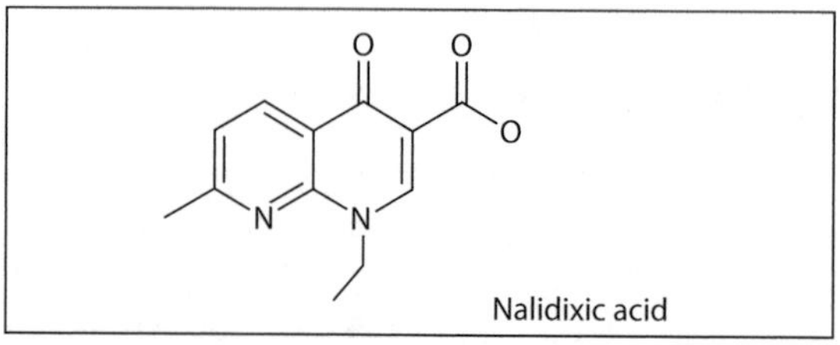

Tetracycline

Figure 34.12 Chemical structure of tetracycline.

Nalidixic acid

Figure 34.13 Chemical structure of nalidixic acid.

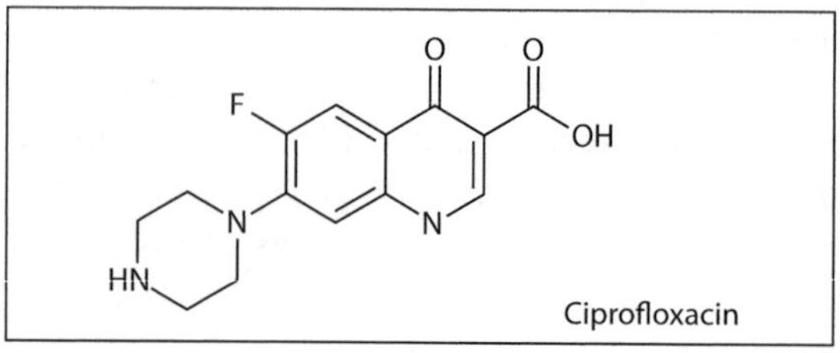

Ciprofloxacin

Figure 34.14 Chemical structure of ciprofloxacin.

- Pregnancy: trimethoprim may be teratogenic, sulphonamides may cause neonatal haemolysis
- Drug interactions: warfarin (enhanced anticoagulant effect), methotrexate (increased risk of haematological toxicity), clozapine (increased risk of agranulocytosis)

Aminoglycosides

Aminoglycosides such as gentamicin, neomycin and tobramycin are active against Gram-negative organisms, including *Pseudomonas* spp., with some activity against staphylococci. Tobramycin is two to four times more active against *Pseudomonas* spp., than gentamicin.

- They are not absorbed from gut and parenteral administration is required for systemic effect; available for topical administration (eye/ear drops, creams/ointment)
- Poor penetration into the cerebrospinal fluid
- Major side-effects that are concentration related are ototoxicity and nephrotoxicity due to tubular destruction
- Narrow therapeutic index. Serum drug concentration monitoring recommended in paediatrics, older persons and patients with renal disease
- Caution: renal impairment
- Contraindication: myasthenia gravis
- Pregnancy: they cross the placenta and may damage the fetus.

Chloramphenicol

- Broad-spectrum activity
- Reserved for life-threatening infections due to toxicity
- Side-effects when administered systemically: blood disorders, peripheral neuritis, optic neuritis.

Clindamycin

- Active against Gram-positive cocci and anaerobes, especially *Bacteroides fragilis*.
- Used for acne, and staphylococcal joint and bone infections such as osteomyelitis.
- Serious side-effect that may occur: pseudomembranous colitis (antibiotic-associated colitis) especially in middle-aged and elderly women; patient should be advised to discontinue treatment if diarrhoea occurs.

Fusidic acid

- Narrow spectrum; used in infections caused by penicillin-resistant staphylococci
- Available for oral, parenteral and topical administration.

Mupirocin

- Effective for skin infections, particularly those due to Gram-positive bacteria
- Available for topical administration only.

Glycopeptide antibiotics

Glycopeptide antibiotics such as vancomycin and teicoplanin have bactericidal activity against aerobic and anaerobic Gram-positive bacteria, especially meticillin-resistant *Staphylococcus aureus* (MRSA).

- Vancomycin: administered intravenously, caution since a rapid intravenous administration may cause histamine release resulting in red man syndrome (fever, chills, rash and hypotension)
- Excreted by the kidney, may cause nephrotoxicity, monitoring of serum drug concentration required in patients with renal disease.

Antituberculous drugs

These include rifampicin, isoniazid, streptomycin, pyrazinamide and ethambutol. Treatment of tuberculosis should be undertaken within a specialised team due to occurrence of resistance and the involvement of other organs outside the respiratory system.

The occurrence of infection caused by resistant strains of *Mycobacterium tuberculosis* is quite common in immunocompromised patients such as HIV-positive patients. Culture to establish the type of strain involved and drug sensitivity tests is required.

Antifungals

The azole antifungals (imidazole and triazole antifungal drugs) inhibit fungal cytochrome P450 enzymes responsible for synthesis of ergosterols that are essential for fungal cell membrane. Due to the interaction with the cytochrome P450 enzyme they are associated with possible drug interactions. Other antifungals are the polyene antifungals and terbinafine.

Imidazole antifungals

The imidazole antifungals clotrimazole, ketoconazole and miconazole are used for local treatment of vaginal candidiasis and for dermatophyte infections. Miconazole is available as an oral gel for treatment of oral candidiasis. Ketoconazole (Figure 34.15) is absorbed when administered orally.

- Monitor: signs of liver disorder (anorexia, nausea, vomiting, fatigue, abdominal pain, jaundice or dark urine)
- Advice: to be taken with or after food
- Chemical structure: consist of a five-membered aromatic ring (azole characteristic) that contains two nitrogens, which is attached to a side-chain that contains at least one aromatic ring.

Triazole antifungals

Examples include fluconazole, itraconazole, posiconazole and voriconazole. They are absorbed after oral administration. Fluconazole and itraconazole are used for the management of systemic mycoses (e.g. tinea pedis, tinea corporis, pityriasis versicolor, mucosal and vaginal candidiasis). Posiconazole and voriconazole are used in life-threatening infections.

- Itraconazole (Figure 34.16): caution when used in patients at high risk of heart failure, monitor for liver toxicity; to be taken with food.

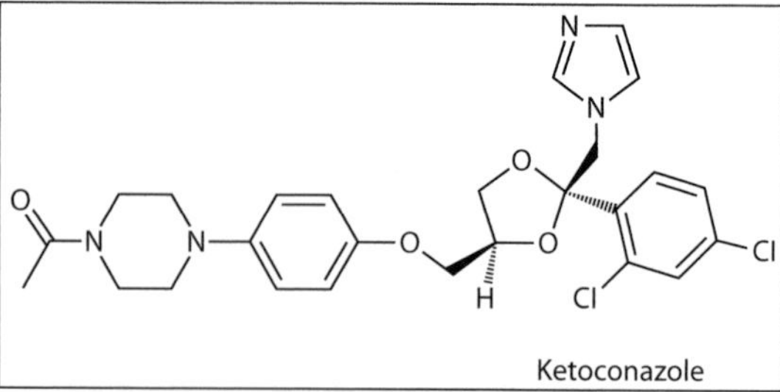

Figure 34.15 Chemical structure of ketoconazole.

- Chemical structure: consist of a five-membered aromatic ring (azole characteristic) that contains three nitrogens, which is attached to a side chain that contains at least one aromatic ring.

Drug interactions

Examples of drug interactions are listed in Table 34.4.

Polyene antifungals

- Amphotericin may be administered intravenously
- Nystatin may be administered orally or topically
- Not absorbed when given by mouth but produce a topical effect in the gastrointestinal tract.

Terbinafine

- Used for dermatophyte infections of the nail, tinea pedis and tinea corporis
- Available for oral and topical treatment.

Antiviral agents

Antiviral agents are required for the management of:

- HIV infection (see Chapter 35)
- herpes virus infections
- viral hepatitis (see Chapter 36)
- influenza (see Chapter 54).

Herpes virus infections

Aciclovir and famciclovir are effective against the virus but do not eradicate it. They interfere with viral

Itraconazole

Figure 34.16 Chemical structure of itraconazole.

Table 34.4 Examples of drug interactions with azole antifungals

Triazoles:	
Warfarin	Enhanced anticoagulant effect
Clarithromycin	Plasma concentration of itraconazole increased
Celecoxib	Plasma concentration of celecoxib increased with fluconazole
Statins	Increased risk of myopathy when given with atorvastatin or simvastatin
Imidazoles:	
Warfarin	Enhanced anticoagulant effect
Antidiabetics	Miconazole increases plasma concentration of sulphonylureas
Statins	Increased risk of myopathy when given with atorvastatin or simvastatin

nucleic acid replication. Aciclovir (Figure 34.17) is a synthetic analogue of deoxyguanosine. Famciclovir (Figure 34.18) is a synthetic purine nucleoside analogue related to guanine and has a longer half-life than aciclovir.

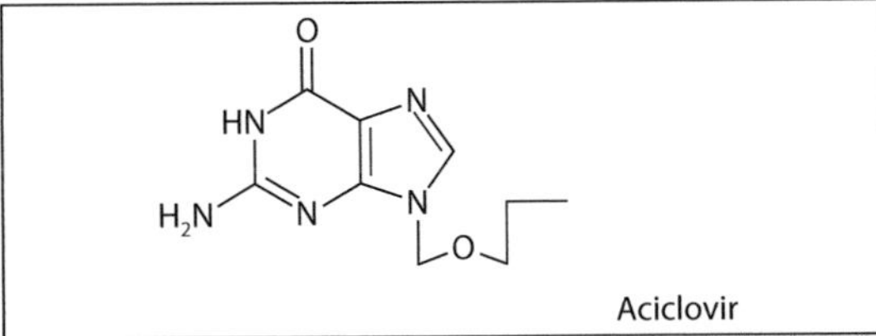

Figure 34.17 Chemical structure of aciclovir.

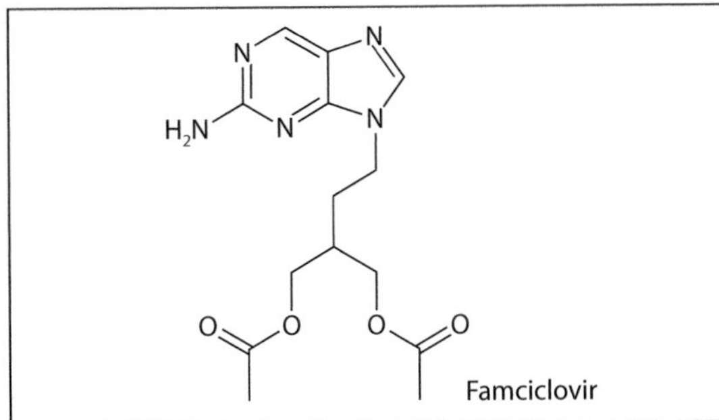

Figure 34.18 Chemical structure of famciclovir.

- Used early in the occurrence of infection
- Used for generalised or systemic infection, skin and mucous membrane infections.

Antiprotozoal agents

These include metronidazole.

- Side-effects: mild headache, gastrointestinal disturbances
- Adverse reaction with alcohol may occur – advise patient to refrain from alcohol consumption during treatment.

Anthelmintic drugs

An example is mebendazole.

- Available for oral administration but a topical effect in the gastrointestinal tract is achieved
- Advantage: it is specific to helminth tissue
- Side-effects: may cause gastrointestinal disturbance.

Anti-infective agents in surgery

These are used to decrease risk of wound infection, infection in implanted material and occurrence of endocarditis in patients with damaged or prosthetic heart valves.

- Risk factors for infection: type of surgery (e.g. abdominal surgery increases risk), occurrence of bacterial contamination during surgery, post-operative wound exposure, patient characteristics – age, obesity, cigarette smoking, malnutrition, comorbidities (e.g. diabetes), concomitant drug therapy (e.g. immunosuppressive therapy).
- Anti-infectives are started before surgery since it is important to have antibacterial drug blood levels at the time of wound incision. Depending on the duration of the surgery and the antibacterial agent used, administration of the antibacterial during the intervention may need to be considered to maintain adequate antibacterial drug concentrations. Doses are continued for a few days after the intervention.
- Route of administration: parenteral administration in the preoperative stage is preferred to ensure required drug blood levels; oral administration may be considered in the post-operative phase once the patient is in a position to take drugs orally.
- Drugs considered: cefuroxime, metronidazole.

Signs of infection

- Monitoring for signs of infection at incision site should be carried out
- Signs of infection: red, inflamed, purulent.

Clean surgical procedures such as cardiac interventions, vascular, orthopaedic and neurosurgery are associated with a lower risk of surgical wound infection than interventions such as gastrointestinal surgery, caesarean section, hysterectomy.

Practice summary

- Factors to be considered in the choice of anti-infective agents include spectrum of activity, possibility of adverse events and pharmaceutical dosage forms.
- Avoid using anti-infective agents unnecessarily or for prolonged periods.
- Healthcare professionals should collaborate to establish treatment protocols for the use of anti-infective agents
- Consider therapeutic drug monitoring where necessary (e.g. aminoglycosides).
- The possibility of drug interactions with azole antifungals should be assessed when other drugs are being used concomitantly.

Questions

1. What side-effects could be expected when an antibacterial drug is administered?
2. What type of antibacterial agent is gentamicin? What is a disadvantage in the administration of gentamicin when used for a systemic effect? What side-effects could occur with the use of gentamicin?
3. Explain the term beta-lactam-containing antibiotics. What are the clinical implications of occurrence of beta-lactamases?
4. Describe spectrum of activity of macrolides.

Answers

1. Hypersensitivity reactions, direct toxicity, superinfections.
2. Gentamicin is classified as an aminoglycoside. The main disadvantage of gentamicin when used for a systemic effect is that it is not absorbed from the gastrointestinal tract and therefore cannot be given orally so the parenteral route is required. Side-effects of gentamicin include ototoxicity and nephrotoxicity.

3 Beta-lactam antibacterials (penicillins and cephalosporins) contain the beta-lactam ring as the basis of their structure. Bacteria that produce beta-lactamases will disrupt the beta-lactam ring and render the antibacterial inactive. For antibacterials to be effective they need to be resistant to beta-lactamase-producing strains of bacteria (e.g. the clavulanic acid component in co-amoxiclav).

4 The macrolide antibacterials have an antibacterial spectrum that is similar but not identical to that of penicillins. They are active against Gram-positive bacteria (including some penicillinase-producing strains), *Chlamydia* and *Mycoplasma* spp.

Further reading

Schwartzberg E (2006). Cost-effective use of antibiotics in hospitals. *Hosp Pharm Eur* May/June: 13–15.

35

Human immunodeficiency virus infection

Learning objectives:

- To appreciate the impact of antiretroviral agents in HIV
- To develop skills to prepare individualised patient therapy and to monitor patients receiving treatment
- To identify risks associated with antiretroviral agents.

Background

Current antiretroviral regimens for human immunodeficiency virus (HIV):

- are complex
- cause several side-effects
- create difficulties in achieving patient adherence to treatment.

Objectives of treatment in HIV

The objectives are to:

- achieve maximal and durable suppression of HIV replication by reducing viral load to <50 copies/ mL
- restore immunological function
- improve patient quality of life
- reduce HIV-related morbidity and mortality
- reduce the progression from HIV infection to AIDS and death.

Patient individualised therapy

- Assess capability of patient to cope with tablet burden and dosing frequency especially if patient is also receiving other drug therapy
- Which side-effects and drug interactions need to be avoided?
- Patient condition: if patient is asymptomatic, to achieve better patient compliance, the least complex regimen is preferred. Consider concomitant disease (e.g. protease inhibitors should be avoided in patients with cardiovascular disease or hepatitis B or C)
- Identify viral sensitivity, prevent the development of resistance and preserve future treatment options.

The factors to be considered in choosing HIV treatment are outlined in Figure 35.1.

Highly active antiretroviral therapy (HAART)

This has improved the prognosis of HIV-infection therapy by controlling HIV replication, but it does

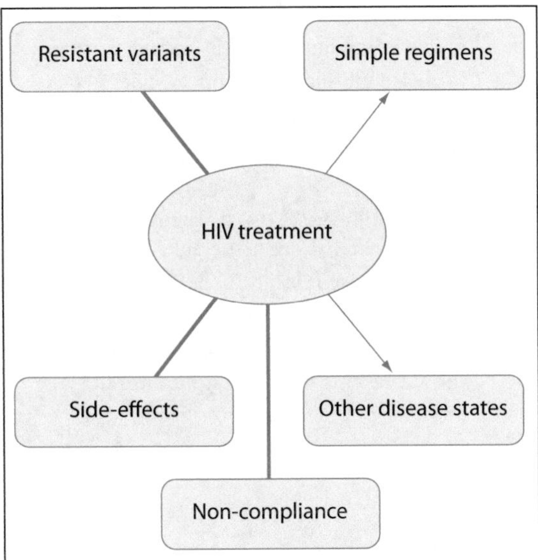

Figure 35.1 Factors to be considered in choosing HIV treatment.

not eradicate the infection and therefore life-long therapy is required.

- Issues: cumulative toxicity, emergence of HIV drug resistance
- Treatment to be started in all symptomatic patients and in asymptomatic patients depending on CD4 lymphocyte cell count, so that therapy is started before the immune system is irreversibly damaged. (Decline in CD4 lymphocyte count leads to the development of AIDS)
- In 1994–1995: dual treatment commenced
- In 1996: triple therapy confirmed
- In 2006: four-drug regimen – has not shown significant different plasma HIV levels.

> 'The message now is that if you want to start treatment, then two drugs are better than one. We still do not know when it is best to start treatment but our data show that if a patient already has AIDS it is not too late to treat.'
>
> Dr Tim Peto, Consultant in Infectious Diseases, Oxford (*Pharm J* 1995; 255: 411)

Triple antiviral therapy in HIV

- Two nucleoside reverse transcriptase inhibitors + one protease inhibitor

or

- Two nucleoside reverse transcriptase inhibitors + one non-nucleoside reverse transcriptase inhibitor

Therapy should be changed with treatment failure or due to intolerance or toxicity.

Antiviral agents and HIV

Nucleoside reverse transcriptase inhibitors

Nucleoside reverse transcriptase inhibitors such as abacavir, didanosine, emtricitabine, lamivudine, stavudine, tenofovir and zidovudine should be used with caution in patients with chronic hepatitis B or C due to increased risk of hepatic side-effects. This is very relevant since patients with HIV may present with concomitant hepatitis B or C.

- Caution: hepatic impairment, particularly obese women with hepatomegaly, patients with alcohol abuse, renal impairment, pregnancy
- Side-effects: gastrointestinal disturbances, anorexia as well as peripheral neuropathy, pancreatitis, lactic acidosis or lactic steatosis. Lactic acidosis is due to mitochondrial toxicity and is presented with gastrointestinal symptoms and dyspnoea; if it occurs, treatment should be withdrawn.

Protease inhibitors

Examples include amprenavir, atazanavir, indinavir, lopinavir, ritonavir, saquinavir and tipranavir. Ritonavir is used in low doses to boost the plasma concentrations of other protease inhibitors.

- Caution: hyperglycaemia and diabetes due to lipodystrophy syndrome, haemophilia due to increased risk of bleeding, hepatic impairment and patients with chronic hepatitis B or C, pregnancy

- Renal impairment: atazanavir, darunavir, fosamprenavir and tipranavir do not require dose adjustments as required with other protease inhibitors
- Contraindications: porphyria, breast-feeding
- Side-effects: gastrointestinal disturbances, anorexia, hepatic dysfunction, pancreatitis, lipodystrophy syndrome and metabolic effects
- Patient monitoring: since these drugs affect glucose metabolism, lipid profile and blood glucose monitoring are required in patients with diabetes and hyperlipidaemia
- Patient advice: patient should be advised on necessary dietary modifications. Risk of myocardial infarction increases by 26% for each year of exposure
- Statin therapy should be considered in patients receiving protease inhibitors.

Non-nucleoside reverse transcriptase inhibitors

Non-nucleoside reverse transcriptase inhibitors such as efavirenz and nevirapine show better patient acceptability than the nucleoside reverse transcriptase inhibitors and protease inhibitors.

- Side-effect that is common to both drugs is skin rash
- Hepatoxicity with nevirapine which may be fatal may occur. This warrants monitoring of liver function in patients receiving nevirapine especially since they are likely also to be receiving a nucleoside reverse transcriptase inhibitor
- Neuropsychological effects and increased plasma cholesterol concentration may occur with efavirenz.

- Lipodystrophy syndrome is used to describe side-effects associated with antiretroviral therapy which include fat redistribution, insulin resistance and dyslipidaemia. Fat redistribution presents with development of a buffalo hump and breast enlargement and is associated with protease inhibitors and nucleoside reverse transcriptase inhibitors. Stavudine and zidovudine are associated with a higher risk.
- Dyslipidaemia, insulin resistance and hyperglycaemia are associated particularly with protease inhibitors. Before initiating therapy with protease inhibitors baseline levels of plasma lipids and blood glucose should be carried out and monitored thereafter.

When to start?

- Before becoming ill
- Not too early: to avoid patient getting side-effects and to decrease occurrence of drug resistance
- Criteria: symptomatic or CD4 cell count <200.

Viral sensitivity and resistance

- Resistance is decreased by using combination therapy.
- Drug resistance can occur with treatment when viral suppression is not optimal.
- Viral genotyping and phenotyping may be carried out to evaluate mutations in the virus and the ability of the virus to grow in the presence of antiretroviral agents respectively.
- Patient may present with a resistant strain prior to initiation of treatment and therefore it is recommended to identify viral sensitivity before starting therapy.
- Occurrence of viral resistance should be considered when starting or changing therapy. When changing treatment due to therapy failure, the new regimen should contain antiretroviral agents that were not used previously in the patient.

Patient compliance

HAART is effective if patient knows how to take medications and adhers to therapy.

Causes of non-compliance in HIV patients

- Patient may be asymptomatic and feel that drug therapy is not necessary.
- Social factors: patient education, personality
- Stigma
- Multiple therapy makes drug regimen complex and difficult for the patient to follow
- Lack of information on drugs and how to take them
- Side-effects.

Improving compliance in HIV patients

- Labelling: large (font size), clean (printed), simple
- Packaging: while maintaining stability, prepare drugs in compliance aids to help patient recognise when to take drug therapy
- Pharmacist intervention during dispensing: provide patient knowledge and education, use pictograms during dispensing (e.g. to identify drugs that need to be taken with food, such as atazanavir)
- Improve patient–pharmacist–doctor rapport.

Pregnancy

- Treatment is considered to minimise viral load and disease progression in the mother and to prevent transmission of infection to the neonate
- However, teratogenic potential is unknown and usually institutions select drug therapy on the basis of previous shared experience.

Breast-feeding

- Risk that infant develops HIV infection is about 10%
- Avoidance of breast-feeding is recommended when breast milk substitutes are feasible and affordable to the mother.

Patients with HIV are at an increased risk of developing other conditions, particularly infective conditions caused by bacteria, fungi and mycobacteria. These conditions can prove difficult to treat and fatal. Also, they are susceptible to neoplastic disease such as lymphoma and Kaposi's sarcoma.

Practice summary

- Evaluate CD4 cell count, viral load and viral resistance.
- Assess clinical signs and symptoms.
- Monitor for co-infections (hepatitis, tuberculosis) and other medical conditions.
- Treatment requires combination therapy.
- Assess adherence to therapy.
- Monitor for occurrence of toxicity of medications: gastrointestinal side-effects are common to all classes of antiretroviral drugs and their occurrence may impact negatively on patient's quality of life and on patient compliance.
- Patients with HIV should receive advice on the use of barrier methods of contraception to reduce risk of transmission of HIV. Women should be informed of the interactions with oral contraceptives (e.g. contraceptive effect reduced with efavirenz, metabolism of oestrogens accelerated by ritonavir).

Question

1 Compare stavudine and atazanavir.

Answer

1 Stavudine is a nucleoside reverse transcriptase inhibitor indicated in HIV infection in combination with other antiretroviral drugs. Atazanavir is a protease inhibitor used in HIV infection in combination with other

antiretroviral drugs. Side-effects of stavudine include peripheral neuropathy, pancreatitis, lactic acidosis or lactic steatosis. If lactic acidosis presents with gastrointestinal symptoms and dyspnoea, treatment should be withdrawn. Atazanavir causes gastrointestinal disturbances as the main side-effect. It also affects glucose metabolism and lipid profile and therefore monitoring is required in patients with diabetes and hyperlipidaemia.

Further reading

Beck E J (2003). HIV costs: individual and population perspectives. *Hosp Pharm Eur* April/May: 48–50.

Cohen C J (2006). Successful HIV treatment: lessons learned. *J Manag Care Pharm* 12(7): S6–S11.

Gellaitry G, Cooper V, Davis C, Fisher M, Leake Date H and Horne R (2005). Patients' perception of information about HAART: impact on treatment decisions. *AIDS Care* 17: 367–376.

Hammer S M, Saag M S, Schechter M, Montaner J S G, Schooley R T, Jacobsen D M *et al.* (2006). Treatment for adult HIV infection: 2006 recommendations of the International AIDS Society – USA Panel. *JAMA* 296: 827–843.

Zabinski R A (2006). Evidence-based health benefits management: Strategies to optimize antiretroviral medication adherence and outcomes in HIV/AIDS. *J Manag Care Pharm* 12(7): S12–S16.

36

Viral hepatitis

Learning objectives:

- To identify characteristics of different hepatitis infections
- To review management of chronic hepatitis.

Background

Five human hepatitis viruses have been identified (A–G):

- Hepatitis A–E affect the liver and may lead to liver damage including hepatocellular necrosis.
- Mode of transmission is primarily by the faecal–oral route (including food borne) for hepatitis A and E and is blood borne for hepatitis B, C and D.
- Prophylaxis is available for hepatitis A and B (see Chapter 61).
- Hepatitis may occur as an acute condition where jaundice or increased serum aminotransferase concentrations occur and the condition is limited to a few months not exceeding 6 months.
- Chronic hepatitis involves hepatocellular necrosis for 6 months or more after the onset of acute illness. Chronic hepatitis is mostly associated with hepatitis B and C.

Hepatitis A

Hepatitis A is transmitted mainly via faecal-contaminated water or food (e.g. shellfish). Its occurrence in different countries is highly related to the levels of sanitation and quality of water supply. The incubation period is 14–45 days.

- Prophylaxis: hepatitis A vaccination presents an active form of immunisation. It should be considered for travellers to high-risk countries, homosexuals, intravenous drug users, people at occupational risk, people with clotting disorders and patients with chronic liver disease.

Clinical signs and symptoms

- Twenty-five per cent of patients are asymptomatic.
- Characteristic symptoms include malaise, fatigue, anorexia, abdominal pain, nausea and vomiting. Sometimes patients present with fever, headache, arthralgias, myalgias and diarrhoea.
- About 66% of patients develop jaundice during the acute attack.
- Diagnosis is based on serological detection of the viral antigen and antibody as well as elevated liver enzymes.

Treatment

- Supportive therapy; patient should be advised to avoid exhaustion

- Ensure rehydration due to nausea and vomiting
- Refrain from alcohol consumption
- Use drugs that are hepatically eliminated with caution; try to switch drug therapy or where not possible use lowest recommended dose.

Hepatitis B

This condition is transmitted via contaminated blood or blood products and sexual contact. Persons at risk of developing the condition are those who engage in different heterosexual contacts, homosexuals, injecting drug abusers, those who undergo acupuncture and tattooing, and people who have an occupational risk.

Education on sexual behaviour, needle handling and use of blood products is a key factor in prophylaxis. Vaccination should be recommended to individuals at high risk of contamination, namely healthcare workers, staff at nursing institutions, recipients of blood products, haemodialysis patients, drug abusers, homosexuals and inmates of long-term correctional facilities. In addition most countries currently require vaccination for all infants.

Clinical signs and symptoms

In acute infection symptoms are very similar to hepatitis A infection and include fatigue, anorexia, nausea and vomiting. Acute liver failure may occur and this presents with hepatic encephalopathy, lethargy, confusion and cerebral oedema, and may ultimately lead to coma.

Chronic infection occurs in 5–10% of patients and leads to cirrhosis and liver failure. Hepatocellular carcinoma may develop.

Diagnosis is based on serological detection of antigen and antibody. In chronic disease, monitoring of liver function tests and liver biopsy are indicated.

Treatment

- During the acute phase, supportive therapy and patient monitoring for the development of complications are recommended.
- Liver transplantation may need to be considered in patients with chronic disease.
- Treatment in chronic hepatitis is discussed as a separate section.

> In hepatitis A and B supportive therapy is the mainstay of treatment during the acute phase.

Hepatitis C

Hepatitis C has greater infectivity than the HIV virus. It is commonly transmitted due to intravenous drug abuse and sharing of needles as well as due to sexual activity.

Clinical signs and symptoms

- Acute infection is mostly asymptomatic.
- Chronic infection occurs in about 85% and patients present with fatigue, nausea, anorexia, abdominal pain and depression.
- Patients with the chronic condition may develop intractable ascites, gastrointestinal or oesophageal bleeding, and encephalopathy. In addition, extrahepatic symptoms such as corneal ulcers, idiopathic pulmonary fibrosis and rheumatoid arthritis may occur.
- Between 20% and 30% of patients progress to end-stage liver disease and a smaller percentage develop hepatocellular carcinoma.
- The genotype of the infecting hepatitis C virus should be determined since treatment outcome depends on genotype.
- Diagnosis is based on detection of antibodies and a liver biopsy may be undertaken to estimate the extent of liver injury. In chronic disease, monitoring of liver function tests and viral load is required.

Treatment of chronic hepatitis

In chronic hepatitis B, patients may be asymptomatic and present with minor elevations in liver enzymes. In this scenario treatment is not started and the patient is monitored every 3–6 months. Once patients are symptomatic, treatment should be initiated to decrease viral replication, limit hepatocellular damage and decrease the risk of long-term negative impact on liver function.

In chronic hepatitis C patients, the aims of treatment are to eradicate the virus, decrease morbidity by improving clinical symptoms, decrease mortality, and prevent progression to cirrhosis, hepatocellular carcinoma and end-stage liver disease. A combination of interferon and ribavirin is usually recommended. Ribavirin as monotherapy is not effective.

In some chronic hepatitis patients there is limited response to treatment and relapse after treatment withdrawal is frequent. Pharmacoeconomic implications of chronic hepatitis are the high cost of therapy and the costs incurred in managing the long-term sequelae in addition to lost patient years.

Interferon

- Interferons are used in the management of chronic hepatitis.
- Peginterferon alfa, with the addition of a polyethylene glycol molecule, is preferred over interferon alfa because it has a longer half-life and thus requires a lower weekly dosing frequency. A disadvantage of pegylated interferons is that the occurrence of cytopenias and injection site reactions is higher than with interferon.
- Sustained action reduces the incidence of viral replication and leads to prolonged virological response.
- Caution: patients who are receiving immunosuppressant therapy.
- Side-effects commonly include anorexia, nausea, influenza-like symptoms (fever, chills, myalgias, fatigue), lethargy. These tend to decrease in occurrence with repeated drug administration.
- Patient monitoring is required to monitor for the development of late-onset side-effects, namely bone marrow suppression, alopecia, thyroid disorders, hyperglycaemia and hypertriglyceridaemia.

Chronic hepatitis B

Drugs used in the treatment of chronic hepatitis B include:

- lamivudine*
- adefovir, dipivoxil and entecavir (used in lamivudine resistance)
- telbivudine (should not be used in patients who present with resistance to lamivudine due to possibility of cross-resistance)
- tenofovir* (used as part of HAART in patients who require treatment for HIV and hepatitis).

*These are antiviral agents used in HIV (see Chapter 35).

Chronic hepatitis C

In treating chronic hepatitis C the aim is to achieve clearance of virus sustained for at least 6 months after treatment is stopped. Peginterferon is used in combination with ribavirin (antiviral agent).

Practice summary

- Education on prophylaxis of hepatitis is necessary to prevent spread of infection.
- The acute phase of the conditions may be asymptomatic.
- There are concerns about the development of chronic hepatitis with hepatitis B and C due to long-term sequelae.
- In the treatment of chronic hepatitis due to hepatitis B and C, interferon plays an important role. Interferon may cause worsening of liver function.

Questions

1 What is the relevance of the genotype of the hepatitis C virus in clinical practice?
2 What is the standard measurement of effectiveness of treatment in the management of hepatitis C?

Answers

1. Before starting treatment, the genotype of the infecting hepatitis C virus should be determined and the viral load measured as this may affect the choice and duration of treatment.
2. The viral load is the standard measurement of effectiveness of treatment in the management of hepatitis C. The aim of hepatitis C treatment is to achieve clearance of virus, sustained for at least 6 months after treatment is stopped.

Further reading

Knighton S (2008). Hepatitis C infection: clinical features and diagnosis. *Hosp Pharm* 15: 411–412.

Knighton S (2008). Hepatitis C infection: current and future treatment. *Hosp Pharm* 15: 413–419.

Nickless G (2008). An overview of hepatitis: Part 1. *Pharm J* 280: 411–414.

Nickless G (2008). An overview of hepatitis: Part 2. *Pharm J* 280: 477–480.

Spooner L M (2009). The critical need of pharmacist involvement in the management of patients with hepatitis C. *J Manag Care Pharm* 15: 151–153.

37

Thyroid disorders

Learning objectives:

- To appreciate presentation of hypothyroid and hyperthyroid states
- To develop skills for management of patients with thyroid disorders.

Background

Thyroid gland synthesises, stores and secretes thyroxine (T_4) and triiodothyronine (T_3). Hormone secretion is controlled by thyroid-stimulating hormone (TSH) or thyrotrophin which is released by the anterior pituitary gland, which in turn is triggered by thyroid-releasing hormone (TRH) secreted from the hypothalamus. The process is controlled by negative and positive feedback.

Function of thyroid hormones

Thyroid hormones probably activate mRNA transcription processes and promote protein synthesis or protein catabolism. Their function relates to:

- growth and development
- the cardiovascular system
- the central nervous system
- the musculature
- sleep
- lipid metabolism.

Thyroid function tests

Commonly used thyroid function tests are described in Table 37.1.

Hyperthyroidism

- Associated with the production and secretion of excessive amounts of thyroid hormones
- Females are affected about ten times more than males
- Various aetiology: genetic predisposition is strong.

Clinical manifestations

- Increased metabolism of all body systems due to excess thyroid hormones
- Increased adrenergic activities, especially cardiovascular and neurological systems.

Signs and symptoms

The signs and symptoms of hyperthyroidism are listed in Table 37.2.

Table 37.1 Thyroid function tests

Thyroid function test	Hypothyroidism	Hyperthyroidism
Serum resin triiodothyronine (RT_3U)	Decreased (<35%)	Increased (>45%)
Serum total thyroxine (TT_4)	Decreased (<5 micrograms/dL)	Increased (>12 micrograms/dL)
Serum total triiodothyronine (TT_3)	Decreased (<80 ng/dL)	Increased (>180 g/dL)
Free thyroxine index (FTI)	Decreased (<5.5)	Increased (<10.5)
Serum thyrotrophin (TSH)	Increased (>6 microunits/mL)	Decreased (<0.5 microunits/mL)

Table 37.2 Signs and symptoms of hyperthyroidism

Skin and appendages	Skin problems associated with increased sweat production and heat intolerance Thinning or loss of hair Bulging eyes and lid retraction Increased sweating Heat intolerance
Nervous system	Anxiety, irritability, lack of sleep and excitation
Musculoskeletal	Osteoporosis Muscle weakness Tremor
Gastrointestinal	Weight loss with increased appetite Frequent bowel movements
Cardiovascular	Palpitations, tachycardia Shortness of breath on exertion Angina
Other	Amenorrhoea

Management of hyperthyroidism

- Antithyroid drugs
- Surgery – partial thyroidectomy
- Radioactive iodine.

Factors influencing choice of treatment

- Large goitre causing obstruction; in this case surgery is preferred
- Severe heart failure where surgery is to be avoided
- Pregnancy and neonates where risk:benefit ratio of the use of antithyroid drugs has to be considered
- Previous iodine exposure may limit repeat of radioactive iodine therapy
- Poor compliance with oral antithyroid drugs might necessitate consideration of surgery or radioactive iodine
- Age (e.g. elderly patients where due to comorbid conditions some of the lines of therapy might not be appropriate).

Carbimazole

- Inhibits synthesis of hormones. A disadvantage is the low incidence of remission after discontinuation of therapy
- Side-effects: rashes, bone marrow suppression (agranulocytosis)
- Patient advice: to report symptoms and signs suggestive of infection especially sore throat
- Monitoring: thyroid function tests, white blood cell count (to be performed if there is evidence of infection), assess improvement in clinical symptoms
- Caution: should be stopped promptly if there is clinical or laboratory evidence of neutropenia
- It crosses the placenta and may cause neonatal hypothyroidism. Decision to use in pregnancy depends on risk:benefit ratio for mother and baby.

Carbimazole

- Initial dose: 15–40 mg daily as a single dose
- T_4 checked every 4 weeks until a maintenance dose between 5 and 15 mg daily is reached

- Once maintenance therapy is achieved, measure T_4 and TSH every 3 months
- Duration of treatment is usually 6–24 months; however some patients require longer periods of treatment, especially those who are not eligible for other treatment modalities.

Beta-blockers

- Provide relief from palpitations, anxiety, sweating, tremor and diarrhoea
- Indicated for short-term use since they do not control underlying condition
- Used prior to surgery or radioactive iodine therapy to reduce heart rate and decrease risk of thyroid storm.

Pharmaceutical care plan in hyperthyroidism

Phase	*Action*
Pre-treatment	Baseline thyroid function tests Baseline white blood count
Initiation of treatment	Patient education: goals, duration of therapy Thyroid function tests every 4 weeks
During treatment	Thyroid function tests Liver function tests Monitor for signs of hyperthyroidism Monitor for signs of neutropenia, request white blood cell count

Counselling points for patients on antithyroid drugs

- Anticipated duration of treatment
- Tapering to maintenance dose
- Explain use of adjuvant therapy (beta-blockers)
- Emphasise importance to report skin rashes, sore throat and mouth ulcers
- Emphasise need for regular review
- Educate on management of relapse.

Surgery

- Preferred when obstructive symptoms due to large goitre are present or where malignancy is suspected.
- Use of beta-blockers and antithyroid drugs prior to surgery to render patient euthyroid. Propranolol is used to achieve pulse of 80 bpm. This approach adopted so as to avoid thyroid storm.
- Outcomes of surgery:
  - recurrent hyperthyroidism: 1–3% of patients, risk decreases with time
  - hypothyroidism: 5–40%, risk increases with time
  - hypoparathyroidism: occurrence may be delayed up to 3 months postoperatively; monitor serum calcium levels to identify its occurrence; intravenous calcium gluconate is used to correct it.

Radioactive iodine

- Easy to administer and effective
- Used in patients where antithyroid drugs cannot be used (e.g. cardiac disease, elderly patients) or where compliance is a problem and in patients who were on carbimazole therapy and suffered a relapse
- Contraindicated in pregnancy and children
- May lead to hypothyroidism
- Withdraw antithyroid drugs 1 week before.

Treatment of complications: eye symptoms

- Eye complications: grittiness, early morning soreness due to protrusion of the eyeball
- Management: use hypromellose eye drops.

Thyroid crisis

- Hyperpyrexia, tachycardia
- Precipitated by infection, stress, surgery.

Example of management during acute thyroid crisis

- Propranolol 5 mg intravenously four times daily or 80 mg orally twice daily
- Carbimazole 20 mg orally three times daily
- Potassium iodide orally 15 mg three times daily
- Dexamethasone 2 mg intravenously four times daily.

Hypothyroidism

The most common cause is a secondary one due to radioactive iodine therapy or surgery for hyperthyroidism. Other causes include congenital disease, hypopituitarism and hypothalamic disorders.

Signs and symptoms of hypothyroidism

- Skin and appendages: dry, cool, flaking skin, faint yellow colour, coarse, brittle hair
- Nervous system: poor memory, somnolence, depression, slow speech
- Muscle: muscle cramps, pain and weakness
- Gastrointestinal: weight gain with decreased appetite, abdominal distension, constipation, loss of taste and smell
- Cardiovascular: reduced cardiac output, bradycardia, cardiac enlargement
- Other: fatigue, sluggishness, dyspnoea, cold intolerance, heavy menstrual periods.

Thyroxine sodium

- Dose taken before breakfast to avoid insomnia and excitability late in the day
- Monitor cardiac function, thyroid function tests, occurrence of clinical symptoms
- Side-effects: too rapid increase in metabolism leading to diarrhoea, vomiting, angina pain, arrhythmias, palpitation, tachycardia, tremor, restlessness, excitability, insomnia.

Hypothyroidism may cause changes in the ECG that mimic cardiac ischaemia. Before initiating therapy, baseline ECG should be taken.

Risks of thyroxine treatment

- Worsening of angina, occurrence of myocardial infarction in patients with a history of angina
- Accelerated rate of bone loss, caution in postmenopausal women; consider use of prophylaxis for osteoporosis.

Thyroxine replacement during pregnancy

- Treatment should be continued during pregnancy.
- Increase in dosage may be required since thyroid hormone requirements are increased.

Drug–disease interaction with thyroxine

- Potentiation of hypoprothrombinaemic effect of warfarin
- In diabetic patients, dose adjustment (increase) of antidiabetic agent may be necessary with initiation of thyroxine.

Hypothyroidism and the elderly patient

- Hypothyroidism is a common endocrine disease in the elderly which can easily go undiagnosed.
- Only 33% of patients exhibit typical signs and symptoms.
- Non-specific symptoms occur such as stumbling, incontinence and falls, which may lead to misdiagnosis such as being mistaken for parkinsonism.
- Correction of hypothyroid state may lead to improvement in lipid profile and a subsequent reduction in cardiac risks. Hypothyroidism may predispose to an adverse lipid profile.
- Use of thyroxine sodium at a starting dose of 25 micrograms and increasing every 3–4 weeks by 25 micrograms.
- Caution: care in compromised coronary artery circulation; thyroxine may unmask underlying cardiac disease.

Pharmaceutical care plan in hypothyroidism

Phase	*Action*
Pre-treatment	Baseline thyroid function tests Baseline ECG
Initiation of treatment	Patient education: goals, duration of therapy Thyroid function tests every 6–8 weeks
During treatment	Thyroid function tests Monitor for signs of hypothyroidism Monitor for signs of toxicity: diarrhoea, tachycardia, tremors, insomnia

Drugs associated with thyroid dysfunction

Amiodarone

- Used in the treatment of arrhythmias
- Contains iodine and may cause thyroid disorders (hypothyroidism or hyperthyroidism)
- See also Chapter 19.

Lithium

- Used in the treatment of bipolar disorder
- It inhibits secretion of T_4 and T_3 and may cause hypothyroidism
- See also Chapter 27.

Patients receiving amiodarone or lithium should have thyroid function tests performed prior to initiation of treatment and every six months.

Practice summary

- Patients with thyroid disorders should be monitored regularly to assess their thyroid state.
- Patients require education on relevance of drug therapy and side-effects to be expected.
- Patients with thyroid disorders who are also receiving warfarin require careful monitoring of their international normalised ratio (INR) since response to warfarin therapy may vary according to thyroid status.

Question

1 Describe a pharmaceutical care plan for a patient newly diagnosed with hyperthyroidism who is started on carbimazole therapy.

Answer

1 (a Identification of patient needs: to educate patient on condition, to advise patient on carbimazole treatment (dosing and tapering of dose, advice to report any signs of infection).

(b) Patient monitoring: parameters to be measured include thyroid function tests and liver function tests; identify any signs of infection and carry out white blood cell count when appropriate.

Further reading

Demirkan K, Stephens M A, Newman K P and Self T H (2000). Response to warfarin and other oral anticoagulants: effects of disease states. *South Med J* 93: 448–455.

MacFarlane I (2000). Thyroid disease. *Pharm J* 265: 240–244.

Rehman S U, Cope D W, Senseney A D and Brzezinski W (2005). Thyroid disorders in elderly patients. *South Med J* 98: 543–549.

Weetman A P (2007). Radioiodine treatment for benign thyroid diseases. *Clin Endocrinol* 66: 757–764.

38

Diabetes mellitus

Learning objectives:

- To describe presentation of diabetes
- To review drug therapy options
- To develop skills to be able to manage drug therapy, provide patient education on drug therapy and manage drug therapy failures
- To describe long-term complications of diabetes
- To appreciate prophylactic therapy in diabetes and patient monitoring.

Background

Diabetes is a heterogeneous group of disorders characterised by varying degrees of insulin hyposecretion and/or insulin insensitivity. It leads to hyperglycaemia.

Classification of diabetes mellitus and allied categories of glucose intolerance

There are two main forms of diabetes:

- insulin-dependent diabetes mellitus *Type 1* or *diabetes:* occurs as a result of insulin hyposecretion due to autoimmune destruction of beta cells in the pancreas.
- non-insulin-dependent diabetes mellitus *Type 2* or *diabetes:* is further subdivided into forms in non-obese and obese patients. It occurs as a result of decreased insulin secretion or due to insulin insensitivity. Despite the nomenclature, some patients may require insulin therapy in due course.

Other related conditions:

- impaired glucose tolerance (IGT)
- gestational diabetes mellitus (GDM)
- malnutrition-related diabetes mellitus (MRDM).

Other types of diabetes are associated with certain conditions and syndromes including pancreatic disease, diseases of hormonal aetiology, and drug-induced and genetic syndromes.

Clinical manifestations

- Polyuria and polydipsia as a consequence of osmotic diuresis secondary to sustained hyperglycaemia
- Blurred vision due to change in refraction as a result of hyperosmolar state
- Weight loss despite normal or increased appetite.

Type 1 diabetes mellitus

- Genetic features are important but do not explain fully the development of the disease.

- A strong immunological component is suspected as a final event which precipitates onset of clinical diabetes (e.g. an infection).
- The condition is characterised by acute onset of signs and symptoms.

Clinical manifestations of IDDM

- Dehydration, anorexia, nausea and vomiting
- If diagnosis is not made when common manifestations of hyperglycaemia occur, diabetic ketoacidosis may occur
- A significant elevation in glycated haemoglobin confirms long-standing hyperglycaemia.

Type 2 diabetes mellitus

- Stronger genetic relationship than with type 1 diabetes
- Obesity associated with hyperinsulinaemia and marked insulin insensitivity and a decrease in number of insulin receptors
- Insidious onset of hyperglycaemia
- Patients, especially obese patients, may have few or none of the classic symptoms
- Commonly presents with chronic skin infections, general pruritus and vaginitis in females.

Investigations

- Fasting blood glucose level greater than 6.7 mmol/L or a random value of more than 10 mmol/L
- Glucose tolerance test: in clinical practice used only in patients who have borderline results
- Urine testing not suitable due to the wide inter-individual variation in renal threshold
- See also Chapter 11.

Risk factors

- Family history
- Obesity
- Age: 45 years and older
- Impaired fasting glucose
- Hypertension
- Hyperlipidaemia
- Gestational diabetes.

Metabolic syndrome

This is a cluster of metabolic abnormalities including insulin resistance, hyperglycaemia, hypertension, reduced high-density lipoprotein-cholesterol levels and increased triglyceride levels.

Risk factors

- Genetic factors
- Obesity
- Physical inactivity
- High carbohydrate diet.

Aims of treatment in diabetes

- Relieve immediate signs and symptoms of diabetes
- Prevent the development or slow the progression of the long-term complications namely:
  - nephropathy
  - retinopathy
  - increased risk of open-angle glaucoma, cataracts
  - neuropathy
  - myocardial infarction
  - peripheral vascular disease
  - cerebrovascular events
  - skin infections: foot problems.

Management

1. Carbohydrate and total calorie restriction, increased fibre intake, decreased fat intake and increased physical activity to cause weight loss and produce normoglycaemia.
2. In patients with type 2 diabetes oral hypoglycaemic agents may be required. Some patients with type 2 diabetes will eventually require insulin therapy.
3. All patients with type 1 diabetes require a diet

containing controlled amounts of carbohydrate and insulin therapy.

In obese type 2 diabetic patients, where achieving weight reduction through diet and physical exercise is not successful, the use of weight-reducing products such as orlistat and sibutramine may be considered.

Sulphonylureas

- Sulphonylureas increase insulin secretion.
- They may be used in combination therapy with other antidiabetic agents.
- Glibenclamide has a shorter elimination half-life than first-generation drugs (e.g. chlorpropamide) but shows a prolonged biological effect possibly due to slower distribution. Consequently glibenclamide is associated with occurrence of hypoglycaemia more than the shorter-acting drugs such as gliclazide, which are preferred especially in the older patients.
- Caution: obese patients since they encourage weight gain, the elderly, hepatic and renal impairment.
- Contraindications: severe hepatic and renal impairment, pregnancy, breast-feeding.
- Gliclazide modified-release tablets taken at breakfast, between one and four tablets a day. Modified-release tablets 30 mg should achieve better glucose control than conventional formulation.
- Side-effects:
  - hypoglycaemia: most common, may be severe; risk factors include reduced food intake, weight loss
  - gastrointestinal: affects 2%; may induce nausea and vomiting; advise patient to take medication with or after food
  - dermatological: affects 1–3%; usually occurs within first 2–6 weeks of therapy and includes photosensitivity and pruritus.

Factors influencing choice of sulphonylurea

There is little or no difference in clinical efficacy between the different agents. The choice usually lies on three factors:

- duration of action
- cost
- prescriber's experience and personal preference.

Biguanides: metformin

- Metformin decreases gluconeogenesis and increases peripheral utilisation of glucose.
- It is used when strict dieting and sulphonylurea treatment have failed to control diabetes. May be used in combination with other antidiabetic agents.
- Compared with sulphonylureas, it is associated with a lower incidence of weight gain and therefore is the drug of choice in obese type 2 diabetic patients.
- Hypoglycaemia is not usually a problem.
- Side-effects: gastrointestinal (anorexia, nausea, vomiting, diarrhoea, abdominal pain), metallic taste.
- Doses (up to three times daily) to be taken with food to minimise gastrointestinal side-effects.
- Cautions:
  - may cause lactic acidosis especially in renal impairment
  - suspend 2 days before surgery and restart when renal function is normalised
  - stop when iodine-containing X-ray contrast media are used and restart after normal renal function
  - monitor renal function.

Acarbose

- Acarbose is an alpha-glucosidase inhibitor. These enzymes are present in enterocytes of the small intestine and are responsible for breaking down carbohydrates. Inhibition of the enzymes results in delayed carbohydrate digestion and absorption.

- It is usually used in combination with other antidiabetic agents.
- Tablets are taken at the start of each main meal.
- Side-effects: gastrointestinal disturbances particularly flatulence, soft stools, abdominal distension, diarrhoea (incidence of side-effects is increased if tablets are not taken with food).

Thiazolidinediones: pioglitazone, rosiglitazone

- Thiazolidinediones decrease peripheral insulin resistance.
- They may be used in combination with oral antidiabetic agents; when combined with insulin therapy risk of heart failure is increased.
- They should be taken with meals.
- Cautions: cardiovascular disease, increased risk of bone fractures in females, monitor liver function.
- Contraindications: hepatic impairment, history of heart failure, pregnancy and breast-feeding.
- Monitor for signs of heart failure, occurrence of liver dysfunction and bone density in women.

Meglitinides: repaglinide, nateglinide

- These drugs stimulate release of insulin from beta cells in pancreas.
- They have a rapid onset of action and short duration of action; to be taken up to 30 minutes before meals and dose should be skipped if meal is not taken.
- They can be used in combination with metformin.
- Cautions: the elderly, debilititated patients, moderate hepatic impairment for nateglinide, moderate renal impairment for repaglinide.
- Contraindications: ketoacidosis, pregnancy, breast-feeding, severe hepatic impairment.
- Side-effects: hypoglycaemia, hypersensitivity reactions; may cause weight gain.

Incretin mimetics/enhancers

Sitagliptin

- Inhibitor of dipeptidylpeptidase-4 which results in increased insulin secretion and decreased glucagon level
- Used as adjunct therapy with metformin or thiazolinediones
- It does not affect weight and does not induce hypoglycaemia
- Side-effects: gastrointestinal disturbances, peripheral oedema, respiratory tract infections, pain, osteoarthritis.

Exenatide

- An incretin mimetic which results in increased insulin secretion, suppression of glucagon secretion and slowing of gastric emptying
- Administered as subcutaneous injections twice daily before meals
- Used as adjunct therapy with metformin or sulphonylureas
- Side-effects: gastrointestinal disturbances, headache, dizziness, asthenia, hypoglycaemia, increased sweating, injection-site reaction.

Insulin

- Insulin is a polypeptide hormone which will be destroyed if administered orally.
- It is given by subcutaneous injection. Patient is advised to use a different site for each injection to minimise fat hypertrophy at injection sites.
- Product should be stored in a refrigerator.
- Dose may need to be reviewed in relation to change in diet or increased exercise.
- Side-effects: local reactions and fat hypertrophy at injection site, increase in body weight, hypoglycaemia.

Insulin design

- Human insulin analogues are preferred to the insulin extracted from pork pancreas.
- Short-acting insulin (e.g. insulin aspart and insulin lispro) has a rapid onset of action.

- Intermediate- and long-acting insulin (e.g. isophane insulin, which is a suspension of insulin in protamine, or insulin zinc suspension, which includes addition of a suitable zinc salt) has a slower onset of action but action is of longer duration.
- Mixtures of short-acting and intermediate-acting insulin (e.g. in the proportion of 30% to 70%, which is administered twice daily) may be used. A short-acting insulin may be required before meals to avoid excessive post-prandial hyperglycaemia.

Insulin administration

- Subcutaneous injection (needles, syringes)
- Injection devices ('pens') are convenient to use; preferred to the conventional administration especially for patients with impaired vision, limited manual dexterity and children. The insulin is supplied in cartridges for the re-usable pens
- Continuous subcutaneous infusion using a portable infusion pump.

Continuous subcutaneous infusion of insulin

This is a method of administering continuous insulin release and bolus doses for example at mealtimes. It is appropriate for patients who suffer recurrent or unpredictable hypoglycaemic attacks or high blood glucose levels in the morning despite appropriate drug therapy. The patient needs to receive training on handling the device and on the requirement to monitor blood glucose concentration.

> Diabetic patients receiving treatment, especially insulin, should be advised to keep a supply of sugar (e.g. dextrose tablets or sweets) so that if symptoms of hypoglycaemia occur they can take some sugar which is rapidly absorbed and corrects the hypoglycaemic state.

Examples of drugs that increase hypoglycaemic effects

- Angiotensin-converting enzyme (ACE) inhibitors
- Alcohol
- Beta-blockers
- Salicylates
- Sulphonamides.

Examples of drugs that increase hyperglycaemia

- Atypical antipsychotics
- Beta-agonists
- Beta-blockers
- Ciclosporin
- Corticosteroids
- Diuretics
- Oestrogen
- Phenytoin
- Protease inhibitors.

Hypoglycaemia

Signs and symptoms

- Anxiety
- Blurred vision
- Confusion
- Hunger
- Numbness
- Sweating
- Tingling
- Tremor.

> The occurrence of nocturnal hypoglycaemia should be addressed with care since, if patient does not recognise signs, the condition may progress to coma. Symptoms at night include nightmares, restless sleep, profuse sweating, morning headache and morning hangover.

Management

Patient should be advised to consume a rapidly absorbed carbohydrate (e.g. dextrose tablets or non-sugar-free sweets or soft drinks) immediately until symptoms subside. If patient is unconscious then patient requires administration of glucagon and glucose.

Warning signs of hypoglycaemia may be minimised in patients who are taking beta-blockers and those who are experiencing increased frequency of hypoglycaemic attacks.

Conditions that may lead to loss of blood glucose control

- Fever
- Trauma
- Infection
- Surgery: patients receiving oral antidiabetic agents who undergo elective surgery are switched to insulin from the day before the intervention and continued on insulin until they start to eat and drink.
- Stress.

Diabetic nephropathy

- Incidence increasing in type 2 diabetes
- Presents with albuminuria, proteinuria and reduced glomerular filtration rate
- Hypertension and oedema develop
- Management: ACE inhibitors ± diuretic or calcium channel blockers
- Target blood pressure in diabetics is 120/80 mmHg.

Retinopathy

- Most common microvascular complication
- Accumulation of sorbitol which cannot be metabolised by cells in the retina takes place and this leads to oedema
- Damage to existing vessels and formation of new unstable vessels
- Precipitated with hypertension, hyperlipidaemia and pregnancy
- Signs: haemorrhage, spots, venous changes on retina.

Blood pressure control in diabetics is important to reduce cardiovascular risk and decrease occurrence of nephropathy and retinopathy. Blood pressure should be maintained at 120/80 mmHg.

Peripheral neuropathy

- Characterised by paresthesia and pain in the lower extremities, and decreased sensation which may contribute to foot injuries
- Management: pain – paracetamol or NSAIDs are first line of treatment. Tricyclic antidepressants particularly amitriptyline and imipramine are used in patients where analgesics alone are not sufficient. Carbamazepine and gabapentin may also be considered. Other antiepileptic drugs, namely lamotrigine and topiramate, have been shown to be effective.

Diabetic ketoacidosis

In diabetic ketoacidosis patients present with moderate-to-high blood glucose levels together with water and electrolyte depletion. This is because, when hyperglycaemia occurs and is sustained, osmotic diuresis occurs resulting in water and electrolyte excretion.

- Signs and symptoms: hyperglycaemia (consistently elevated blood glucose), thirst, excessive urination, fatigue, blurred vision, fruity breath odour, deep and difficult breathing, dehydration (dry mouth, dry skin), nausea, vomiting, stomach pains and loss of appetite.
- Management:
  - fluid replacement: use of 0.9% saline
  - insulin: continuous intravenous infusion of insulin and monitor blood glucose level
  - electrolytes: potassium supplementation is started once elevated potassium levels begin to drop and good urine outflow is achieved. In acidosis, serum potassium level may be high initially.

Patient monitoring

- Blood pressure monitoring
- HbA1c (glycated haemoglobin) 6.5–7.5%: provides an indication of glycaemic control over the previous 3 months
- Blood glucose levels
- Lipid profile
- See also Chapter 11.

Peaks and troughs in blood glucose should be avoided. Peaks, especially when they are sustained, are associated with long-term complications while troughs are associated with occurrence of hypoglycaemia. Continuous blood glucose monitoring may be undertaken to establish blood glucose control, especially during the night, and review medication accordingly.

Prophylactic treatment

Drugs that should be considered in diabetics to reduce cardiovascular risk include:

- ACE inhibitors
- aspirin
- lipid-regulating drugs.

Patient education checklist

Points to consider in patient education are listed in Table 38.1.

Practice summary

- Hypoglycaemia may develop in:
  - insulin overdosage
  - increased work or exercise
  - omission or delay of a meal
  - vomiting, diarrhoea.

Table 38.1 Patient education checklist

About the condition	Signs, symptoms, causes
Lifestyle	Exercise, driving
Hyper-hypoglycaemia	Causes, signs, management
Nutrition	Food intake, patterns
Monitoring	Blood glucose, HbA1c, blood pressure, lipid profile, body weight
Medication	Insulin/oral therapy intake
Action during illness	Diarrhoea, vomiting, fever
Care of the feet, eyes	
Self-monitoring	Glucose testing: technique and interpretation of results

- Patient self-monitoring: to maintain blood glucose level between 4 and 7 mmol/L before meals and less than 9 mmol/L after meals.
- Monitoring for eye disease (yearly ophthalmic check-ups), vascular complications (care with injuries especially injuries in the feet), kidney disorders (routine check of kidney function tests).
- Skin and infections: to refer immediately to health professional; anti-infective therapy is considered.
- Exercise: test blood glucose level before, during and after exercise. Occurrence of hypoglycaemia is more likely in patients taking insulin than those taking sulphonylureas.
- Travelling: patients should be advised to take enough drug therapy and blood testing supplies for the journey. Meal regularity and lifestyle measures should be maintained (e.g. requesting meals for diabetics on flights). If travelling across time zones blood glucose should be tested more frequently.
- Lifestyle measures:
  - body weight control
  - reduce intake of fat and complex carbohydrates
  - foods for diabetics: limited intake; may contain sorbitol which may cause diarrhoea
  - physical activity.

Questions

1 List two factors that could indicate diabetic nephropathy.
2 Which classes of drugs are used to manage diabetic nephropathy?

Answers

1 Factors that indicate diabetic nephropathy include albuminuria, proteinuria and decreased creatinine clearance which may be identified through renal function tests. Hypertension and oedema occur.
2 Angiotensin-converting enzyme inhibitors such as perindopril and calcium channel blockers such as amlodipine are used in diabetic patients with nephropathy who usually also require strict blood pressure control.

Further reading

Azzopardi L M, Serracino Inglott A, Zarb Adami M and Zerafa N (2006). Patient education in diabetes. *Clin Pharm Eur* 2: 45–46.

Eugenio K R and Eugenio Clark L M (2004). Community pharmacists' counselling about metformin-associated lactic acidosis. *J Am Pharm Assoc* 44: 629–632.

Hogan E G, Leal S, Slack M and Apgar D (2006). Diabetes drug management: pharmacists vs physicians. *Hosp Pharm Eur* July/August: 16–17.

Peel E, Douglas M and Lawton J (2007). Self monitoring of blood glucose in type 2 diabetes: longitudinal qualitative study of patients' perspectives. *BMJ* 335: 493.

39

The menopause and hormone replacement therapy

Learning objectives:

- To appreciate characteristics of the menopause
- To develop skills so as to estimate risks and benefits of hormone replacement therapy (HRT)
- To appreciate patient monitoring required with the use of HRT.

Background

Menopause is signalled by the last menstrual period. This can be diagnosed retrospectively and is usually confirmed following 12 months of blood-free interval. Cessation of menstruation is caused by a loss of ovarian follicular activity resulting from decrease in the female steroid hormone oestrogen.

Menopause is characterised by vasomotor symptoms, localised atrophy of the genitalia, psychological symptoms and osteoporosis. Table 39.1 shows ovarian hormone secretion after the onset of a normal menstrual cycle.

Vasomotor symptoms

- Hot flushes
- Headaches
- Insomnia
- Faintness.

Advice: avoid foods and drinks that cause vasodilatation.

Atrophy of genitalia

- Vaginal dryness
- Vaginal discharge and bleeding

Table 39.1 Changes in hormone secretion wih onset of menopause

	Premenopausal	Perimenopausal	Postmenopausal
Oestrogens	+++	++	+, −
Progesterone	+++	+	−
Androgens	+	+	+,−
FSH		↑	↑↑
LH		↑	↑↑

LH, luteinising hormone; FSH, follicle-stimulating hormone.

- Urinary incontinence, urgency of micturition, recurrent symptoms of cystitis.

Psychological symptoms

- Depression
- Irritability
- Exhaustion
- Poor concentration and memory
- Panic attacks.

> 'With the recent publication of data from trials designed to assess the long-term risks and benefits of HRT, and which considered the associated risks of cardiovascular disease and breast cancer in particular, pharmacists will be approached by women with questions about the use of HRT.'[1]

Hormone replacement therapy (HRT)

Hormone replacement therapy is used to relieve the symptoms of oestrogen deficiency. When used to prevent osteoporosis:

- the duration of therapy should be at least 5 years
- the patient should be informed of increased incidence of cardiovascular disease and breast cancer shown in studies
- the benefits of treatment over risks should be re-assessed every year
- other options of pharmacotherapy for osteoporosis should be considered (see Chapter 46).

Contraindications and cautions

- Presence of oestrogen-dependent tumour
- Liver disease
- Deep vein thrombosis.

Oestrogen therapy

The naturally occurring oestrogens, estradiol, estrone and estriol, are rapidly inactivated by the liver and so cannot be administered orally. The attachment of an ethinyl group to the 17α position of estradiol leads to ethinylestradiol (Figure 39.1) which undergoes slower metabolism in the liver, allowing for oral administration. In addition to oral administration there are other routes of administration.

Oestrogen transdermal patch (e.g. estradiol patch)

- Maintains estradiol:estrone physiological ratio and achieves a constant reservoir of hormone levels
- Patches present estradiol either alone or in combination with a progestogen
- Patch should be applied to non-hairy skin of the lower body and should be placed away from breast tissue
- Does not require daily change.

Oestrogen implant (e.g. estradiol implants)

- Provides a constant level of oestrogen for up to 6 months
- Maintains estradiol:estrone physiological ratio
- Upregulation of oestrogen receptors may occur
- Convenient for the patient. However, once inserted it cannot be readily removed and levels take at least a month to fall following removal. This may present a problem when drug therapy needs to be withdrawn either due to side-effects or, for example, due to surgery.

Vaginal creams

- Preferred when symptoms are limited to vaginal area such as atrophic vaginitis.

Nasal formulation of estradiol

- A spray that presents estradiol 150 micrograms/puff

Figure 39.1 Chemical structure of ethinylestradiol.

- Dose: 1–4 puffs into each nostril daily at the same time of day continuously or for 21–28 days
- In severe blocked nose: administer double the usual dose between cheek and gum of upper jaw.

Choice of product

- Oestrogen therapy alone is suitable for long-term continuous therapy in a *woman without a uterus*.
- A *woman with a uterus* requires oestrogen with cyclical progestogen for the last 10–13 days of the cycle to limit risk of endometrial hyperplasia and endometrial carcinoma.

In women with a uterus the progestogen therapy can be administered either cyclically or as continuous combined therapy.

Cyclical HRT given sequentially

- Oestrogen is taken continuously
- Progestogen used for the last 10–13 days of the 28 days
- Regular withdrawal bleeding occurs upon cessation of the progestogen intake
- Indicated for perimenopausal or borderline women
- Patient pack either presents two different types of tablets (one containing oestrogen only and another containing the combination of oestrogen and progestogen) or consists of a calendar pack that presents two tablets to be taken during the last days of cycle.

Continuous combined HRT

- Combination of oestrogen and progestogen is taken throughout 28 days (continuous)
- Avoids withdrawal bleeding
- Irregular bleeding may occur for the first 6 months
- Indicated for postmenopausal women since it avoids occurrence of withdrawal bleeding.

See also Chapter 40 for a discussion on progestogens.

It is essential to advise patient to follow calendar pack when available since the tablets may vary or there may be a requirement for varied tablet-taking pattern.

Start-up effects to HRT

- Breast tenderness and nipple sensitivity
- Headaches
- Increased appetite
- Calf cramps.

Side-effects

- Weight gain
- Venous thrombosis
- Breast cancer
- Stroke.

Venous thrombosis

The risks associated with HRT may exceed the benefits in women who have predisposing factors to venous thrombosis, such as a personal or family history of deep vein thrombosis or pulmonary embolism, severe varicose veins, obesity, surgery, trauma or prolonged bed rest.

Risk of deep vein thrombosis especially in flights longer than 5 hours' duration should be considered. Patient should be advised to use elastic hosiery and where appropriate use aspirin prophylaxis. In patients undergoing major surgery, orthopaedic and vascular leg surgery, HRT should be stopped 4–6 weeks before surgery and should be started after full patient mobilisation.

Risk of cancer

The increased risk of breast cancer is related to the duration of HRT use and this excess risk disappears within about 5 years of drug withdrawal.

Some studies have indicated that during HRT the risk of ovarian cancer is increased.[2]

Tibolone

Tibolone (Figure 39.2) is a synthetic steroid with oestrogenic, progestogenic and androgenic effects.

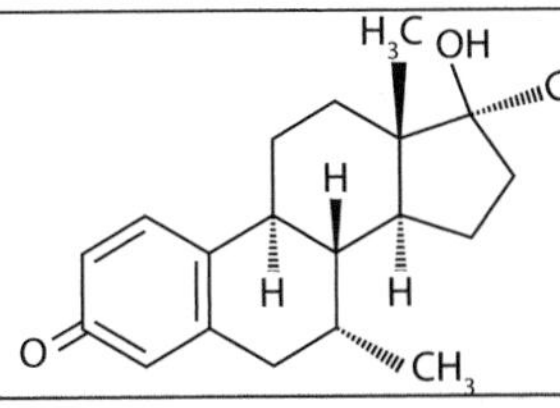

Tibolone

Figure 39.2 Chemical structure of tibolone.

- Given continuously
- Not suitable for women within 1 year of menopause
- Protective against osteoporosis and suitable for the treatment of vasomotor symptoms
- Long-term cardioprotective effect, which is experienced with oestrogen-based HRT, is questionable
- Increases risk of breast cancer to a lesser extent than combined HRT. Associated with a risk of stroke.

The Women's Health Initiative Study was stopped because of safety concerns about HRT with oestrogen and progestogen. There was an increase in breast cancer, but this was not greater than the increase reported in observational studies. Although there was an increase in vascular events, many of the women in the study had pre-existing risk factors for cardiovascular disease. No long-term trials of combined HRT are continuing, so the balance between benefit and harm will remain uncertain.[3] These findings emphasise the importance for the need for continued use to be reviewed annually for each individual patient.

Recommendations for use of HRT

- HRT is associated with an increased risk of endometrial cancer (reduced by progestogen) and, after some years of use, possibly an increased risk of breast cancer.
- It is appropriate for women whose lives are inconvenienced by vasomotor instability and in patients with early natural or surgical menopause (before 45 years) since these patients are at high risk of osteoporosis. In these patients HRT is continued for 5–10 years.
- In menopausal women with a uterus the risks may outweigh benefits if used for longer than 5 years.

- Before initiating therapy, a physical examination should be carried out.
- Assessment of bone mineral density needs to be undertaken regularly.
- Baseline and monitoring of serum electrolytes and liver function tests are necessary.
- Patient should be advised to undertake routine cervical smear test and mammography.
- Initially, patient is reviewed after 3 months of therapy, then reviewed periodically every 6–12 months.

Other products

- Phyto-oestrogens: plant-based products that exert mild oestrogenic effects such as isoflavones in soy products
- Oil of evening primrose
- Herbal preparations such as valerian, kava: effective to counteract psychological effects of menopause.

Practice summary

- HRT is used to control menopausal symptoms and improve quality of life.
- Patients should be advised about the mixed risks and benefits of HRT.
- Women with a uterus should not receive oestrogen alone; a progestogen component needs to be included either as a continuous therapy (with each tablet) or a cyclical therapy (during the last 10–13 days of the 28-day cycle).
- Where urogenital symptoms predominate, local vaginal oestrogen is preferred.

- HRT is not advocated for treatment or prevention of cardiovascular disease, the risk of which is higher in postmenopausal women than in premenopausal women.
- HRT therapy should be reviewed yearly to determine benefit and time for cessation of treatment.
- After 4–5 years of therapy it is appropriate to opt for a trial period off HRT and to identify whether vasomotor, genital and psychological symptoms still interfere with the patient's quality of life.

Question

1 What is tibolone and when is it indicated?

Answer

1 Tibolone is a synthetic steroid with oestrogenic, progestogenic and androgenic effects. It is indicated for the short-term treatment of vasomotor symptoms of oestrogen deficiency (including women being treated with gonadotrophin-releasing hormone analogues) and osteoporosis prophylaxis in women at risk of fractures (second line). It is given continuously and is not suitable for women within 1 year of menopause.

Further reading

Azzopardi L M, Serracino-Inglott A, Zarb Adami M and Galea F (2003). HRT in practice: helping women make the right choice. *Nurs Pract* May/June: 67–68.

Bath P M W and Gray L J (2005). Association between hormone replacement therapy and subsequent stroke: a meta-analysis. *BMJ* 330: 342–345.

Mcintosh J and Blalock S J (2005). Effects of media coverage of women's health initiative study on attitudes and behaviour of women receiving hormone replacement therapy. *Am J Health-Syst Pharm* 62: 69–74.

Tanna N (2003). Hormone replacement therapy: risks and benefits. *Pharm J* 271: 646–648.

References

1 Tanna N. Hormone replacement therapy: an overview. *Pharm J* 2003; 271: 615–617.

2 Beral V, Million Women Study Collaborators. Ovarian cancer and hormone replacement therapy in the Million Women Study. *Lancet* 2007; 369: 1703–1710.

3 MacLennan A H. Hormone replacement therapy: where to now? *Aust Pres* 2003; 26: 8–10.

40

Menstrual cycle disorders and contraception

Learning objectives:

- To review characteristics of premenstrual syndrome, dysmenorrhoea, menorrhagia, endometriosis and polycystic ovary syndrome
- To appreciate pharmacotherapy in the management of menstrual cycle disorders
- To review use of oral contraceptives and identify patient monitoring required.

Background

The menstrual cycle presents changes in hormonal levels – predominantly oestrogen and progestogen. However, other hormones such as prostaglandins and leukotrienes are involved as well.

Premenstrual syndrome (PMS)

- More common in the 30–40 year age group.
- Symptoms occur a day before menstruation begins and disappear at the onset or shortly after menstruation begins. Symptoms are cyclical and may not be present with each cycle.
- Aetiology: physiological changes in hormone levels. Condition may be exacerbated by other factors (e.g. stress).
- Psychological and behavioural symptoms: depression, tiredness, fatigue, lethargy, tension, irritability, sleep disorders, aggression, food cravings.
- Physical symptoms: breast tenderness, swollen, bloated feeling, weight gain, headache, appetite changes, constipation, diarrhoea, muscle stiffness.

Management of PMS

- Exercise and relaxation techniques.
- Manage fluid retention that is associated with PMS by advising patient to reduce salt intake, increase intake of potassium salts (e.g. banana, nuts, tomatoes) and increase intake of food with diuretic effect (e.g. prunes, figs, celery, cucumber, parsley).
- Advise patient to keep a diary to help identify trigger factors or activities that exacerbate the condition.

Drug therapy of PMS

Pyridoxine

- Dosage regimen requires either daily dosing throughout the month or higher doses that are used 3 days before onset of menstruation and continued for 2 days after start of menstruation

- Helps against mood changes, headache and breast discomfort.

Evening primrose oil

- Treatment needs to be on a regular basis
- Helps against breast tenderness and mood changes.

Combined oral contraceptive

See page 246.

Bromocriptine

- Stimulates central dopamine receptors, inhibits release of prolactin
- Counteracts breast tenderness, mood changes, fluid retention.

Danazol

- Synthetic steroid with antioestrogenic and antiprogestogenic activity combined with weak androgenic activity
- Provides relief of breast tenderness and mood changes
- Occurrence of side-effects (e.g. nausea, weight gain, acne, muscular pain, photosensitivity, nervousness, mood changes and anxiety) limits its use.

Prostaglandin synthesis inhibitor – mefenamic acid

- Take 250 mg three times daily 12 days before menstruation or 500 mg three times daily 9 days before menstruation
- Continued up to third day
- Helps in counteracting general aches and pain, headache, tension, irritability and depression.

Antidepressants

- Use of selective serotonin re-uptake inhibitors (SSRIs) and other antidepressants may be considered when depression is clinically significant.

Dysmenorrhoea

Primary dysmenorrhoea

- Occurs in young patients
- Presents with lower abdominal pain that radiates to back and thighs, nausea, vomiting, diarrhoea, headache
- Probably higher concentration of prostaglandins occurs which in turn favours increased myometrial contractility.

Secondary dysmenorrhoea

- Occurs in women 30–40 years old as a consequence of other pelvic pathology (e.g. endometriosis)
- Pain starts before menstruation and continues for the duration of menses
- Characteristic symptoms are abdominal bloating, backache and feeling of heaviness.

Management

- NSAIDs: decrease prostaglandin synthesis
- Combined oral contraceptives
- Antispasmodics: however, these are thought to have a negligible effect on the uterus.

In secondary dysmenorrhoea the underlying pathology should be identified. If the underlying cause includes endometriosis this may impact negatively on fertility, which may be an issue in this age group.

Menorrhagia

Average menstrual blood loss is estimated to be 35–80 mL per cycle. Menorrhagia is a condition where there is blood loss in excess of 80 mL. This is difficult to quantify and hence diagnosis is based on:

- increase in flow relative to former pattern
- iron-deficiency anaemia (Hg <12 g/dL)
- intermenstrual bleeding.

Causes

- Dysfunctional uterine bleeding
- Endometriosis
- Pelvic inflammatory disease
- Uterine or ovarian tumours
- Hypothyroidism
- Platelet problems.

Treatment

The occurrence of menorrhagia should be investigated and, once secondary conditions are eliminated, treatment options include:

- combined oral contraceptives
- danazol
- NSAIDs
- tranexamic acid: an antifibrinolytic drug which is contraindicated in thromboembolic disease
- gonadorelin analogues (e.g. goserelin, buserelin, nafarelin, triptorelin)
- surgery: undertaken when patient is in her perimenopausal state and where this is not going to interfere with family planning.

Gonadorelin analogues inhibit production of androgen and oestrogen. They are used in patients with infertility and endometriosis. Treatment should not exceed six months. Side-effects: menopausal-like symptoms (hot flushes, increased sweating, vaginal dryness), decrease in bone mineral density, headache and hypersensitivity reactions.

Endometriosis

This is a condition characterised by the occurrence of endometrial tissue outside the uterus (e.g. in the cervix, ovaries, peritoneum, small intestine, genitourinary tract). Symptoms include:

- dysmenorrhoea
- menstrual irregularities including menorrhagia
- infertility.

Management

Endometriotic tissue is oestrogen-dependent and therefore drug therapy is aimed at opposing effects of oestrogens:

- combined oral contraceptives
- danazol
- gonadorelin analogues.

Polycystic ovary syndrome

This is associated with a hyperandrogenic state and symptoms include:

- amenorrhoea/oligomenorrhoea
- hirsutism
- alopecia
- acne
- obesity.

Management

- Oestrogen + anti-androgen (e.g. cyproterone)
- Low-dose combined oral contraceptives, particularly those containing drospirenone as the progestogen component
- Progestogen (e.g. dydrogesterone)
- Metformin: in patients experiencing insulin resistance, use of insulin sensitisers lowers testosterone blood levels and increases ovulation
- Clomifene.

Clomifene is an anti-oestrogen and it induces gonadotrophin release by occupying oestrogen receptors in the hypothalamus. Cautions to its use include risk of ovarian cancer (recommendation that therapy should be limited to six cycles); cysts may enlarge during therapy and multiple births. Side-effects: hot flushes, abdominal pain. Withdraw therapy if visual disturbances or ovarian hyperstimulation occur. It is used in polycystic ovary syndrome (PCOS) particularly where infertility is an issue. It is also used in the treatment of infertility.

Progestogens

Progestogens can be classified into two: progesterone analogues and testosterone analogues.

Progesterone analogues

These are less androgenic than the testosterone analogues. Examples include dydrogesterone and medroxyprogesterone.

- Dydrogesterone (Figure 40.1): used in infertility, recurrent miscarriage, menstrual cycle disorders (PMS, dysmenorrhoea, endometriosis, amenorrhoea)
- Medroxyprogesterone (Figure 40.2): used in malignant disease, menstrual cycle disorders (amenorrhoea, endometriosis).

Testosterone analogues

Testosterone analogues include norethisterone, which is used in the postponement of menstruation and in menstrual cycle disorders (PMS, dysmenorrhoea, endometriosis), and other progestogens (e.g. norgestrel, levonorgestrel (Figure 40.3), desogestrel, gestodene, norgestimate) which are included in combination products with oestrogens for hormone replacement therapy and combined oral contraceptives.

Oral contraceptives

Oral contraceptives may contain an oestrogen together with a progestogen component and these are referred to as the combined oral contraceptives (COCs). COCs are usually taken for 21 days followed by a 7-day pill-free period or inactive tablet taking during which withdrawal bleeding occurs. When COCs are used for the treatment of a pathological condition, treatment may be given continuously.

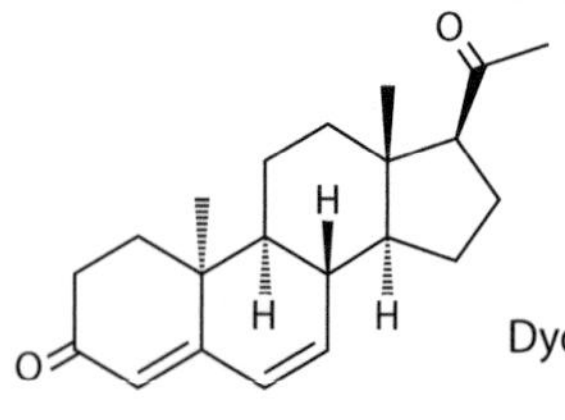

Dydrogesterone

Figure 40.1 Chemical structure of dydrogesterone.

Progestogen-only (POP) oral contraceptives are also available. They are used when oestrogens are contraindicated (e.g. due to a history or predisposition to venous thrombosis) and when breast-feeding since they do not affect lactation.

Criteria by which contraceptive methods are judged for contraceptive effect

- Effectiveness
- Patient acceptability
- Side-effects.

Effectiveness is reported in terms of pregnancy rates:

$$\text{Pregnancy rate per 100 woman-years} = 1200 \times \frac{\text{Total no. of conceptions}}{\text{Total months of exposure}}$$

Various methods of contraception are compared in Table 40.1.

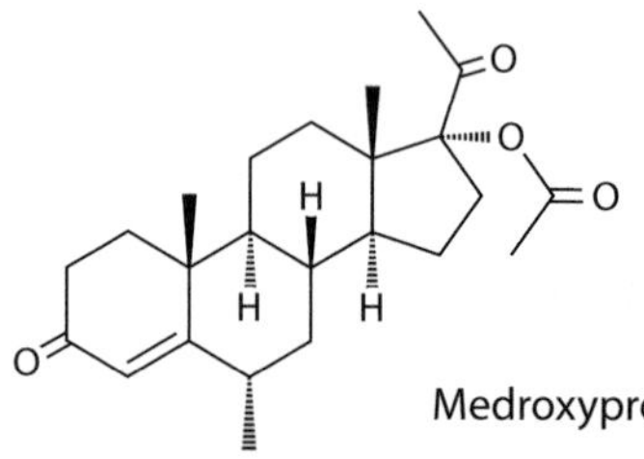

Medroxyprogesterone

Figure 40.2 Chemical structure of medroxyprogesterone.

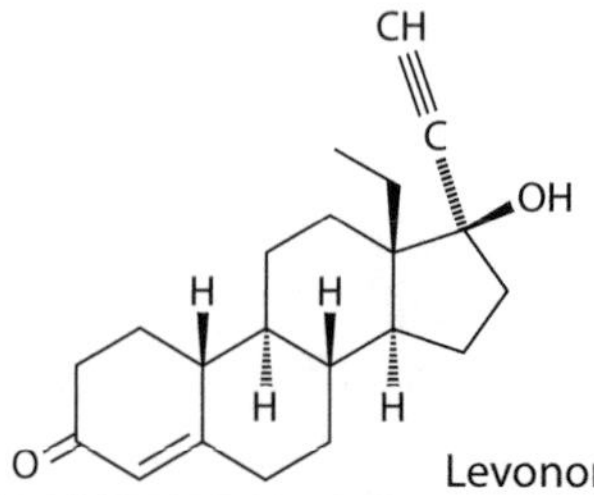

Levonorgestrel

Figure 40.3 Chemical structure of levonorgestrel.

Table 40.1 Comparison of contraceptive methods

Method of contraception	Pregnancies/100 woman-years
Oral contraceptives	
>35 micrograms ethinylestradiol	<1
Progestogen only	3
Rhythm: calendar method, temperature method, mucus method	<1–47
Mechanical/chemical condoms	3–36
Intrauterine device	<1–6

Advantages of combined oral contraceptives

- Reliability for contraceptive effect
- Avoidance of dysmenorrhoea and menorrhagia (lower occurrence of iron-deficiency anaemia)
- Avoidance of premenstrual tension.

The starting routine for COCs to achieve a contraceptive effect is shown in Table 40.2.

Classification of preparations of COCs

The different preparations may be classified according to the strength of the oestrogen component. For each patient the lowest strength oestrogen product that gives the desired clinical outcome should be used to keep occurrence of side-effects to a minimum.

- Low-strength preparations: 20 micrograms ethinylestradiol
- Standard-strength preparations: 30–35 micrograms ethinylestradiol
- High-strength preparations: 50 micrograms ethinylestradiol or mestranol.

Progestogens and COCs

The progestogens included in COCs are testosterone analogues which can be divided into second-generation progestogens (e.g. norethisterone and levonorgestrel) and third-generation progestogens (e.g. desogestrel, gestodene, norgestimate and drospirenone).

COCs containing desogestrel and gestodene should be used only by women who are intolerant of other COCs since they are associated with an increased risk of venous thromboembolism.

Drospirenone is a derivative of spironolactone and hence has anti-androgenic activity together with anti-mineralcorticoid activity. For this reason, COCs containing drospirenone may be preferred in the management of PCOS. It may cause an increase in serum potassium.

Table 40.2 Starting routine for combined oral contraceptives to achieve a contraceptive effect

Circumstance	Start date (day of cycle)	Requirement for extra precautions for 7 days
Menstruating	Day 1	No
	Day 2	Yes
Postpartum:		
No lactation	Day 21	No
Lactation	Progestogen-only preferred	No
Amenorrhoea	Any day	Yes

Phased preparations of COCs

COCs may present varying amounts of oestrogens and progestogens depending on the stage of the cycle. Such preparations are termed biphasic (two different types of tablets) or triphasic (three different types of tablets). Patient adherence to the calendar pack is important so that the different tablets are taken according to the stage of the cycle. Preparations that contain the same amount of oestrogen and progestogens are termed monophasic and do not require special patient advice to ensure a specific pattern in taking the tablets.

> Patient compliance with COCs is essential to ensure contraceptive effect. Patients should be advised on factors that may occur during the cycle which may interfere with the contraceptive effect. They should also be advised to take the tablets at the same time of the day each day.

Missed pill

When patients forget to take the tablet, this could lead to loss of contraceptive effect for the cycle. The risk is increased if the missed tablet occurs at the beginning or end of a cycle.

Patients should be advised that if they forget a dose they should take it as soon as possible and the next one at the normal time. If tablet taking is delayed by more than 24 hours and occurs for two or more pills in a cycle, then contraceptive effectiveness may be lost. The patient should continue normal pill taking but will not be protected for the next 7 days. If these 7 days run beyond the end of the packet, the patient should start the next packet at once, skipping the 7-day pill-free period or the seven inactive tablets.

Conditions that affect absorption of COCs

In oral administration, factors that interfere with the absorption of oestrogen and progestogen from the gastrointestinal tract may lead to loss of the contraceptive effect.

- Nausea and vomiting, diarrhoea: when the conditions last for more than 24 hours, additional contraceptive protection is required.
- Antibiotics, namely ampicillin, amoxicillin and related penicillins, tetracyclines and cephalosporins disturb normal gut flora which split oestrogen metabolites, entering the bowel, and reduce reabsorption of re-activated oestrogen. If patient is taking such antibacterial agents, she should be advised that the contraceptive effect of COCs may be lost.

Interactions with COCs and POP

The effectiveness of COCs and POP is reduced when they are taken together with drugs that act as hepatic enzyme inducers such as carbamazepine, phenytoin, griseofulvin, rifampicin and St John's wort. Hence a high-dose oestrogen COC preparation is preferred or else alternative methods of contraception should be considered.

Causes of breakthrough bleeding with COCs

Occurrence of bleeding during tablet taking (breakthrough bleeding) should be investigated since it may occur as a result of changes in tablet-taking patterns or may indicate pathological conditions. Minimal amount of bleeding is referred to as spotting. If breakthrough bleeding occurs with initiation of treatment, this may resolve on its own. Breakthrough bleeding in patients who have been taking the medication for a while should be investigated.

Causes include:

- missed pills
- disturbance of absorption due to drugs or gastrointestinal problems
- infection
- cervical disease.

When no underlying pathology is detected with breakthrough bleeding, strategies that may be considered include:

- switching from a monophasic to a triphasic preparation

- increasing progestogen dose: if bleeding is occurring in late cycle
- increasing oestrogen component: if bleeding is occurring in early cycle.

Tricycling

Tricycling is when the patient takes three or four packets of monophasic preparations without the 7-day pill-free period in between. It is adopted when:

- cyclical symptoms occur during pill-free period
- there is a predisposition to reduced efficacy (e.g. missed tablets at end of cycle)
- heavy painful withdrawal bleeding occurs
- the woman requests it to avoid withdrawal bleeding during a holiday or an activity
- maintenance treatment for endometriosis is required.

Extended and continuous cycle COCs

New formulations of COCs that are termed extended cycle or continuous cycle have been developed lately. They provide a means of changing a woman's withdrawal bleeding associated with COCs. An example of such a formulation consists of ethinylestradiol and drospirenone which provides 24 days of therapy and 4 days of placebo and is associated with a lighter flow which is of shorter duration when compared with a traditional formulation. Other formulations where treatment is given over 84 days leading to four withdrawal bleedings per year are available. Currently these formulations are associated with a higher risk of breakthrough bleeding and spotting. They are useful for patients where withdrawal bleeding is causing distress (e.g. menstrual migraine).

Cautions

- Patients at risk of developing venous thromboembolism, arterial disease and migraine
- Personal or family history of hypertriglyceridaemia, hyperprolactinaeamia
- History of severe depression, undiagnosed breast mass and inflammatory bowel disease including Crohn's disease.

COCs should not be considered for patients where the risks associated with therapy are greater than the expected benefits. Before starting use of these products, individual assessment should consider the personal history of venous or arterial thrombosis, heart disease associated with pulmonary hypertension or risk of embolus, history of transient ischaemic attacks, liver disease, systemic lupus erythematosus, pregnancy and breast-feeding, among others. They should not be used in patients who have been diagnosed with breast cancer and within 5 years of evidence of disease.

Side-effects due to relative oestrogen excess

- Nausea
- Headache
- Dizziness
- Irritability
- Bloating, cyclical weight gain
- Vaginal discharge
- Breast pain
- Benign breast disease
- Endometriosis
- Fibroids.

Side-effects due to relative progestogen excess

- Vaginal dryness
- Sustained weight gain
- Depression
- Lassitude
- Breast tenderness
- Acne, seborrhoea
- Hirsutism.

Major side-effects of COCs

- Increased risk of cardiovascular disease: blood clots, heart attacks and stroke
- Risk is increased in:
  - smokers

- patients over 35 years of age
- patients with hypertension, history of arterial or venous thrombosis, ischaemic heart disease
- patients undergoing surgery: COCs should be discontinued 4 weeks before major elective surgery and all surgery to the legs; it is recommended to start therapy 2 weeks after full mobilisation
- patients undertaking travel, particularly travel over 5 hours: patient should receive advice on prophylaxis of travel-related deep vein thrombosis (see also Chapter 61).

Practice summary

- COCs are used in the management of menstrual cycle disorders where fertility is not an issue.
- Patients taking COCs should be advised to take the tablet at the same time each day, adhere to the schedule to visit the prescriber and to report immediately any of the following symptoms:
  - sudden severe pain in chest
  - sudden breathlessness
  - severe pain in calf of one leg
  - severe pain in stomach
  - unusual, severe prolonged headache.

Question

1 Compare the use of metformin and clomifene in polycystic ovary syndrome.

Answer

1 *Metformin* is used in polycystic ovary syndrome in patients experiencing insulin resistance. Use of insulin sensitisers lowers testosterone levels and increases ovulation. *Clomifene* is an anti-oestrogen. It induces gonadotrophin release by occupying oestrogen receptors in the hypothalamus. Cautions: risk of ovarian cancer (recommendation that therapy should be limited to six cycles), cysts may enlarge during therapy, multiple births. Side-effects include: hot flushes, abdominal pain. Withdraw therapy if visual disturbances or ovarian hyperstimulation occur. It is used in patients who are considering a pregnancy.

Further reading

Hendelmalm K and Samuelsson E (2005). Fatal venous thromboembolism associated with different combined oral contraceptives. *Drug Safety* 28: 907–916.

Shrader S P and Dickerson L M (2008). Extended- and continuous-cycle oral contraceptives. *Pharmacotherapy* 28: 1033–1040.

Upadhya K and Trent M (2007). Effects of polycystic ovary syndrome on health-related quality of life. *Exp Rev Pharmacoecon Outcomes Res* 7: 597–603.

41

Genito-urinary disorders

Learning objectives:

- To appreciate characteristics of benign prostatic hyperplasia and urinary frequency and incontinence
- To understand principles of drug therapy in benign prostatic hyperplasia and urinary frequency and incontinence
- To compare drugs used for each condition.

Background

The drugs that are considered in this section are drugs used for urinary retention (mainly due to benign prostatic hyperplasia) and drugs used for urinary frequency, enuresis and incontinence.

Benign prostatic hyperplasia

- Enlarged prostate compresses urethra and produces lower urinary tract symptoms and symptoms of bladder obstruction.
- Symptoms: weak urinary flow, sense of incomplete bladder emptying, delay in starting urination, need to urinate frequently, urgency, nocturia, urge incontinence and urinary leakage.
- Occasionally may result in acute retention of urine, warranting catheterisation.
- The occurrence of chronic urinary retention increases the risk of urinary tract infection which is otherwise very rare in males.

Diagnosis

- Measurement of flow rate: uroflow which records peak flow (25 mL/s) and average flow (12 mL/s)
- Digital rectal examination to assess size and presence of a tumour
- Measurement of prostate-specific antigen (PSA): PSA is a glycoprotein which is normally detected in minimum levels in all males. PSA levels greater than 10 ng/mL indicate a high probability of prostate cancer and require further assessment
- Scoring systems can be used to assess degree of hypertrophy in benign prostatic hypertrophy. Factors that are considered include occurrence of nocturia, daytime frequency, hesitancy, intermittency, terminal dribbling, urgency, impairment of size and force of urinary stream, dysuria and sensation of incomplete voiding.

Management

- Surgery: transurethral resection of the prostate is one method that could be adopted. Surgery is preferred when the hypertrophy is large or in the presence of a tumour. Immediate complications associated with surgery include failure to void, haemorrhage and urinary tract infections. Long-term complications include erectile dysfunction, urinary incontinence and bladder neck contractures.

- Drug therapy: alpha-blockers and anti-androgens.

Alpha-blockers

- Selective alpha$_1$-adrenergic receptor blockers (e.g. alfuzosin, prazosin, terazosin)
- Result in relaxation of smooth muscle
- Produce an increase in urinary flow rate and an improvement in obstructive symptoms
- Produce a rapid onset of action with clinical effects noticeable within weeks of initiation of therapy
- Cautions: hypotension, older persons, hepatic and renal impairment
- Side-effects: dizziness, hypotension (first-dose phenomenon), headache, asthenia, dry mouth, gastrointestinal disturbances.

Anti-androgens

- Dutasteride and finasteride inhibit 5α-reductase which is responsible for metabolising testosterone into dihydrotestosterone
- Result in improvement in urinary flow and in obstructive symptoms; delay in positive outcome of about 6 months
- Preferred to alpha-blockers in significantly enlarged prostate
- Finasteride in low doses is also used in male pattern baldness (see Chapter 47)
- Caution: decrease serum concentration of PSA (may interfere with PSA test result); not to be handled by women of childbearing potential; excreted in semen
- Side-effects: impotence, decreased libido, reduced ejaculatory volume, breast tenderness and enlargement.

> - Alpha-blockers produce symptomatic relief within weeks and have an impact on symptoms of chronic urinary retention due to benign prostatic hyperplasia.
> - Anti-androgens reduce prostate volume, are less effective for symptomatic improvement than alpha-blockers and have a lag time to produce the expected effect of a few months.
> - Combination of alpha-blockers with anti-androgens could be considered.

Overactive bladder

- Primary symptoms: frequency, urgency, urinary incontinence
- Urgency and frequency are more prevalent.

Definitions

- Urgency: sudden compelling need to pass urine which is difficult to defer
- Frequency: need to pass urine eight or more times in a 24-hour period
- Nocturia: awakening at night two or more times to pass urine.

Impact

- Negative impact on quality of life – interference with physical, sexual, occupational and social activities, psychological impact
- Direct costs – cost of drug therapy
- Indirect costs – cost of reduced productivity of patient, cost of health professionals' time.

Aetiology

- Acetylcholine stimulates muscarinic receptors (M_2 and M_3) on the detrusor muscle
- Involuntary contractions of the detrusor muscle result as the bladder fills.

Risk factors

- Age: more common in older persons
- Female gender: the decline in oestrogen levels during the postmenopausal stage can precipitate symptoms of urinary incontinence
- Uncontrolled diabetes
- Neurological conditions: e.g. stroke, Parkinson's disease, dementia
- Functional factors: pelvic injury, hysterectomy

- Medications: diuretics, alpha-adrenergic agonists and antagonists, anticholinergics, neuroleptics.

Incontinence

- Urge incontinence: involuntary leakage due to urgent need to pass urine. Conditions that may lead to its occurrence include cystitis, urethritis, outflow obstruction and neurological disorders such as stroke, dementia, parkinsonism and spinal cord injury.
- Stress incontinence: bladder leakage during exercise, coughing, sneezing, laughing or body movements which put pressure on bladder; most common in elderly women.

Management of urinary frequency, enuresis and incontinence

- Bladder training
- Pelvic floor exercises
- Pharmacotherapy: antimuscarinic agents and inhibitors of serotonin and noradrenaline re-uptake for stress incontinence.

Antimuscarinic agents

- Bladder contraction is mediated by muscarinic receptors in the bladder wall.
- M_3 receptors are the main muscarinic receptors.
- Antimuscarinic agents reduce bladder contractions and increase bladder capacity.
- Cautions: older patients, cardiovascular disease, prostatic hypertrophy, glaucoma.
- Contraindications: myasthenia gravis, significant bladder outflow obstruction or urinary retention, severe ulcerative colitis, toxic megacolon and in gastrointestinal obstruction or intestinal atony.
- Side-effects: dry mouth, constipation, blurring of vision, difficulty in micturition, sedation.

Comparative approach for antimuscarinics

- Oxybutynin relaxes urinary smooth muscle through a direct antispasmodic action on smooth muscle of the bladder.
- Flavoxate has a direct smooth muscle relaxation effect with very weak antimuscarinic activity, fewer side-effects but is less effective than oxybutynin.
- Tolterodine (Figure 41.1) offers functional uroselectivity and efficacy and side-effects are similar to those of modified-release oxybutynin. Side-effects may also include dyspepsia, fatigue, flatulence, chest pain, dry eyes, peripheral oedema.
- Darifenacin, propiverine, solifenacin and trospium (Figure 41.2) are newer products. Darifenacin and solifenacin have specific activity at the M_3 receptors. Propiverine also exhibits calcium channel-blocking effects.
- Oxybutynin and tolterodine are tertiary amines while trospium is a quaternary amine. Compounds with a quaternary ammonium structure present with unreliable absorption after oral administration. In fact trospium should be administered before food.

> - Oxybutynin has a short half-life. Modified-release preparations are preferred.
> - Flavoxate is less used. Tolterodine and trospium are preferred; both drugs require a twice daily dose administration.
> - Newer products (e.g. solifenacin and darifenacin) that are selective M_3 antimuscarinics have a lower probability of side-effects. They have a long half-life and are administered once daily.

H_3C CH_3 H_3C N CH_3 HO CH_3

Tolterodine, tertiary amine

Figure 41.1 Chemical structure of tolterodine.

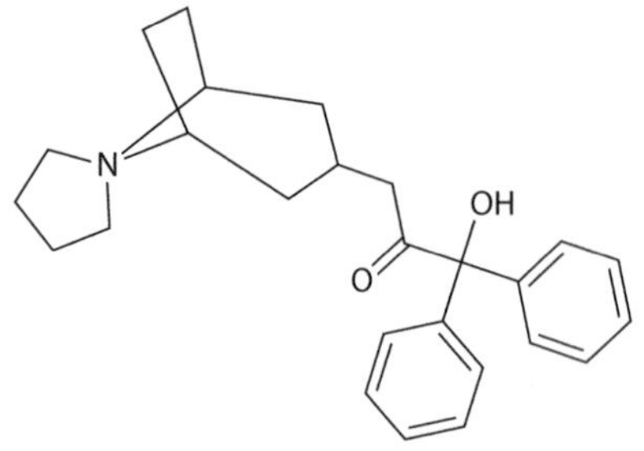

Figure 41.2 Chemical structure of trospium.

Other medications

- Antidepressants (e.g. imipramine) are used for nocturnal enuresis. They reduce bladder contractility and have a sedative effect.
- Oestrogen therapy including topical vaginal preparations may improve symptoms in postmenopausal women.

Duloxetine

- Indicated for stress urinary incontinence
- Is a serotonin–noradrenaline re-uptake inhibitor
- Used in conjunction with pelvic floor exercises
- Caution: cardiac disease, hypertension, history of mania/seizures, glaucoma, increased risk of bleeding
- Side-effects: nausea, vomiting, dyspepsia, constipation or diarrhoea, dry mouth, hot flushes, insomnia or drowsiness, anxiety, headache, dizziness, tremor, anorexia. Rarely urinary retention may occur.

Practice summary

- Review medication history, problem could be originating from drug therapy.
- Patient education and monitoring for adherence to therapy.
- Monitoring of occurrence of side-effects.
- Monitoring for effectiveness.
- Recommend use of absorbent products where necessary.

Question

1 Compare the use of oxybutynin and solifenacin in urinary incontinence.

Answer

1 Involuntary detrusor contractions cause urgency and urge incontinence, usually with frequency and nocturia. Antimuscarinic drugs reduce these contractions and increase bladder capacity. Oxybutynin has a direct relaxant effect on urinary smooth muscle. Side-effects limit the use of oxybutynin but they may be reduced by starting at a lower dose. A modified-release preparation of oxybutynin is effective and has fewer side-effects; a transdermal patch is also available. Solifenacin is a newer antimuscarinic drug selective to the M_3 receptor and is licensed for urinary frequency, urgency and incontinence. Since both oxybutynin and solifenacin are antimuscarinic drugs, cautions, contraindications and side-effects are similar. Cautions: the elderly, autonomic neuropathy, glaucoma, hiatus hernia, reflux oesophagitis, hepatic and renal impairment, cardiovascular disease, hyperthyroidism and prostatic hypertrophy. Contraindications: myasthenia gravis, significant bladder outflow obstruction or urinary retention, severe ulcerative colitis, toxic megacolon, gastrointestinal obstruction or intestinal atony. Side-effects: dry mouth, constipation, blurred vision, difficulty in micturition, sedation. Dosage regimen: oxybutynin is administered two to three times daily unless the modified-release preparation is used, while solifenacin is administered once daily.

Further reading

Gulliford G and Bidmead J (2001). Management of incontinence. *Pharm J* 267: 230–232.

Herbruck L F (2008). Stress urinary incontinence: an

overview of diagnosis and treatment options. *Urol Nurs* 28: 186–198.

Lee M and Weberski J (2005). Options for treatment of overactive bladder. In: *Pharmacy Today: Topics in patient care*. Washington DC: American Pharmacists Association.

National Institute for Health and Clinical Excellence (2006). Urinary incontinence: the management of urinary incontinence in women. http://www.nice.org.uk/cg40.

Thor K B and Viktrup K L (2007). Serotonin and noradrenaline involvement in urinary incontinence, depression and pain: scientific basis for overlapping clinical efficacy from a single drug, duloxetine. *Int J Clin Pract* 61: 1349–1355.

42

Cancer chemotherapy and palliative care

Learning objectives:

- To appreciate side-effects of cytotoxic chemotherapy agents
- To develop skills for patient advice and monitoring.

Background

Cancer represents a group of diseases including leukaemias, lymphomas and solid tumours. Treatment options include:

- surgery
- radiotherapy
- chemotherapy
- combined treatment modalities.

Lymphomas

These malignant tumours of lymph nodes or other lympathic tissue are classified into Hodgkin's disease and non-Hodgkin's disease.

- Clinical features: painless enlargement of lymph nodes especially in the neck, fever and weight loss.

Leukaemia

Haematological malignancy classified according to cell morphology (e.g. chronic lymphoid leukaemias).

- Clinical features: weakness, lethargy, anaemia, bleeding

Solid tumours

Can affect any organ. It represents a population of cells that have a growth regulatory defect.

- Ten commonest causes of solid tumour death: lung, breast (females), colon, prostate (males), stomach, oesophagus, pancreas, rectum, bladder, ovary (females)
- Clinical features: non-specific complaints (weight loss, bleeding, malaise, pain), presence of a painless lump
- Average number of tumour cells when clinically detectable: 10^8–10^9
- Average number of tumour cells in terminal stages of disease: 10^{12}.

Risk factors for cancer

- Occupational exposure: asbestos (lung)
- Environmental: ionising radiation (leukaemia, breast), UV radiation (skin)

- Lifestyle: tobacco (lung)
- Viruses: human papillomavirus (cervix)
- Genetic: breast, ovary, colon
- Iatrogenic: cytotoxic drugs (various).

Complications due to the malignant state include malnutrition, mechanical obstruction, pain, increased risk of venous thromboembolism and anaemia.

Diagnosis and treatment

Figure 42.1 shows the diagnostic process.

Performance status scales

These are physical rating scales applied before treatment to help in the prognosis and to indicate the patient's ability to withstand aggressive chemotherapy (e.g. Karnofsky's Performance Index and WHO Performance Scale).

Treatment objectives

- To cure: achieve remission, patient is completely disease free and has a normal life expectancy
- To provide palliation: bring disease under control with the hope of relieving disease symptoms and achieving a worthwhile increase in survival time
- To provide symptom relief: treatment has no antitumour effects (e.g. analgesics).

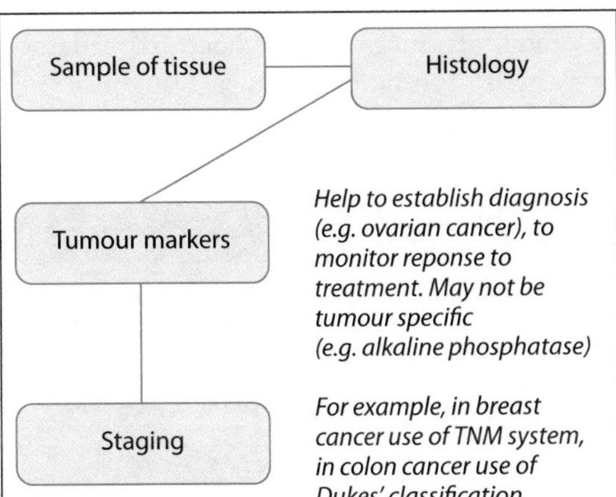

Figure 42.1 Diagnostic process.

Cytotoxic chemotherapy

In the 1950s it was demonstrated that chemotherapy was more effective when two or more drugs were used in combination regimens to achieve additive or synergistic effects (e.g. CMF – cyclophosphamide, methotrexate, fluorouracil combination for breast cancer). In combination chemotherapy, drugs included should have different mechanisms of action and minimal overlapping toxicities.

In the 1990s studies were started with regard to *in vivo* administration of high-dose chemotherapy with haematopoietic growth factors (e.g. epoietin) which counteract the bone marrow depression, a dose-limiting side-effect of cytotoxic drugs (see also Chapter 43).

Adjuvant chemotherapy

This follows definitive treatment of primary disease (e.g. surgery) and is adopted when the risk of subclinical metastatic disease is known to be high.

Neo-adjuvant chemotherapy

This is given before local therapy to reduce the primary tumour size, thereby rendering local therapy less destructive, more effective and easier.

Most cytotoxic drugs are teratogenic and all may cause life-threatening toxicity.

Guidelines on cytotoxic drug handling

- Reconstitution should be carried out in designated areas where a biological safety cabinet is available.
- Protective clothing should be worn (e.g. gloves, protective goggles).

Administration of cytotoxic drugs

- Dose of cytotoxic drugs is calculated for the individual patient based on body surface area.
- Some drugs have a maximum cumulative dose (e.g. doxorubicin: if total dose administered throughout the treatment is higher than 550 mg/m^2 risk of cardiomyopathy is increased).
- Treatment is given in cycles (e.g. up to six cycles with a 3- to 4-week interval between each cycle).
- Most drugs are administered parenterally and extravasation may be a problem.
- Extravasation: severe local tissue necrosis if leakage into the extravascular compartment occurs. If pain occurs during administration, administration is stopped and canula resited somewhere in another vein. Products that are associated with a risk of pain on extravasation include doxorubicin and the vinca alkaloids, such as vincristine and vinblastine.

Pharmacist intervention in cytotoxic chemotherapy administration

- Prevention of chemotherapy toxicity: managing nausea and vomiting, monitoring for bone marrow suppression
- Symptom management: advice on how to counteract symptoms, use of supportive therapy such as paracetamol and lifestyle modifications (e.g. good oral hygiene to decrease stomatitis)
- Provide appropriate verbal advice specific to the individual patient and provide written information about treatment.

Side-effects of chemotherapy

- Chemotherapy agents are not specific to tumour cells and hence cause toxicity to host tissues and organs where renewal of cell population is high (e.g. lymphoid tissue, bone marrow and epithelium of the gastrointestinal tract and skin).
- Chemotherapy may increase risk of venous thrombosis, especially in patients who have restricted mobility.
- Hypersensitivity reactions to cytotoxic chemotherapy agents (e.g. bleomycin, cisplatin, daunorubicin, paclitaxel, rituximab, trastuzumab) may occur. For drugs at high risk of hypersensitivity reactions, corticosteroids are administered intravenously simultaneously with drug administration.

Type of cancer, patient characteristics, other disease states and concomitant drug therapy may impact on the side-effect profile presented by individual patients.

The occurrence of side-effects in chemotherapy is summarised in Table 42.1.

Nausea and vomiting

Nausea and vomiting as a consequence of chemotherapy may be classified as:

- acute – occurring within 24 hours of treatment
- delayed – first incident occurring later than 24 hours after treatment

Table 42.1 Occurrence of side-effects

Immediate (hours)	Early (days)	Delayed (weeks)	Late (months/years)
Phlebitis due to extravasation	Ototoxicity	Pulmonary fibrosis	Sterility
Nausea, vomiting	Diarrhoea	Peripheral neuropathy	Premature menopause
Fever, chills	Stomatitis	Hyperpigmentation	Secondary malignancies
	Alopecia	Anaemia	
	Myelotoxicity		

- anticipatory – occurring prior to subsequent dose, very much related to occurrence of anxiety.

Occurrence varies depending on patient susceptibility; the risk is higher in women, patients under 50 years and anxious patients. It is also related to the emetic potential of drugs (Table 42.2).

Prevention of acute symptoms of nausea and vomiting

- Intravenous administration during treatment with $5HT_3$ serotonin antagonists (e.g. ondansetron) ± dexamethasone
- Pre-treatment with oral treatment: metoclopramide, domperidone, prochlorperazine.

Prevention of delayed symptoms of nausea and vomiting

- Oral metoclopramide is usually preferred with or without dexamethasone or prochlorperazine. Serotonin antagonists are less effective for delayed symptoms.

Prevention of anticipatory nausea and vomiting

- Oral metoclopramide started before treatment.
- Lorazepam (orally or intravenously) is helpful because it has a sedative, anxiolytic and amnesic effect.
- Good control of acute and delayed symptoms of nausea and vomiting decreases occurrence of anticipatory nausea.
- See also Chapter 18.

Granisetron vs ondansetron

- Granisetron has a longer half-life.
- Granisetron is more effective than ondansetron in combination with dexamethasone in preventing acute and delayed vomiting with highly emetogenic chemotherapy. This is of particular significance in offering better control on day 2 when patient is most likely to suffer from nausea and vomiting and is usually at home.

Table 42.2 Emetic potential of drugs

High	Moderate	Low
Cisplatin	Cyclophosphamide	Bleomycin
Dacarbazine	Doxorubicin	Fluorouracil
Ifosfamide	Mitozantrone Paclitaxel	Methotrexate Vincristine

Bone marrow suppression

- Occurs 7–10 days after treatment when white blood cell count is at *nadir* (lowest level), then recovery occurs after 20 days and this explains why treatment is given in cycles of 3–4 weeks.
- Before each treatment cycle, blood count is checked and if it is too low treatment has to be delayed.
- Patients should be advised to report immediately occurrence of fever and, if patient is neutropenic, antibacterial treatment is required.
- Consider use of granulocyte colony-stimulating factors (see Chapter 43).

See Table 42.3 for patient counselling on expected side-effects.

Chemotherapy agents

Cyclophosphamide

- An alkylating agent
- Administration by mouth or intravenously
- A urinary metabolite of cyclophosphamide, acrolein, may cause haemorrhagic cystitis and so advise patient to increase fluid intake for 24–48 hours after administration.

Antimetabolites

Methotrexate

- Administration by mouth or intravenously
- It has a folate-antagonist action and folinic acid (calcium folinate) is used to counteract this action and speed recovery from methotrexate-induced mucositis

Table 42.3 Patient counselling on expected side-effects

Bone marrow suppression	Expect tiredness Report bleeding Report signs of infection Good oral care
Alopecia (particularly occurs with doxorubicin, paclitaxel, vincristine, vinblastine)	Hair re-grows after treatment
Mucositis (particularly occurs with doxorubicin, fluorouracil, methotrexate)	Oral care: use of mouthwash Drink fluids and eat soft foods
Nausea and vomiting	Take tablets before meals Eat small frequent meals Avoid spicy and fried food

- Calcium folinate is given 24 hours after methotrexate, every 6 hours for two to eight doses, depending on dose of methotrexate used.

Capecitabine

- Metabolised to fluorouracil, an antimetabolite drug that is administered by intravenous injection since oral administration of fluorouracil is associated with unpredictable absorption
- Administered orally
- Monotherapy for metastatic colorectal cancer and breast cancer, and can also be used in combination therapy.

Pemetrexed and ralitrexed

- Inhibit thymidylate transferase
- Pemetrexed is used in lung cancer while ralitrexed is used in colorectal carcinoma
- Characteristic side-effects are myelosuppression and gastrointestinal toxicity.

Vinca alkaloids

- Vincristine, vinblastine, vinorelbine, which is a semi-synthetic vinca alkaloid
- Vincristine and to a lesser extent vinblastine and vinorelbine cause neurological toxicity: peripheral or autonomic neuropathy that is manifested as a tingling sensation and with constipation
- Myelosuppression occurs to a lesser extent with vincristine
- Vinorelbine is available for parenteral and oral administration. Vincristine and vinblastine are available only for parenteral administration.

Cytotoxic antibiotics

Bleomycin

- May cause hyperpigmentation and progressive pulmonary fibrosis, which is manifested as breathlessness
- Patient should be monitored for signs of lung disease.

Doxorubicin, daunorubicin

- May cause cardiomyopathy; monitor for occurrence of breathlessness, tiredness and malaise.

Liposomal formulations of doxorubicin

- Long-circulating pegylated liposomal formulation which is comparable in efficacy to doxorubicin
- Reduction in incidence of cardiotoxicity and lower potential for local necrosis
- Occurrence of hand–foot syndrome (painful, macular, reddening skin eruptions) after two to three treatment cycles. May be dose limiting. Prevention: cooling of hands and feet, avoid tight-fitting footwear for 4–7 days after treatment.

Platinum compounds

Cisplatin, carboplatin and oxaliplatin

- Commonly used for ovarian cancer and testicular teratoma
- Nephrotoxicity may occur: to avoid ensure pre-treatment hydration and prolonged hydration with intravenous fluids, monitor kidney function
- Ototoxicity may occur.

Taxanes

Palcitaxel and docetaxel

- Used for ovarian cancer and secondary treatment for breast cancer
- Hypersensitivity reactions can occur, peripheral neuropathy, cardiac conduction defects with arrhythmias, muscle pain, alopecia, oedema.

Topoisomerase I inhibitors

Irinotecan and topotecan

- Used for colorectal cancer and ovarian cancer respectively as a secondary line of treatment
- Gastrointestinal side-effects, particularly diarrhoea, and asthenia, alopecia and anorexia may occur.

Protein kinase inhibitors

Imatinib, dasatinib

- Tyrosine kinase inhibitors
- Used in leukaemia
- Available for oral administration.

Erlotinib

- A tyrosine kinase inhibitor that is available for oral administration; licensed for the treatment of pancreatic and lung cancer.

Sunitinib

- A tyrosine kinase inhibitor that is available for oral administration; licensed for the treatment of renal cell carcinoma.

Sorafenib

- An inhibitor of multiple kinases which is licensed for renal cell and hepatocellular carcinoma.

Trastuzumab

- For metastatic breast cancer with tumours overexpressing the human epidermal growth factor receptor 2 (HER-2)
- May be used in combination with paclitaxel
- Caution: cardiotoxicity may occur, special care when used in combination with anthracyclines (e.g. doxorubicin).

Pharmacists are engaged in:

- developing standard dosage systems (e.g. CMF in breast cancer), which leads to efficient utilisation of pharmacy staff time
- collating evidence for specific treatment regimens in different types of cancers
- developing treatment protocols on evidence-based care (e.g. all women with early breast cancer should receive 3–6 months of adjuvant polychemotherapy)
- estimating costings and identifying priorities of funding within a National Health Service scheme.

Palliative care

- Care of patients where disease is not responsive to curative treatment
- Attention to physical, emotional and spiritual needs of the patient and close carers
- Assessment of symptoms and needs of the patient
- Drug treatment: minimise number of drugs, adjust dose and pharmaceutical dosage form, ensure accessibility to medication.

Pain management in palliative care

- Analgesics are more effective in preventing pain than in the relief of established pain. The aims are to prevent occurrence of pain using analgesics.
- Consider use of non-opioid (paracetamol) and opioid analgesics.

- Initiation of opioid analgesics should not be delayed by concerns of dependence.
- Consider managing side-effects of opioid drugs particularly nausea and constipation by using antiemetic agents and laxatives when opioid analgesia is started.

Practice summary

- In the management of cancer, education and support of patient and carers are essential to ensure good quality of life of patients.
- Monitoring of occurrence of side-effects: nausea and vomiting, bone marrow suppression, liver function (e.g. doxorubicin to reduce dose; methotrexate and paclitaxel to avoid in severe hepatic impairment), renal failure (e.g. cisplatin and ifosfamide to avoid; methotrexate and cyclophosphamide to reduce dose).
- Pharmacogenetic implications in the selection of drug therapy (e.g. trastuzumab).
- Future considerations: chronotherapy leading to appropriate timing of administration of antineoplastic agents may improve efficacy and diminish toxicity due to variation in enzyme levels in circadian rhythm (e.g. irinotecan and capecitabine are prodrugs), bioactivation depends on enzyme activity (carboxyesterases). Consider use of programmable automatic drug delivery systems.
- In palliative care, patient access to medications that encompass different systems (e.g. opioid analgesics, antidepressants, laxatives, antiemetics, adjuvant analgesics) should be ensured.

Questions

1. Explain the rationale of using liposomal formulations of doxorubucin. Describe side-effects that may occur with the administration of this product.
2. Explain the rationale of applying pharmacogenetic principles when considering trastuzumab therapy in metastatic breast cancer. What cautions are required when administering trastuzumab?
3. Giving reasons for your answer, explain when opioids are used in palliative care. List factors that should be considered in pain management in palliative care.
4. What are the disadvantages associated with the use of morphine sulphate solution in patients with terminal cancer?

Answers

1. Liposomal formulations of doxorubicin have comparable efficacy with doxorubicin. However, they have a decreased risk of cardiotoxicity and local necrosis. Side-effects that may occur with the administration of doxorubicin (including the liposomal formulations) include nausea and vomiting, alopecia and bone marrow suppression.
2. Trastuzumab is effective in patients who respond positively to a test to identify tumours that overexpress human epidermal growth factor receptor 2 (HER-2). When administering trastuzumab cardiotoxicity may occur and risk is increased if administered with anthracyclines (e.g. doxorubicin). Concomitant use with anthracyclines should be avoided.
3. Palliative care is the care of patients where disease is not responsive to curative treatment and where attention is given to the physical, emotional and spiritual needs of the patient and close carers. In palliative care both non-opioid and opioid analgesics are used and the initiation of opioids should not be delayed by concerns of dependence. Analgesics are more effective in preventing pain than in the relief of established pain and therefore it is imperative that analgesia is provided to prevent the occurrence of pain. When considering drug treatment in palliative care it is important to assess the symptoms and needs of the patient and to minimise the number of drugs used, adjust doses and pharmaceutical dosage forms and ensure accessibility to medication. Common side-effects of opioid analgesics are nausea and constipation. These side-effects should be managed, for example nausea with metoclopramide and constipation with an osmotic laxative such as lactulose or a stimulant laxative such as senna.

4 Side-effects of opioids include nausea and vomiting and constipation. The occurrence of these side-effects requires the use of antiemetics such as metoclopramide and laxatives such as lactulose. The unwanted effect of dependence is not an issue that should limit use of morphine in terminally ill patients. However, occurrence of tolerance requires dose adjustments so as to maintain the patient pain free.

Further reading

Mader R M and Schwarz U (2004). Safety concerns in oncology pharmacy – an evidence based approach. *Eur J Hosp Pharm* 6: 28.

Wiela-Hojenska A and Orzechowska-Juzwenko K (2004). Optimisation and individualization of anticancer chemotherapy. *Eur J Hosp Pharm* 6: 24–25.

43

Anaemia and drug-induced blood dyscrasias

Learning objectives:

- To review presentation and management of iron-deficiency anaemia and megalobastic anaemia
- To appreciate occurrence and management of anaemia in chronic disease and malignancy
- To identify drugs that cause blood dyscrasias
- To review use of drugs in the management of neutropenia.

Background

Anaemia is a group of disorders where there is either:

- a decrease in haemoglobin synthesis which may be due to lack of nutrient or bone marrow failure OR
- an increase in haemoglobin loss due to haemorrhage or haemolysis.

Diagnostic tests

- Full blood count (FBC)
- Red blood cell count
- Red blood cell indices
- Haemoglobin
- White blood cell count
- Platelet count.

Red blood cell (RBC) count

- Male 4.7–6.1 $\times$ 10^6/mm^3, female 4.2–5.4 $\times$ 10^6/mm^3
- Level is decreased: anaemia, haemorrhage, bone marrow failure, renal disease, pregnancy
- Level is increased: dehydration, chronic obstructive pulmonary disease (COPD), congenital heart disease.

Haemoglobin

- Male 14–18 g/dL, female 12–16 g/dL (reduced in the elderly)
- Drugs that may lower level: antibiotics, aspirin, sulphonamides.

Red blood cell indices

- Mean corpuscular volume (MCV):
  - increased in pernicious anaemia
  - decreased in iron-deficiency anaemia, anaemia of chronic illness
- Mean corpuscular hameoglobin concentration (MCHC):
  - decreased in iron-deficiency anaemia.

Iron-deficiency anaemia

Causes of iron-deficiency anaemia

- Chronic blood loss: gastrointestinal disease, drug induced, menstrual loss
- Increased requirements: pregnancy
- Malabsorption
- Dietary deficiency.

Clinical presentation of iron-deficiency anaemia

- Pale skin and mucous membranes
- Glossitis
- Angular stomatitis
- Koilonychia
- Dysphagia
- Pica
- Atrophic gastritis.

It is important to exclude any underlying cause of anaemia that warrants further investigation (e.g. gastrointestinal bleeding due to cancer).

Iron

- Oral administration is the preferred method of administration
- Patient monitoring: haemoglobin level, clinical symptoms
- Side-effects: gastrointestinal irritation (nausea, pain), constipation or diarrhoea
- Caution: patients with inflammatory bowel disease may present with an exacerbation of diarrhoea, diverticular disease
- Patient advice: may discolour stools, absorption is better if taken on an empty stomach, take after meals if gastrointestinal side-effects occur
- Also available in combination with folic acid as an oral dosage form, intended for use during pregnancy.

Factors influencing which product to use

- Efficacy: absorption
- Patient acceptability: side-effects, frequency of administration (modified-release formulations are available but these may be associated with poor absorption)
- Cost.

Parenteral iron therapy

This may be considered in the case of:

- excessive adverse effects from oral iron or with poor patient compliance
- malabsorption of oral iron
- continuing severe blood loss.

It may cause anaphylactic reactions, hypersensitivity reactions (urticaria, hypotension).

Iron dextran injection

This is a complex of iron and dextrans administered by deep intramuscular injection. Staining at the intramuscular injection site can occur due to leakage of iron along the needle track.

Iron sucrose injection

This is a complex of iron and sucrose that may be administered as slow intravenous injection or by intravenous infusion.

Iron prophylaxis

This is indicated in patients at high risk of iron deficiency, such as those with gastrointestinal conditions leading to malabsorption (previous gastrointestinal surgery), menorrhagia, pregnancy, haemodialysis or poor diet.

Megaloblastic anaemia

Causes of megaloblastic anaemia

- Vitamin B_{12} deficiency: malabsorption, pernicious anaemia – lack of gastric intrinsic factor
- Folate deficiency: inadequate intake, malabsorption, increased demands
- Drugs: anticonvulsants, trimethoprim, methotrexate.

> Vitamin B_{12} prophylaxis should be considered in patients who have undergone partial or total gastrectomy or total ileal resection.

Clinical features of megaloblastic anaemia

- Glossitis
- Angular stomatitis
- Altered bowel movements
- Anorexia
- Jaundice.

Dietary sources

- Vitamin B_{12}: meat, fish, eggs, cheese, milk
- Folic acid: fruit, green vegetables, yeast.

Treatment of vitamin B_{12} deficiency: hydroxycobalamin

- Large doses of folic acid can reverse the megaloblastic anaemia caused by vitamin B_{12} deficiency but do not reverse the neurological damage of vitamin B_{12} deficiency. It is important that in patients with vitamin B_{12} deficiency folic acid monotherapy is not adopted.
- Hydroxycobalamin is retained in the body for longer than cyanocobalamin and treatment can be given every 3 months.
- Given by intramuscular injection.
- Initial dose: 1 mg every 2–3 days for five times.
- Maintenance dose: given every 3 months.

Treatment of folic acid deficiency anaemia

- In deficiency, folic acid replacement therapy of 5–15 mg a day for about 4–6 months replenishes depleted stores.
- In pregnancy daily supplementation reduces the occurrence of neural tube defects. Women at low risk of neural tube defects should take 400 micrograms daily pre-conception and during pregnancy.
- Women at high risk of neural tube defects should take 5 mg daily pre-conception and during pregnancy. Risk is increased when either partner has a neural tube defect or a family history of neural tube defects, coeliac disease, diabetes or sickle cell anaemia, or are taking antiepileptic medicines.

Glucose-6-phosphate dehydrogenase deficiency anaemia

- Leads to haemolytic anaemia
- Triggered by certain drugs (e.g. quinolones, nalidixic acid, sulphonamides, aspirin).

Anaemia and chronic renal failure

Anaemia occurs due to reduced renal erythropoietin production and the accumulation of toxic metabolites which lead to reduced red blood cell lifespan.

Management

- Recombinant human erythropoietins (epoetin alfa and beta).
- Erythropoiesis-stimulating factor darbepoetin alfa has a longer half-life therefore less frequent administration than epoetin is required.
- Methoxy polyethylene glycol-epoetin beta (pegzerepoetin alfa) – a continuous erythropoietin receptor activator – has a longer duration of action than epoetin.
- Administered by intravenous or subcutaneous injection.

- Caution: overcorrection of haemoglobin concentration; such a situation may increase the risk of thrombosis.
- Patient monitoring: blood pressure, haemoglobin level.
- Side-effects: peripheral oedema, hypertension, arrhythmias, flu-like symptoms, nausea and vomiting.
- Note: pure red cell aplasia may occur due to formation of neutralising anti-erythropoietin antibodies (severe anaemia resistant to epoetin which may develop after 3–67 months of treatment). Patients who develop pure red cell aplasia should not be switched to other erythropoietins.

Use of corticosteroids in anaemia

- Oral prednisolone is used in autoimmune haemolytic anaemia
- Slows or stops haemolysis
- Monitor haemoglobin levels.

Anaemia due to chronic illness

- Occurs in conditions of chronic infections, chronic inflammation, malignancy
- Develops after 1–2 months of the disease
- Cytokine release from neoplastic cells or injured cells results in reduced production of red blood cells
- Activation of macrophages which results in reduced lifespan of red blood cells
- Consider use of erythropoietins in patients presenting with anaemia in malignancy who are receiving chemotherapy.

Drugs that can cause pancytopenia

- Chloramphenicol
- Anticonvulsants
- Carbimazole
- Meprobamate
- Tricyclic antidepressants
- Phenothiazines
- Cytotoxic drugs.

Drugs that can cause neutropenia

- Antihistamines
- H_2-receptor blockers
- Captopril
- Metronidazole
- Mianserin
- Sulfasalazine.

Drugs that can cause thrombocytopenia

- Carbamazepine
- Meprobamate
- Methyldopa
- Thiazide diuretics
- Tetracyclines
- Paracetamol.

Drugs used in neutropenia

- Recombinant human granulocyte colony-stimulating factor (rhG-CSF): filgrastim, lenograstim, pegfilgrastim (pegylated derivative of filgrastim which presents a longer duration of action)
- Stimulate the production of neutrophils
- Used in specialist scenario in congenital neutropenia, chemotherapy-induced neutropenia, bone marrow transplantation
- Administration: subcutaneous route
- Caution: malignant myeloid conditions, pulmonary infiltration
- Side-effects: gastrointestinal disturbances, headache, asthenia, fever, musculoskeletal and bone pain, rash, alopecia and leukocytosis
- Monitor: temperature, full blood count, cardiac function
- Do not use 24 hours before or after cytotoxic agents.

Practice summary

- Occurrence of anaemia is a sign of an underlying condition which should be assessed.
- Oral administration of iron is preferred. Patient

should be advised to take preparation before food to increase absorption.

- Use of erythropoietins and recombinant human granulocyte colony-stimulating factors require patient monitoring.
- Erythropoietins may be used to shorten the period of symptomatic anaemia in patients receiving cytotoxic chemotherapy but should not be used in patients with anaemia associated with cancer since data indicate that there is a risk of increased mortality and tumour progression.

Questions

1. Name two factors that could lead to iron-deficiency anaemia.
2. Describe side-effects that could occur with administration of filgrastim and outline patient monitoring required.

Answers

1. Heavy menstrual flow, perforated peptic ulcer.
2. Side-effects include gastrointestinal disturbances, headache, asthenia, fever, musculoskeletal and bone pain, rash, alopecia and leukocytosis. Patient monitoring: full blood count, body temperature, blood pressure and pulse rate.

Further reading

Ardevol M, Fontsere N, Casals M, Bonal J, Garcia L, Gabas J *et al.* (2006). A feasibility cost-analysis study of recombinant human erythropoietin and darbepoetin alfa in ambulatory haemodialysis patients during current clinical practice. *Eur J Hosp Pharm Sci* 12: 47–51.

Macdougall I C (2006). The treatment of anaemia in renal disease. *Eur J Hosp Pharm Pract* 12: 46–48.

Mughal T I (2006). The use of erythropoietin in cancer patients. *Hosp Pharm Eur* March/April: 52–53.

44

Rheumatoid arthritis

Learning objectives:

- To characterise presentation of rheumatoid arthritis and its management
- To appreciate the use of disease-modifying antirheumatic drugs and biologic agents in the management of rheumatoid arthritis
- To develop skills required to ensure patient safety and to plan patient monitoring required.

Background

Rheumatoid arthritis is a chronic systemic inflammatory disease characterised by joint involvement as well as extra-articular manifestations. Chronic inflammation of synovial tissue lining of joints (pannus) causes proliferation and erodes the bone surface and cartilage.

The extra-articular features of rheumatoid arthritis are listed in Table 44.1.

Table 44.1 Extra-articular features of rheumatoid arthritis

Common	Uncommon
Anaemia	Pleural effusion
Muscle wasting	Pulmonary fibrosis
Dry eyes	Pericarditis
Depression	Systemic vasculitis
Osteoporosis	Mitral valve and conduction defects
Leg ulcers	
Lymphadenopathy	

Epidemiology

- Most common chronic inflammatory disease of the joint
- Two per cent of males and 5% of females over the age of 55 years have rheumatoid arthritis
- Age of onset reaches its peak in the fourth decade.

Clinical presentation

- Fatigue, weakness, swelling of soft tissues around joints
- Stiffness and muscle aches, especially morning stiffness
- Joint involvement is symmetrical
- Haematologic tests: anaemia, thrombocytosis, increased erythrocyte sedimentation rate (ESR), increased C-reactive protein, rheumatoid factor positive.

Diagnostic criteria

- Morning stiffness
- Arthritis of three or more joint areas (e.g. wrists, elbows, shoulders, knees)

- Arthritis of hand joints
- Symmetrical swelling of same joint areas
- Serum rheumatoid factor
- Radiographic features of rheumatoid arthritis
- Rheumatoid nodules.

Prognosis

- 20% of patients achieve remission with no further disease
- 25% obtain remission with mild residual disease
- 45% have persistent activity with variable progressive deformity
- 10% progress to complete disability.

Goals of treatment

- Relieve symptoms of pain, swelling and stiffness
- Preserve joint function
- Prevent further disease progression
- Improve quality of life of patient
- Deal with extra-articular manifestations.

In rheumatoid arthritis, patients may present with chronic joint pain and inflammation. This may lead to decreased activity which can result in loss in range of motion, atrophy and weakness of affected limb or joint. Non-pharmacotherapeutic recommendations such as appropriate physical therapy and the use of prosthetic devices may help to maintain mobility.

Drug therapy

- NSAIDs
- Steroids
- Drugs that suppress the disease process:
  - disease-modifying antirheumatic drugs (DMARDs)
  - gold
  - antimalarials: hydroxychloroquine
  - immunosuppressants: methotrexate, sulfasalazine, leflunomide
  - biologic agents: adalimunab, anakinra, etanercept, infliximab.

Figure 44.1 shows the treatment approach.

Disease-modifying antirheumatic drugs

DMARDs are used to interfere with the progression of the disease. A full therapeutic response may not be obtained before 2–6 months of therapy. Hence, drug therapy changes should not be undertaken within a few weeks of initiation of therapy.

Sulfasalazine and methotrexate are usually the preferred first-line DMARDs because they are better tolerated than penicillamine and gold. A combination of two or more DMARDs may be considered in patients where monotherapy is not leading to the therapeutic objective.

The DMARDS used to treat rheumatoid arthritis are summarised in Table 44.2.

Methotrexate

- Suitable for moderate-to-severe disease
- Onset of action within 4–6 weeks

Conventional	Current trend
NSAIDs	Since joint destruction develops within the first 2 years of disease early treatment with disease-modifying anti-rheumatic drugs (DMARDs) is recommended
DMARDs	Combination therapy with different DMARDs and consideration of the use of biologic agents

Figure 44.1 Treatment approach.

Table 44.2 Disease-modifying antirheumatic drugs used to treat rheumatoid arthritis

Drug	Dose schedule	Side-effects	Monitoring
Sulfasalazine (oral)	Initially 500 mg once daily increasing to 1 g three times daily	Nausea, reversible male infertility, rashes, bone marrow suppression, hepatitis	FBC and LFTs monthly for first 3 months and then every 3 months. If stable for 1 year every 6 months, renal function tests and electrolytes every 6 months
Methotrexate (oral)	5–25 mg once weekly	Rashes, nausea, stomatitis, marrow suppression, hepatitis, pneumonitis	FBC and LFTs fortnightly until 4 weeks after last dose increase, thereafter every 6 months; renal function tests and electrolytes every 6 months
Sodium aurothiomalate (gold, IM) auranofin (gold, orally)	10 mg IM test dose then 50 mg weekly until signs of remission and then reduce to monthly dose	Gastrointestinal disturbances, stomatitis, diarrhoea rashes, marrow suppression, proteinuria	FBC, urinalysis prior to each dose since it may cause proteinuria, annually chest X-ray
Hydroxychloroquine (oral)	Initially 400 mg in divided doses, maintenance of 200–400 mg daily to be taken with or after food and not at the same time as indigestion medicines	Gastrointestinal disturbances, headache, skin reactions, ECG changes, visual disturbances, convulsions, blood disorders	Renal function tests, LFTs, visual acuity, FBC, ECG
Ciclosporin (oral)	2.5 mg/kg per day in two divided doses	Hirsutism, gingival hyperplasia, hypertension, renal impairment	Every 15 days: U&Es, BP, urinalysis then 1–2 monthly
Azathioprine (oral)	1.5–2.5 mg/kg per day	Gastrointestinal disturbances, diarrhoea, marrow suppression	Every 15 days for 2–3 months: FBC, U&Es, LFTs and then 1–2 monthly

BP, blood pressure; FBC, full blood count; LFTs, liver function tests; U&Es, urea and electrolytes.

- Single weekly oral dose is the most common dosage regimen. May be administered subcutaneously or intramuscularly
- Avoid alcohol intake to reduce risk of hepatic fibrosis and liver toxicity
- Monitor liver function, full blood count, renal function
- Nausea and stomatitis can be managed by addition of folic acid dose once every week, a day after the administration of the methotrexate dose
- Patient education on dosage regimen and symptoms to be reported to health professionals is required. Patients should be advised to seek advice if dyspnoea or cough (symptoms of pulmonary toxicity), if easy bruising or bleeding (symptoms of thrombocytopenia), if sore throat or fever (symptoms of neutrophilia) develop. The rationale for using methotrexate, which patients may associate with the treatment of cancer, needs to be explained since otherwise patients may be hesitant to take the drug as it is an anticancer agent
- Patients should not take aspirin or other NSAIDs on same day of administration of methotrexate, since concomitant administration reduces methotrexate elimination from the body, leading to increased toxicity
- Teratogenic: discontinue 6 months before planned conception.

Leflunomide

- As effective as methotrexate and sulfasalazine, and may present better quality of life to patients

who cannot achieve stabilisation in their condition with these two agents
- Presented as oral therapy but is more expensive than methotrexate and sulfasalazine
- Side-effects: gastrointestinal disturbances, headache, hypertension, alopecia, rash, bone marrow toxicity, rarely potentially life-threatening hepatoxicity, increased risk of malignancy
- Cautions: renal and hepatic impairment
- Contraindications: a history of tuberculosis, impaired bone marrow function
- Patient monitoring: liver function tests, full blood count, blood pressure, monitor for signs of thrombocytopenia (easy bruising, bleeding) and neutropenia (sore throat, fever)
- Leflunomide has an active metabolite that has a long half-life and therefore this has to be taken into consideration with the occurrence of adverse effects, stopping the treatment, and when switching to other DMARDs
- Teratogenic: in patients planning to conceive, leflunomide treatment has to be withdrawn for 2 years in women and 3 months in males before conception.

Biologic agents

- These products are more expensive than other DMARDs. They are used in patients resistant to conventional DMARDs.

> In rheumatoid arthritis, patients are reviewed periodically and adjustments to drug therapy are required according to clinical presentation. Effectiveness of the conventional DMARDs may diminish as the disease progresses or due to unacceptability of the treatment regimen. Patient monitoring relies on identifying occurrence of side-effects, monitoring clinical parameters that may be affected by the drug, measuring patient's quality of life and discussing specific issues such as family planning.

- Adalimumab, etanercept and infliximab inhibit the activity of tumour necrosis factor alpha (TNFα). TNFα is believed to mediate inflammation in rheumatoid arthritis.
- They are used in combination with methotrexate or leflunomide except in patients where methotrexate is contraindicated or cannot be tolerated.
- Caution: administration has been associated with occurrence of infections, including tuberculosis, septicaemia and hepatitis B reactivation. Therefore before starting treatment, screen for infections including tuberculosis (chest X-ray, tuberculin skin test) and hepatitis B. Before planning a pregnancy, women should consult with health professionals when taking these drugs or immediately after stopping the drugs.
- Side-effects: predisposition to infections, nausea, abdominal pain, worsening of heart failure, hypersensitivity reactions, fever, headache, depression, antibody formation, pruritus, injection site reaction, blood disorders.
- Patient monitoring: monitor for infections, symptoms of heart failure and hypersensitivity reactions.

The routes of administration for biologic agents are shown in Table 44.3.

Anakinra

- An interleukin-1-receptor antagonist
- Interleukin 1 appears to mediate bone and cartilage destruction
- Side-effects: development of severe infections and neutropenia commonly reported
- Patient monitoring: full blood count should be done routinely to monitor for neutropenia; assess

Table 44.3 Routes of administration for biologic agents

Drug	Route of administration
Adalimumab	Subcutaneous injection
Etanercept	Subcutaneous injection
Infliximab	Intravenous infusion

occurrence of symptoms suggestive of neutropenia such as fever, sore throat and infection.

Abatacept

- Prevents full activation of T lymphocytes
- Is used in combination with methotrexate but should not be used in patients receiving TNF inhibitors
- Similar to the other biologics, it increases predisposition to infection and may cause blood dyscrasias
- Side-effects: abdominal pain, diarrhoea, dyspepsia, nausea, flushing, hypertension, cough, dizziness, fatigue, headache, infection, rhinitis, rash.

Corticosteroids

Patients receiving DMARDs and biologic agents should be advised to report immediately signs of bone marrow suppression such as easy bruising or bleeding (in thrombocytopenia) and sore throat or fever (in neutrophilia). With biologic agents risk of serious infections is higher and patients should be monitored for occurrence of these signs and educated to contact immediately a health professional should signs of an infection develop.

- Corticosteroids in rheumatoid arthritis provide a rapid anti-inflammatory response in contrast to the slow response given by DMARDs.
- Side-effects associated with long-term high doses limit their place in therapy. If long-term therapy is required, monitor bone mineral density and consider using calcium supplementation and prophylactic therapy for osteoporosis (see Chapter 46).
- Usually oral prednisolone is used for temporary relief during a flare-up or as a bridge therapy until DMARD therapy becomes effective and then the corticosteroid dose is tapered off slowly.
- Administration of oral dose may be carried out in divided doses rather than as a single dose in the morning. The advantage of administering corticosteroids orally as a single morning dose is that it mimics early morning physiological secretion of cortisol, reducing hypothalamic–pituitary–adrenal axis suppression. On the other hand, in rheumatoid arthritis a once-daily morning dose may lead to a reduced anti-inflammatory effect during the night, resulting in early morning stiffness when the patient wakes up and is still due for the next dose.

Non-steroidal anti-inflammatory drugs

The use of NSAIDs should be to supplement DMARDs and maintain the patient as symptom free as possible. Their use should be reviewed periodically so as to use them for the shortest time possible (see also Chapter 31).

Some non-selective NSAIDs are listed in Table 44.4.

COX-2 selectivity

- Cyclo-oxygenase-2-selective inhibitors are indicated for patients who are at high risk of developing gastroduodenal ulceration or bleeding. Such patients include the elderly, patients on concomitant medication which increases risk such as on SSRIs and patients with a past medical history of gastroduodenal ulceration or bleeding.
- They are not to be used for routine management and should not be used in combination with low-dose aspirin, which reduces the benefit of COX-2.
- Pulmonary sensitivity to aspirin involves the COX-1 enzyme and therefore use of COX-2 inhibitors can be undertaken with caution in patients who are aspirin sensitive.
- Selective NSAIDs are associated more with increased risk of thrombotic events, namely

Table 44.4 Examples of non-selective non-steroidal anti-inflammatory drugs

Drug	Dose for oral administration
Acetic acids	
Diclofenac	75–150 mg in 3 doses
Anthranilic acids	
Mefenamic acid	1500 mg in 3 doses
Indole derivatives	
Indometacin	50–200 mg in 3 doses
Propionic acids	
Naproxen	500–1000 mg in 2 doses
Ibuprofen	1.2–2.4 g in 3–4 doses
Ketoprofen	100–200 mg in 2–4 doses
Tiaprofenic acid	600 mg in 2 doses
Butanone	
Nabumetone	1–1.5 g in 1–2 doses
Oxicams	
Piroxicam	15–30 mg in 1–2 doses
Meloxicam	7.5–15 mg in 1 dose

myocardial infarction and stroke, compared with the non-selective NSAIDs. However, non-selective NSAIDs may also be associated with this risk.
- Examples: partial selectivity – meloxicam; COX-2 selective – celecoxib.

Factors contributing to response to NSAIDs

- Lipid solubility: more lipid soluble, therefore greater anti-inflammatory activity, analgesia and CNS toxicity (e.g. indometacin)
- Prodrug: may be less nephrotoxic (e.g. sulindac) and produce fewer gastrointestinal side-effects (e.g. nabumetone).

Side-effects

- Gastrointestinal: nausea and indigestion, peptic ulceration
- Renal: reversible acute renal failure
- Respiratory: exacerbation of asthma in patients
- Central nervous system: headache, drowsiness, confusion
- Skin: rashes.

Cautions and contraindications

- To be used with caution in patients with renal impairment since they may cause acute renal failure and in patients with cardiac disease or hepatic impairment since they may cause fluid retention which will impact negatively on the cardiac or hepatic disease.
- For selective NSAID cautions: history of heart failure, left ventricular dysfunction, hypertension, oedema, patients at risk of heart disease.
- Contraindicated in severe heart failure, active peptic ulceration.
- For selective NSAIDs contraindications: ischaemic heart disease, cerebrovascular disease, peripheral arterial disease, moderate-to-severe heart failure.

Drug interactions of NSAIDs are listed in Table 44.5.

When NSAID use is started in patients receiving antihypertensives, the hypotensive effect may be antagonised. This may be witnessed during blood pressure monitoring upon introduction of NSAID therapy.

Factors to consider when choosing a specific NSAID

- Relative efficacy
- Toxicity
- Concomitant drugs

Table 44.5 Drug interactions of NSAIDs

Affected drug	Effect
Oral anticoagulants	Increased risk of gastrointestinal bleeding, antiplatelet effects
Selective serotonin re-uptake inhibitors	Increased risk of bleeding
Ciclosporin	Increased risk of nephrotoxicity
Diuretics	Decreased diuretic effect, increased risk of nephrotoxicity

- Concurrent disease states
- Patient's age
- Renal function
- Dosing frequency
- Cost.

Practice summary

- It is important to check that the patient is taking the correct medicine at the correct dose.
- This is particularly relevant for patients on methotrexate, which is a weekly dose.
- It may be difficult for patients to access medicine (e.g. problems with managing blister packs due to impaired manual dexterity).
- Quantitative tools should be used to assess the effect of condition on patients' activities and joint involvement.
- Regular patient monitoring and follow-up are required and drug therapy should be adjusted accordingly.

Question

1 Name three side-effects that are associated with systemic oral use of methotrexate and discuss pharmaceutical care issues in patients receiving methotrexate.

Answer

1 Side-effects: gastrointestinal (nausea and vomiting, dyspepsia), bone marrow suppression, pulmonary fibrosis. Pharmaceutical care issues: patient education on the inflammatory condition and on the treatment. Patient should be advised to report any signs and symptoms of infection and any symptoms indicating precipitation of the condition. Patient should be advised on drug administration since normally dose is taken once weekly, followed the day after by a dose of folic acid (to prevent oral mucositis). Patient should be advised of the importance of attending scheduled appointments including appointments for blood tests. Patient monitoring required includes evaluation of disease management, identification of drug-related problems and monitoring of renal and liver function and a full blood count. For women of child-bearing age, pregnancy and family planning must be discussed since treatment review may be required if patient is planning a pregnancy.

Further reading

Breedveld F C and Huizinga T W J (2005). Rheumatoid arthritis: what's around the corner? *Eur J Hosp Pharm* 3: 58–59.

Bayraktar A, Hudson S, Watson A and Fraser S (2000). Arthritis. *Pharm J* 264: 57–68.

Doan Q V, Chiou C and Dubois R W (2006). Review of eight pharmacoeconomic studies of the value of biologic DMARDs in the management of rheumatoid arthritis. *Eur J Hosp Pharm* 12: 555–559.

National Institute for Health and Clinical Excellence (2009). Rheumatoid arthritis: the management of rheumatoid arthritis in adults. http://guidance.nice.org.uk/CG79.

Seed M (2009). Development of disease-modifying treatments for rheumatoid arthritis. *Pharm J* 2009; 282: 191–192.

Acknowledgements

Bernard Coleiro, Consultant Physician and Rheumatologist, Department of Medicine, Mater Dei Hospital, Malta

45

Osteoarthritis and gout

Learning objectives:

- To understand rationale for drug therapy and identify characteristics of the drugs used in the management of osteoarthritis and gout
- To develop skills required to provide patient support in the management of osteoarthritis and gout.

Background

In osteoarthritis there is breakdown of articular cartilage that lines the joint surface in weight-bearing areas. Dense bone formation at the base of cartilage lesion occurs.

Clinical presentation of osteoarthritis

- Localised deep aching pain
- Pain on motion
- Stiffness
- Local tenderness
- Bony proliferation
- Occurrence of symptoms may be related to weather.

Therapeutic goals in osteoarthritis

- Pain relief
- Increased mobility
- Reduction of disability and minimisation of disease progression.

Non-drug therapy of osteoarthritis

- Loss of weight in overweight individuals
- Physical therapy: application of heat, exercise programmes
- Avoiding excessive load on the joint involved through use of walking support devices or appropriate shoes.

Drug therapy in osteoarthritis

- Simple analgesia
- NSAIDs (see Chapter 44)
- Steroids: intra-articular corticosteroids
- Chondroprotective agents
- Viscosupplements
- Topical rubefacients.

Simple analgesics

- Paracetamol is now accepted as a first-line therapy, taken on a regular basis (up to 4 g per day) or on an as-required basis. It is not associated with side-effects and is as effective as NSAIDs for the symptomatic pain relief of osteoarthritis.

- Compound analgesics: products containing an opioid analgesic and a non-opioid analgesic. However, the content of opioids may be at somewhat subtherapeutic doses. These products may present with constipation as a side-effect.

Intra-articular corticosteroids

- Used to reduce pain and relieve synovitis associated with acute attacks
- May cause direct cartilage injury and accelerate cartilage loss
- Injection is not carried out more frequently than every 3 months since repeated injections in the same joint may lead to joint damage such as joint capsule calcification and microcrystalline deposits of corticosteroid in the synovial fluid
- Dose differs according to joint (e.g. dose for administration of methylprednisolone acetate to the knee is 20–80 mg).

Chondroprotective agents

- Examples: chondroitin, glucosamine.
- Improve cartilage metabolism, counteracting the destruction of cartilage.
- When used chronically they result in improvement in pain and function in patients with osteoarthritis. Further studies are required to understand mechanism of action.
- For glucosamine it should be used with caution in patients with impaired glucose tolerance and in patients with a predisposition to cardiovascular disease.
- Hypercholesterolaemia may occur as a side-effect. Common side-effects include nausea, abdominal pain, indigestion, diarrhoea, constipation, headache and fatigue.

Viscosupplements

- Examples: hyaluronan and hylan
- Hyaluronan naturally occurs in synovial fluid and is intended to create a viscous medium which will cushion joints and maintain normal function of the joint
- Usually considered when treatment with analgesics and corticosteroids has failed and in those patients who cannot undergo surgical interventions
- They are administered intra-articularly as a parenteral preparation.

Surgery

In cases where there is joint deterioration, surgery may be considered. Examples include hip and knee replacement.

Hip replacement (arthroplasty)

- Surgical procedure in which the diseased parts of the hip are removed and replaced with an artificial joint (prosthesis)
- Full recovery after surgery can take between 3 and 6 months
- Pharmacist intervention: use of heparin to prevent thrombosis, pain management, prevention of infection (see also Chapters 24, 31 and 34).

Other treatments

- Topical agents: application of products containing methylsalicylate or capsaicin may be considered as an adjuvant treatment to simple analgesia
- Application of local heat and cold treatment
- Ultrasound therapy
- Acupuncture
- Hydrotherapy.

The management of osteoarthritis is summarised in Figure 45.1.

Gout and hyperuricaemia

Gout is an abnormality in either the production (associated with neoplastic diseases such as multiple myeloma, leukaemias, lymphomas, Hodgkin's disease and myeloproliferative conditions such as

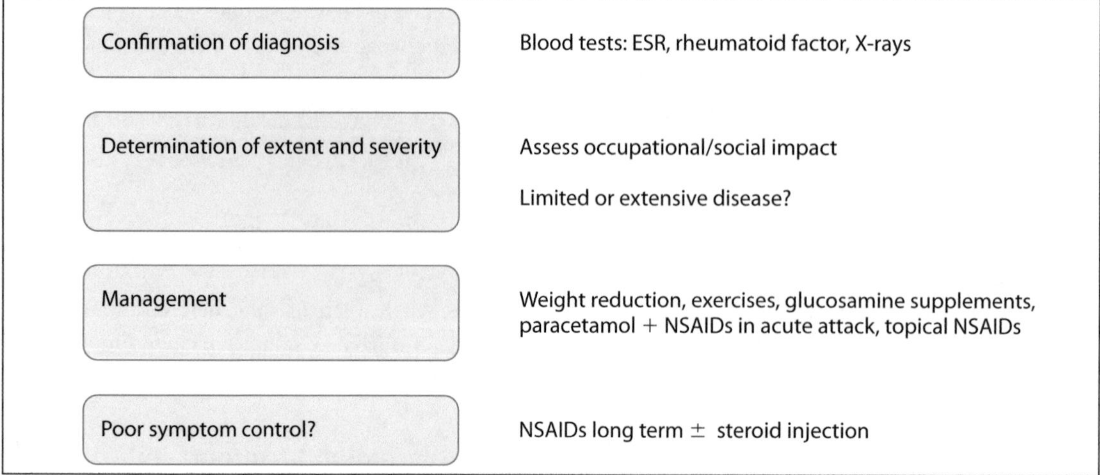

Figure 45.1 Management of osteoarthritis. ESR, erythrocyte sedimentation rate; NSAIDs, non-steroidal anti-inflammatory drugs.

myeloid metaplasia) or the elimination of uric acid or both.

Presentation of gout

- Acute onset of pain which typically occurs at night
- Swelling and inflammation of a single joint which usually involves the first metatarsophalangeal joint, when it is referred to as podagra. Recurrent attacks may be polyarticular
- Occurrence of attacks may be associated with increased episodes of physical exercise.

> Patients presenting with an acute attack of gout should have their blood pressure measured and renal function assessed since hypertension and impaired renal function are common in patients with gout.

Epidemiology of gout

- Affects mostly middle-aged men. If it occurs in premenopausal women or in men younger than 30 years of age, further investigations are required to evaluate underlying pathology.
- May be precipitated by drugs such as diuretics (bumetanide, furosemide, thiazides), ciclosporin, ACE inhibitors (lisinopril, ramipril) and cytotoxic chemotherapy (carboplatin, cisplatin, cyclophosphamide, daunorubicin, vinblastine, vincristine).

Drug treatment of gout

- NSAIDs
- Steroids
- Colchicine
- Allopurinol
- Uricosuric agents.

Management of gout

- Acute attack: high doses of NSAIDs (e.g. diclofenac, naproxen, indometacin), colchicine
- Long-term control: *allopurinol, probenecid, sulfinpyrazone.

*Drugs used for long-term control may precipitate an acute attack when they are introduced. They should not be used to manage an acute attack, they should be started within 2–3 weeks from an acute attack and they are usually given in combination with NSAIDs or colchicine for the first few weeks.

Aspirin is not indicated in gout.

Colchicine

- Used in acute attacks of gout and in the short term in the initial stages of prophylaxis with allopurinol or uricosuric agents
- Its disadvantage is the occurrence of side-effects particularly at high doses. Common side-effects include nausea, vomiting and abdominal pain. Other side-effects are profuse diarrhoea, gastrointestinal haemorrhage, rash, renal and hepatic damage. Rarely peripheral neuritis, myopathy, alopecia, inhibition of spermatogenesis and blood disorders may occur
- It is preferred to NSAIDs in acute attacks in patients where NSAIDs are contraindicated, in patients who cannot tolerate NSAIDs, in patients with heart failure and in patients receiving anticoagulants.

Allopurinol

- Inhibits synthesis of uric acid by competitively inhibiting xanthine oxidase, which is the enzyme catalysing the hypoxanthine–xanthine–uric acid reaction
- Effect is dose related. It is started in a low dose and dose increased according to required outcome
- Administration once daily after meals
- Side-effects: generally well tolerated with gastrointestinal disturbances being the common side-effects. However, occurrence of skin rashes requires monitoring since treatment should be withdrawn if recurrent and if it is due to a hypersensitivity reaction.

Probenecid and sulfinpyrazone are uricosuric drugs and they reduce serum urate concentration by increasing renal excretion of uric acid.

Probenecid

- Low doses used in initial stages of treatment to avoid development of kidney stones. Patient should be advised to maintain good fluid intake
- Side-effects: gastrointestinal disturbances, urinary frequency, headache, flushing, dizziness, alopecia, anaemia, haemolytic anaemia, sore gums, hypersensitivity reactions, rarely nephritic syndrome, hepatic necrosis, leukopenia and aplastic anaemia
- Patient monitoring: renal function tests.

Sulfinpyrazone

- Since it may cause salt and water retention, it should be used with caution in patients with cardiovascular disease
- Side-effects: gastrointestinal disturbances, allergic skin reactions, salt and water retention; rarely: blood disorders, gastrointestinal ulceration and bleeding, acute renal failure, raised liver enzymes, jaundice and hepatitis
- Patient monitoring: full blood counts, renal function tests.

Practice summary

- In osteoarthritis, the use of paracetamol is preferred to compound analgesics and NSAIDs for long-term pain relief.
- Intra-articular corticosteroids reduce the pain and inflammation in the joint affected with osteoarthritis and need to be administered every few months.
- When pain and joint deterioration is considerable, surgery for joint replacement should be considered in patients who are eligible for the intervention (e.g. can undertake anaesthesia, have no other complications).
- Patients receiving treatment for acute attacks of gout or treatment for long-term control of gout should be advised about the importance of ensuring adequate fluid intake.
- Patients should be advised to avoid alcohol and red meat.

Questions

1 Describe the clinical presentation of an acute attack of gout.
2 When is allopurinol indicated in gout and what advice should be given to patients receiving allopurinol?

Answers

1 Acute onset of symptoms with a painful swelling and inflammation of joints, characteristically the metatarsophalangeal joint.
2 Allopurinol is used in the long-term management of gout and should not be used during the acute attack. Patients receiving allopurinol should be advised to take product with or after food with plenty of water.

Further reading

Bayraktar A, Hudson S, Watson A and Fraser S (2000). Arthritis. *Pharm J* 264: 57–68.
Waddell D D and Bricker D C (2007). Total knee replacement delayed with Hylan G-F 20 use in patients with grade IV osteoarthritis. *J Manag Care Pharm* 13: 113–121.

Acknowledgements

Bernard Coleiro, Consultant Physician and Rheumatologist, Department of Medicine, Mater Dei Hospital, Malta.

46

Bone disorders

Learning objectives:

- To appreciate lifestyle measures that are required in the prophylaxis and treatment of osteoporosis
- To develop skills required to counsel patients and monitor patients receiving drugs for prophylaxis and treatment of osteoporosis
- To review background and drug therapy relevant to Paget's disease.

Background

The normal function of bone is to:

- provide structural support
- act as depot for calcium, phosphorus, magnesium, sodium and carbonate.

Composition of bone

- Protein matrix
- Mineral phase
- Bone cells: osteoblasts, osteocytes, osteoclasts.

Types of bone

- Cortical (compact): mid-shafts and outer surfaces of long bones and on surface of flat bones
- Trabecular (cancellous): inner aspect of metaphyses of the long bones.

Calcium-controlling hormones

- Parathyroid hormone: increases calcium levels in circulation by mobilising calcium from bone, increases absorption of calcium from intestine and reduces loss of calcium from kidney
- Vitamin D: metabolised to the active dihydroxy form which increases absorption of calcium and phosphate
- Calcitonin: increases calcium uptake into bone.

Definitions

- Osteopenia: significant decrease in bone mass relative to normal values adjusted for race, age, sex
- Osteomalacia: deficient mineralisation of bone leading to an accumulation of unmineralised osteoid
- Osteoporosis: progressive systemic skeletal disease characterised by low bone mass and micro-architectural deterioration of bone tissue, with a consequent increase in bone fragility and susceptibility to fracture, which typically involves the wrist, spine or hip.

Osteoporosis

This is a common metabolic disease involving a reduction in bone mass per unit volume leading to skeletal weakness and subsequent fracture. A major complication is hip fracture. Preventive strategies are important from an early age: regular exercise (e.g. walking), smoking cessation and calcium supplementation.

Education on the importance of preventing occurrence of osteoporosis particularly in patients with osteopenia should be undertaken, since if osteoporosis occurs this is a progressive disease where the risk of fractures increases. If fractures occur, in a large number of cases they will lead to a degree of immobility and sometimes may be associated with the development of complications.

Risk factors

- Female sex: decline in oestrogen in the postmenopausal phase is associated with accelerated bone loss
- Age >60 years
- Family history of osteoporosis
- Early menopause: due to early decrease in oestrogen levels.
- Low body mass index
- Smoking
- Sedentary lifestyle
- Corticosteroid use >3 months.

Aetiology

- Genetics, family history
- Dietary deficiencies of calcium and vitamin D
- Menopause or irregular periods
- Long-term use of alcohol, tobacco
- Age related
- Medications: corticosteroids, thyroxine, anticonvulsants, lithium, heparin, tamoxifen
- Disease: chronic liver disease, chronic renal failure, hyperthyroidism, primary hyperparathyroidism, Cushing's syndrome, gastrointestinal resection or malabsorption.

In patients taking high doses of corticosteroids for long-term use, prophylaxis of osteoporosis should be considered. This could be undertaken using bisphosphonates, calcitriol or hormone replacement therapy in premenopausal women.

Diagnosis

Diagnosis is based on bone densitometry measured at the hip or spine using dual-energy X-ray absorptiometry (DXA). The result compares a patient's bone mineral density (BMD) with that of a healthy young adult, T score and takes into consideration previous history of fracture. Interpretation of bone density results is shown in Table 46.1.

Clinical features may indicate occurrence of osteoporosis (e.g. loss of height).

Management

Aims

- To reduce and prevent fractures
- To alleviate fracture-related morbidity and decrease risk of further fractures
- To decrease mortality and reduce healthcare costs.

Risk of fractures increases in patients who have a history of fractures, with an alcohol intake of 4 or more units per day, in patients with rheumatoid arthritis and in patients on long-term oral corticosteroids.

Table 46.1 Interpretation of bone density result

Normal	0 to –1
Osteopenia (low bone mass)	Between –1 and –2.5
Osteoporosis	Below –2.5
Severe osteoporosis	Below –2.5 and one or more fragility fractures

Monitoring

- Bone densitometry
- X-rays: back, hip, knees, fingers.

- The treatment plan for patients with osteoporosis should also address modifiable risk factors, namely muscle weakness (increase exercise), abnormality of gait or balance, poor eyesight (prevent falls).
- Avoid drug therapy or limit use of drugs that may increase risks (e.g. drugs that induce sedation such as benzodiazepines, hypnotics, diuretics, antidepressants).
- Ensure management of diseases that affect mobility (e.g. arthritis and neurological diseases such as stroke, Parkinson's disease).

Drugs that prevent further bone loss (bone resorption)

- Bisphosphonates
- Calcium
- Calcitonin
- Calcitriol
- Oestrogens.

Drugs that stimulate bone formation

- Anabolic steroids
- Parathyroid hormone
- Teriparatide
- Fluoride.

Drug that has a dual action: preventing bone loss and promoting bone formation

- Strontium ranelate.

Patients receiving prophylactic therapy or treatment for osteoporosis should be advised to maintain an adequate intake of calcium and vitamin D and to adopt prevention strategies namely decrease smoking and undertake regular non-impact exercise.

Calcium

- Increases net absorption of calcium
- Decreases bone turnover
- Calcium absorption is influenced by level of vitamin D which is necessary for absorption and uptake into bone
- Proposed daily intake 1000–1500 mg daily
- To be taken over several years to provide prophylactic therapy
- Evidence of reduction in fracture rate in patients with osteoporosis is limited.

Calcitriol (hydroxylated derivative of vitamin D)

- Stimulates active transport of calcium
- Acts on bone mineralisation
- Side-effect: occurrence of hypercalcaemia
- Monitor plasma calcium concentration and creatinine levels.

Bisphosphonates

These are analogues of pyrophosphate that have a strong affinity for calcium phosphate. They decrease osteoclast activity by preventing binding of osteoclasts to bone resorption sites, thus decreasing resorption rate.

- Released slowly from the skeleton and therefore have a prolonged action.
- Studies report significant reductions in vertebral and non-vertebral fracture rate in postmenopausal women with osteoporosis after 1 year of treatment.
- Some (e.g. disodium pamidronate) are also used in hypercalcaemia in malignancy and in bone metastases in breast cancer.
- Contraindications: abnormalities of oesophagus, hypocalcaemia, pregnancy, breast-feeding, patients who cannot sit upright for 30 minutes after ingesting the drug.
- Cautions: upper gastrointestinal disorders, history of active gastrointestinal ulceration, renal impairment, hypocalcaemia, vitamin D deficiency, risk factors for osteonecrosis of the jaw: cancer, chemotherapy treatment, corticosteroid therapy, poor oral hygiene.

- Side-effects: oesophageal reactions, abdominal pain, dyspepsia, regurgitation, melaena, diarrhoea or constipation, flatulence, musculoskeletal pain, headache, osteonecrosis of the jaw especially with intravenous administration.
- Counselling: swallow whole with plenty of water in sitting or upright position and remain upright for at least 30 minutes, to be taken on an empty stomach 30 minutes before food, to maintain oral hygiene.
- For oral administration: alendronate 70 mg once weekly, alendronate in combination with calcitriol (bisphosphonates do not work optimally if there is vitamin D deficiency), ibandronic acid 150 mg once a month, risedronate 35 mg once weekly, tiludronic acid 400 mg daily for 12 weeks which may be repeated after 6 months.
- Zoledronic acid 5 mg may be administered intavenously once a year.

> Some patients may be intolerant to oral administration of bisphosphonates due to the persistent occurrence of severe gastro-intestinal disturbances that occur despite patients following drug administration instructions. In these patients other drugs such as strontium ranelate could be considered.

Strontium ranelate

- Reduces bone resorption and increases bone formation
- Caution: predisposition to thromboembolism, renal impairment.
- Side-effect: diarrhoea especially with initial treatment, venous thromboembolism, headache, dermatitis, eczema. Very rarely severe allergic reactions presenting with drug rash, eosinophilia and systemic symptoms (DRESS) which can be fatal have been reported
- Available: granules in sachets and is relatively well tolerated by patients
- Counselling: take daily in water at bedtime. Avoid food intake 2 hours before and after administration. Avoid concomitant administration of calcium-, aluminium- or magnesium-containing tablets. Stop medication and consult a health professional if skin rash develops.

Raloxifene

This is a selective oestrogen receptor modulator (SERM) and is preferred in the prophylaxis of osteoporosis when other menopausal symptoms, namely vasomotor symptoms or genitourinary symptoms, are predominant.

- Has an agonist effect on oestrogen receptors in blood vessels and bone and an antagonist effect on receptors in breast and uterus
- Contraindications: history of venous thromboembolism, undiagnosed uterine bleeding, endometrial carcinoma
- Cautions: venous thromboembolism, breast cancer, history of oestrogen-induced hypertriglyceridaemia
- Side-effects: venous thromboembolism, hot flushes, leg cramps, peripheral oedema, influenza-like symptoms.

Calcitonin

This is a naturally occurring peptide hormone produced by the parathyroid gland which decreases osteoclastic activity. Since it is a polypeptide it cannot be given orally. Route of administration is by injection or as a nasal spray. It has analgesic properties and may be used in acute pain in collapsed vertebrae. It is less effective than bisphosphonates in the prophylaxis of osteoporosis. It is used in Paget's disease and in the treatment of hypercalcaemia associated with malignancy.

- Contraindications: hypocalcaemia
- Patient monitoring: serum calcium level, renal and liver function tests
- Side-effects: nausea, vomiting, diarrhoea, abdominal pain, flushing, dizziness, headache, taste disturbances, musculoskeletal pain.

Hormone replacement therapy

This causes a decrease in bone resorption, an increase in calcitriol concentration and an increase in calcium absorption. It should be used when other options are contraindicated, cannot be tolerated or when there is lack of response (see also Chapter 39).

Treatment with bisphosphonates, strontium, calcitonin and raloxifene is long term and pharmacists should ensure that patient understands the correct dosage regimen (particularly relevant for bisphosphonates which are not taken on a daily basis) and that patient is taking the drug regularly and not attempting to use it for symptomatic relief.

Teriparatide

This is a recombinant fragment of the human parathyroid hormone that promotes bone growth. It is available as a subcutaneous injection administered daily for 18 months for the treatment of osteoporosis and corticosteroid-induced osteoporosis.

- Very expensive therapy
- Contraindications: hypercalcaemia, Paget's disease, previous radiation therapy to the skeleton, skeletal malignancies or bone metastases, unexplained raised alkaline phosphatase, pregnancy and breast-feeding
- Caution: renal impairment
- Side-effects: gastrointestinal disorders: nausea, reflux, haemorrhoids, postural hypotension, dyspnoea, depression, dizziness, vertigo, urinary tract disorders, polyuria, muscle cramps, irritation at injection site.

Parathyroid hormone

Since it is an amino acid peptide, parathyroid hormone cannot be administered orally. Human recombinant parathyroid hormone is available for subcutaneous administration. It requires daily administration and is also available as a pen device to facilitate self-administration.

- Recommended duration of treatment not to exceed 24 months; may be administered intermittently
- Recommended in the treatment of osteoporosis
- Contraindications: hypercalcaemia, metabolic disease including hyperparathyroidism and Paget's disease, previous radiation therapy to the skeleton, unexplained raised alkaline phosphatase, severe hepatic impairment, pregnancy and breast-feeding
- Monitoring: serum or urinary calcium concentration, renal function
- Side-effects: nausea, vomiting, dyspepsia, constipation, diarrhoea, palpitation, headache, dizziness, fatigue, asthenia, transient hypercalcaemia, hypercalciuria, muscle cramp, pain in extremities, back pain, injection site reactions.

After patients have taken maximum therapy with teriparatide or parathyroid hormone, long-term bisphosphonate therapy may be considered.

Fluoride

This increases bone formation in cancellous bone rather than cortical bone. It requires calcium supplementation. However, concomitant administration of fluoride with calcium may adversely affect fluoride

Prophylaxis

- In premenopausal women: HRT (discuss risk – benefit profile with patient)
- In postmenopausal women: bisphosphonates/strontium ranelate.

Treatment

1. Bisphosphonates/strontium ±calcium
2. Calcitriol/calcitonin
3. Teriparatide.

Calcium and vitamin D supplementation to be considered in all scenarios absorption. To date there is limited clinical experience with fluoride.

Paget's disease

This is a condition presenting with bone pain, skeletal deformity, neurological complications or fractures.

- Excessive bone resorption and formation occur
- Disease may have a viral origin
- Drugs used: analgesics, calcitonin and bisphosphonates.

Practice summary

- Lifestyle changes are essential for the prophylaxis and management of osteoporosis.
- Adequate daily calcium supplementation should be ensured for all adults, particularly women.
- Weight-bearing exercises such as climbing stairs and brisk walking help in the prevention and deterioration of the condition.
- Fall and injuries prevention requires attention as much as ensuring patient adherence to drug therapy for the management of osteoporosis. Strategies to make the home safer (e.g. removing rugs, improving lighting, putting up bathroom handles) as well as ensuring that patient undertakes regular eye tests and wears foam shields should be considered.

Questions

1. When should teriparatide be used in osteoporosis? What are the advantages of teriparatide over bisphosphonates? What are the disadvantages of teriparatide?
2. Mention four side-effects that could be expected due to teriparatide.
3. Describe monitoring requirements and lifestyle changes to be suggested in the management of osteoporosis.

Answers

1. Teriparatide is used in patients with severe osteoporosis or patients who did not respond to other drug therapy. The advantage of teriparatide over bisphosphonates is that it promotes bone growth. The disadvantages are that it is available for parenteral administration and treatment is comparatively more expensive.
2. Side-effects include gastrointestinal (nausea, gastro-oesophageal reflux), palpitations, dyspnoea and headache.
3. Monitoring: bone density. Lifestyle modifications: increase calcium intake, take up exercise and prevent falls and injuries at home (e.g. remove carpets, ensure availability of handrails).

Further reading

Cadarette S M, Katz J N, Brookhart A, Sturmer T, Stedman M R and Solomon D H (2008). Relative effectiveness of osteoporosis drugs for preventing nonvertebral fracture. *Ann Intern Med* 148: 537–646.

Ferguson N (2004). *Osteoporosis in Focus*. London: Pharmaceutical Press.

Jarvinen T L, Sievanen H, Khan K M, Heinonen A and Kannus P (2008). Shifting the focus in fracture prevention from osteoporosis to falls. *BMJ* 336: 124–126.

Mulder J E, Kolatkar N S and LeBoff M S (2006). Drug insight: existing and emerging therapies for osteoporosis. *Nat Clin Pract Endocrinol Metab* 2: 670–680.

National Institute for Health and Clinical Excellence (2008). Technology appraisal guidance: Alendronate, etidronate, risedronate, raloxifene and strontium ranelate for the primary prevention of osteoporotic fragility fractures in postmenopausal women. http://www.nice.org.uk/Guidance/TA160.

47

Skin disorders

Learning objectives:

- To consider different dosage forms for topical application in the management of skin conditions
- To understand the use of emollients and barrier preparations
- To appreciate use of antipruritics
- To review presentation of common skin conditions
- To identify use of medications for the treatment and management of particular conditions.

Dosage forms for topical application

Ointments

- Greasy preparations that are normally anhydrous and insoluble in water
- More occlusive than creams
- Suitable for chronic, dry lesions
- Different ointment bases are used.

Ointment bases – fatty bases

- Anhydrous hydrocarbons (e.g. white soft paraffin)
- Very greasy
- Form an occlusive layer on the skin.

Ointment bases – absorption bases

- Examples: wool fat, wool alcohols
- Absorb water and encourage hydration
- Spread easily
- Less occlusive than fatty bases.

Ointment bases – water-soluble bases

- Examples: macrogols
- Freely soluble in water
- Spread well
- Can be washed off easily.

Ointment bases – emulsifying bases

- Examples: surfactants such as cetomacrogol
- Form oil-in-water emulsions.

Creams

- Emulsions of oil and water
- Well absorbed into the skin
- Less greasy and less occlusive than ointments, more cosmetically acceptable
- Less effective at hydrating stratum corneum, less preferred when condition presents as very dry.

Other dosage forms

- Gels: high water content
- Lotions: cooling effect, consider alcohol content, preferred when the required application of a drug is to hairy areas
- Dusting powders.

Choice of product

The following factors should be considered when choosing a product to use:

- efficacy
- cosmetic acceptability
- areas of application
- time of application.

Emollients

- Soothe, smooth and hydrate the skin
- Useful for dry and scaly conditions
- Duration of effect is short and should be applied frequently
- Applied as creams or wash products
- Light emollients (e.g. aqueous cream)
- Greasy emollients (e.g. white soft paraffin, emulsifying wax)
- Considerations: ease of application and appearance, smell, duration of effect, effect on clothing, ease of removal.

Barrier preparations

- Contain a water repellent
- Constituents include dimeticone, zinc oxide
- Used in stomas, bedsores, protection against nappy rash
- Example: zinc and castor oil cream.

Antipruritics

Calamine

- Contains zinc oxide and liquid paraffin
- Contracts tissue
- Causes dryness of area of application and this may be a disadvantage if skin is dry
- Forms a thick dried paste that may not be acceptable to patients.

Topical antihistamines

- Example: mepyramine
- Used in allergic reactions, insect bites
- To be avoided in eczema
- May cause hypersensitivity and photosensitivity reactions.

> **Choice of preparation**
>
> Skin texture and the site of application (size, location).

Topical corticosteroids

Steroids consist of four fused rings of which one is a five-membered cyclopentane ring. Glucocorticoid activity is increased by the addition of a halogen atom on carbon-9 and this is seen in the higher potency for betamethasone (Figure 47.1), clobetasol (Figure 47.2), dexamethasone, diflucortolone, triamcinolone (fluorine) and beclometasone (chlorine) compared with hydrocortisone (Figure 47.3). Products that contain a second halogen atom, such as difluorinated products (difluocortolone, fluorine on carbon-6) and the addition of chlorine atom as a 21-chloro group (clobetasol), result in increased topical glucocorticoid activity compared with the other halogenated compounds.

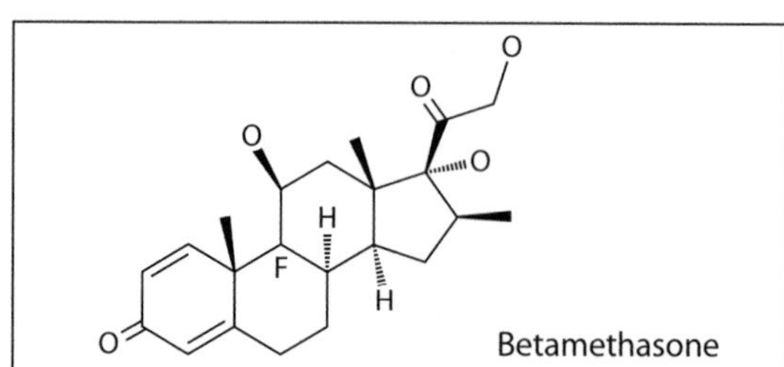

Figure 47.1 Chemical structure of betamethasone.

Figure 47.2 Chemical structure of clobetasol.

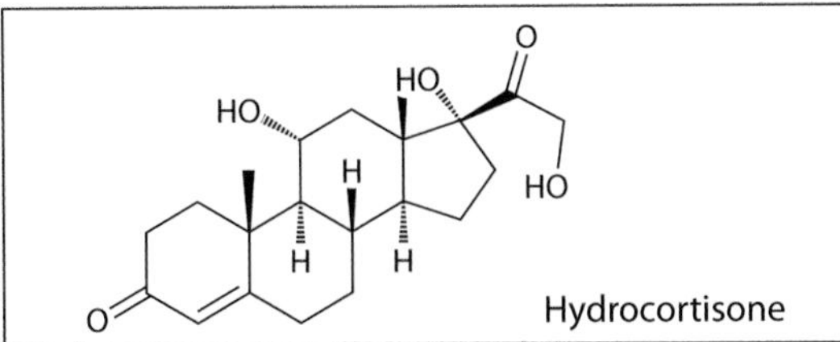

Figure 47.3 Chemical structure of hydrocortisone.

- Suppress inflammatory reaction
- Cautions: avoid prolonged use on face and in children
- Contraindication: untreated infections.

Side-effects

- Local side-effects: spread and worsening of untreated infection
- Thinning of skin
- Irreversible striae and telangiectasia
- Contact dermatitis
- Mild depigmentation
- Hypertrichosis.

- The use of topical corticosteroids should be limited as much as possible to avoid occurrence of unwanted effects.
- The least potent corticosteroid that is effective in controlling the symptoms should be used for the shortest possible period.

Application

- Apply thinly to affected area using least potent formulation; usually once to twice daily application is recommended
- Applied for the least possible period
- May be applied as combination products with antifungals or antibacterial agents
- Avoid occlusion with dressings and plastic nappies (the latter increase systemic absorption)
- Vehicles: ointments increase absorption.

Potencies

- Mild: hydrocortisone 0.1–2.5%
- Moderate: betamethasone 0.025%
- Potent: betamethasone 0.1%, hydrocortisone butyrate 0.1%, beclometasone 0.025–0.05%
- Very potent: clobetasol 0.05%, diflucortolone 0.3%.

Questions to ask patient presenting with skin disorders

- Where is it located?
- Is it widespread or localised?
- How long have you had the symptoms?
- Is it itchy?
- Are there any other symptoms?
- What is your occupational history?
- Are you taking any other medications?

Impetigo

This is an infection caused by *Staphylococcus aureus* or *Streptococcus pyogenes*.

- Development of a sore, clusters or small vesicles or pustules with a honey-yellow crust
- Could occur as a secondary infection
- Use of topical anti-infective agents is required.

Tinea corporis – ringworm

- Central clearing, slightly elevated, reddened edge with sharp margination
- Does not involve face, hands, feet, groin or scalp
- Management: topical application of imidazole creams or terbinafine cream.

Dandruff – pityriasis capitis

- Chronic, relapsing, hyperproliferative skin condition
- Increased occurrence of *Pityrosporum ovale*
- Clinical presentation: dry, itchy and flaky scalp; very much limited to scalp.

Management

- Pyrithione zinc: safe for children; to be used daily until condition clears
- Selenium: not suitable for children under 5 years of age. Avoid if broken or inflamed skin since irritation may occur. Apply twice weekly for 2 weeks, then once weekly for 2 weeks and then as necessary
- Ketoconazole shampoo: acute treatment – twice weekly for 2–4 weeks. Prophylaxis – once every 1–2 weeks. Suitable for use in children.

Dandruff presents with flaky and itchy scalp. However, usually there are no other skin lesions and no redness in the area as may be expected with other skin conditions such as seborrhoeic dermatitis.

Seborrhoeic dermatitis

This is a chronic inflammatory skin disorder confined to areas where sebaceous glands are prominent.

- Yellow–red lesions, oily yellow scales
- Frequent cleansing
- Management: antifungal agents (e.g. ketoconazole shampoo), use of almond oil or olive oil to remove scales, particularly in young children, and topical corticosteroids may be considered for a short time due to the inflammatory reaction.

Contact dermatitis

This presents with a rash that results from skin contact with an allergen or irritant. It is associated with profuse itching.

- Management: calamine lotion, hydrocortisone, antihistamines (systemic administration)
- Identification of allergen to avoid re-occurrence. Examples of allergens include detergents, cosmetic preparations, jewellery, rubber gloves.

Topical corticosteroids and dermatitis

- Indicated for relief of symptoms in acute phase
- May cause skin atrophy, acne-form pustules, spreading of infection, contact dermatitis, striae, mild depigmentation
- Creams indicated for moist lesions, ointments preferred for dry scaly lesions.

Atopic dermatitis

This is a red, dry, scaly rash spreading to the flexures in the neck, wrist, elbows and knees. Scratching due to irritation and itchiness may lead to secondary bacterial infection such as impetigo.

- Dry, crusty thickening of skin
- Management: emollients to address dry skin, topical corticosteroids to reduce inflammation and calcineurin inhibitors.

Topical drugs affecting the immune system

- Calcineurin inhibitors (e.g. tacrolimus and pimecrolimus) result in inhibition of transcription of inflammatory genes
- Used for atopic eczema which is uncontrolled by maximal topical treatment or if there is intolerance to topical corticosteroids
- Can be used in children over 2 years
- Side-effects: application site reactions (burning sensations, rash); less common: herpes simplex virus, skin malignancy.

Emollients and atopic dermatitis

- Emollients hydrate the skin and form an occlusive barrier to prevent evaporation of moisture
- Dosage forms: cream, ointment, emollient wash

- Examples: aqueous cream, white soft paraffin.

Scabies

This condition is caused by the mite *Sarcoptes scabiei*, which is transmitted by physical contact. The female mite burrows in the stratum corneum and deposits eggs, while the faecal pellets left in the burrow cause a local hypersensitivity reaction.

- Incubation period: up to 6 weeks
- Occurrence generally limited to finger webs, sides of fingers and wrists
- Diagnosis: visible signs of the mite, intense itching
- Treatment: permethrin as a topical formulation (e.g. cream)
- Caution: avoid contact with eyes, mouth; do not use on broken skin.

Pruritus occurring with scabies may persist for several weeks after the infestation has been eliminated. Consider use of topical corticosteroids or oral antihistamines.

Hair loss

Factors inducing hair loss

- Stress
- Nutrition: iron deficiency
- Endocrine disorders: hypothyroidism, diabetes, hypopituitarism
- Tinea capitis
- Traction alopecia
- Medicine induced: cytotoxic chemotherapy, warfarin, isotretinoin.

Androgenic alopecia (male-pattern baldness)

- Scalp hair transforms into vellus-like hair follicles which are shorter due to preferential binding by dihydrotestosterone to hair follicle receptors
- Causes hair loss at the front of the head in men and in women causes generalised and diffuse hair loss
- Not associated with other symptoms
- Strongly genetically linked.

Treatment

- Minoxidil, a topical scalp solution, delays and slows hair loss. Baldness returns upon discontinuation of treatment, tailing off of effect occurs and it is effective in a minority of individuals. Applied twice daily.
- Finasteride is an anti-androgen that can be used in men. Oral tablets are given for 3–6 months before evaluation of outcomes can be carried out. Effects are reversed 6–12 months after treatment withdrawal (see also Chapter 41).

Acne

This is a disorder of the sebaceous follicle that has significant psychological impact on the patient. During puberty, increased androgen levels in both males and females stimulate enlargement of the sebaceous follicle resulting in enormous increase in sebum production, leading to seborrhoea and the occurrence of greasy skin.

- Follicular hyperkeratosis may occur, resulting in the characteristic comedo (blackhead) formation
- Excessive proliferation of the commensal bacterium *Propionibacterium acnes* is associated with occurrence of acne.

Benzoyl peroxide

This is a potent bactericidal that acts against *P. acnes*. It is effective in mild-to-moderate acne. Local skin irritation, bleaching of hair and clothing may occur. Start with a low dose and increase strength gradually.

Azelaic acid

This may be preferred to benzoyl peroxide since it is less likely to cause irritation than benzoyl peroxide.

Topical antibiotics

Erythromycin, clindamycin and tetracycline are used. Generally well tolerated, may cause irritation. Bacterial resistance may be reduced by using benzoyl peroxide concomitantly.

Topical retinoids

Topical retinoids such as adapalene and tretinoin can be used.

- Main side-effects: redness and skin peeling which occurs to a lower extent with adapalene
- Teratogenicity: pregnancy
- Avoid contact with eye, mucous membranes, nostrils
- Avoid exposure to sunlight.

Systemic medication

- Tetracylines: oxytetracycline/tetracycline – note interaction with isotretinoin
- Erythromycin: increasing levels of *P. acnes* resistance among acne patients limits its clinical use
- Oral isotretinoin
- Anti-androgens (e.g. cyproterone) used in androgen-induced seborrhoea.
- Combined oral contraceptives: in androgen-induced seborrhoea, oestrogens inhibit sebaceous gland activity.

> When combined oral contraceptives are used, a preparation where the progestogen component is either drospirenone, which is anti-androgenic, or a low-dose progestogen (progestogens have an androgenic effect) should be chosen.

Oral isotretinoin

- Can induce remission and is the most effective treatment
- Treatment period of 4–8 months
- Occurrence of side-effects: facial dermatitis, epistaxis, conjunctivitis, dryness of mucous membranes, psychiatric symptoms
- Prescription-restricted item in many countries
- Teratogenicity: care with women patients; pregnancy testing and contraception advice have to be provided.

> **Monitoring patient outcomes in the management of acne**
>
> Clinical severity assessment using health-related tools such as the American Academy of Dermatology (AAD) classification and the Acne Disability Index may be undertaken to evaluate patient outcomes.

Psoriasis

This is a genetically influenced chronic skin disorder that is characterised by a hyperproliferative condition. It presents with well-demarcated red plaques covered with a silvery-white scale, typically affecting elbows, knees, scalp (scalp psoriasis) and sacrum. It is a chronic relapsing condition that may impact on patient's social life and psychological well-being.

Factors that may aggravate psoriasis

- Infections
- Stress
- Alcohol
- Sunlight
- Trauma
- Drugs (e.g. lithium, antimalarials, beta-blockers, NSAIDs, ACE inhibitors, withdrawal of corticosteroids).

Treatment

- Emollients: improve dryness, scaling and cracking, useful in inflammatory psoriasis, used as adjunct treatment
- Topical corticosteroids: used for specific sites to counteract inflammatory reactions and for the shortest time period possible
- Coal tar: has anti-inflammatory and anti-scaling properties, useful in chronic plaque psoriasis. Available also as shampoos and liquid bath formulations. Disadvantage: smelly and may stain clothing and skin, patient acceptability low
- Salicylic acid: used for its keratolytic properties. Particularly used for psoriasis affecting the scalp
- Dithranol: used in short term since it is associated with skin irritation. To be applied on chronic extensor plaques avoiding small lesions, flexures or the face. Patients should be advised about irritation and possibility of staining of skin and clothing.
- Topical vitamin D derivatives.

Vitamin D and analogues

- Examples: calcipotriol, calcitriol and tacalcitol
- Side-effects: local skin reactions
- Advise patient to wash hands thoroughly after application
- Suspend use during an inflammatory phase
- Maximum application: 100 g weekly
- Indicated for chronic stable plaque psoriasis.

Management of psoriasis

Choice of products depends on site affected.

- Trunks and limbs: emollients, vitamin D analogues, coal tar, topical corticosteroid
- Face, flexures and genitalia: emollients, mild/moderate topical corticosteroid.
  Note: vitamin D analogues to be used with caution
- Scalp: coal tar shampoo, corticosteroid lotion, coal tar–salicylic acid–coconut oil ointment.

Other options

- Oral retinoids (e.g. tazarotene)
- Immunosuppressants (e.g. ciclosporin, azathioprine)
- Phototherapy
- PUVA (psoralen and ultraviolet A): photochemotherapy.

> Patients using tar-based products, dithranol, vitamin D analogues and tazarotene should be advised about the risk of skin irritation and to apply product specifically to the affected areas as advised.

Practice summary

- Differential diagnosis is required to differentiate between skin disorders.
- Choice of dosage form of products used in the management of the skin conditions may depend on vehicles included in the preparation.
- Emollients soothe and hydrate the skin and can be applied freely in any condition that is associated with a dry and scaling presentation.
- Barrier preparations are used to prevent skin deterioration due to increased moisture in the area.
- The use of calamine preparations and topical antihistamines as antipruritics is limited due to ineffectiveness and sensitisation for topical antihistamines.
- Topical corticosteroids are used to relieve symptoms of inflammation associated with acute conditions (e.g. insect bites) or with chronic conditions (e.g. eczema).
- In chronic skin disorders patient participation in the use of medications and dose adjustments (e.g. of topical corticosteroids) during flare-ups is necessary.

Questions

1 What are the distinguishing characteristics of absorption and fatty bases?

2 Compare use of minoxidil and finasteride in male-pattern baldness.
3 Compare the use of clobetasol and tacrolimus in atopic eczema.
4 Discuss treatment of scabies.

Answers

1 Fatty bases are very greasy and form an occlusive layer on the skin. Absorption bases absorb water and encourage hydration, spread easily and are less occlusive than fatty bases.

2 *Minoxidil:*
- vasodilator (previously used to treat high blood pressure)
- available as a topical scalp solution
- delays and slows hair loss, baldness returns upon discontinuation of treatment, tailing off of effect occurs
- effective in a minority of individuals
- applied twice daily.

Finasteride:
- anti-androgen
- available as oral tablets
- effects reversed 6–12 months after treatment withdrawal
- given once daily for 3–6 months before evaluation of treatment outcomes can be carried out.

3 Clobetasol is a very potent topical corticosteroid indicated for relief of symptoms in the acute phase of atopic eczema. It may cause skin atrophy, acne-form pustules, spreading of infection, contact dermatitis, striae and mild depigmentation. Topical corticosteroid creams are indicated for moist lesions while ointments are preferred for dry scaly lesions. It should be applied thinly once or twice times daily for up to 4 weeks. Tacrolimus is licensed for topical use in moderate-to-severe atopic eczema. It is a calcineurin inhibitor that inhibits transcription of inflammatory genes (affects the immune system). Tacrolimus is used for atopic eczema which is uncontrolled by maximal topical treatment or if there is intolerance to topical steroids. In contrast to corticosteroids, calcineurin inhibitors are not indicated for first-line treatment. Treatment should be short term; continuous long-term treatment should be avoided. Side-effects include application site reactions (burning sensation, rash) and less commonly herpes simplex virus and skin malignancy.

4 Permethrin is effective for the treatment of scabies; malathion can be used if permethrin is inappropriate. Aqueous preparations are preferable to alcoholic lotions, which are not recommended owing to skin irritation. Avoid contact with eyes and mouth and do not use formulations on broken skin. Pruritus occurring with scabies may persist for several weeks after the infestation has been eliminated. The use of topical corticosteroids or oral sedating antihistamines at night may be considered.

Further reading

Clark C (2004). How to choose a suitable emollient? *Pharm J* 273: 351–352.

Clark C (2007). Scalp problems in the pharmacy. *Pharm J* 278: 431–434.

Clark C (2009). Acne: causes and clinical features. *Clin Pharm* 1: 163–166.

Clark C (2009). Acne: treatment. *Clin Pharm* 1: 168–172.

Jerram P (2008). Proprietary emollients: why pump dispensers can complicate selection. *Pharm J* 281: 369.

Nathan A (2007). Advising on insect bites and stings. *Pharm J* 278: 557–560.

Seaton R A (2009). Skin and soft tissue infection: diagnosis and management. *Clin Pharm* 1: 13–19.

48

Wound management

Learning objectives:

- To identify characteristics of wound dressings
- To develop skills required in the handling of wound management products and in wound management.

Background

- *Wound:* damage to the skin or mucous membrane which may be caused by elective trauma or accidental trauma
- *Process of healing:* replacement of damaged tissue by new living material.

Classification of wounds

- Degree of tissue loss: e.g. incision or graze?
- Clean or contaminated: e.g. wound occurring after an injury sustained in the fields or wound sustained in the bathroom?
- Depth: e.g. puncture or superficial damage?
- Site of wound: e.g. bed sore occurring in the sacral area, a wound occurring in the periphery in a diabetic patient or wound occurring in the thigh?
- Exudate: dry, necrotic, black or clean exuding (granulating wound) or dry low exudates (epithelialising wound)?

Process of wound healing

- Healing by first intention: healing takes place from the internal layers outwards
- Healing by second intention: scar (granulation) tissue formation.

Stages in the healing process

- Inflammation
- Destruction and removal of debris
- Proliferation and maturation of new tissue
- Contraction
- Epithelialisation.

Necrotic tissue

Necrotic tissue presents as yellowish-brown to black tissue. It is associated with chronic wounds (e.g. pressure sores). The occurrence of necrotic tissue creates concern since it delays healing and promotes infection. It may be removed by debridement. Dressings used should promote rehydration and moisture retention.

Slough

This is accumulation of dead cells in the exudate from wounds. The exudate is yellowish and is removed by desloughing. Dressings should promote fluid and odour absorption if the wound is moist or moisture retention and rehydration if the wound is dry.

Factors influencing wound healing

- Blood supply: compromised blood supply in area of wound delays healing (e.g. in patients with diabetes or in patients with peripheral circulation disorders)
- Nutritional factors: malnourished patients have a delay in wound healing
- Drugs: immunosuppressive drugs, corticosteroids
- Infection: occurrence of infection interferes with process of healing and may lead to gangrene and amputations of extremities
- Hypergranulation: leads to scar formation, some individuals are prone to develop scars and keloids
- Oedema: interferes with healing process
- Incontinence: increases risk of infection and maceration of the area.

Wound management

Dressings must create an environment at the wound surface that promote the process of healing where maximum cell division and replication can occur.

- *Dressing:* material that covers a wound should not interfere negatively with the process of healing
- *Bandage:* used to keep a dressing in place at the site of the trauma (conforming-stretch bandage), to immobilise a dry area or to provide compression (elasticated tubular or support bandages, compression bandages, adhesive bandages)
- *Surgical absorbents:* e.g. swabs applied to the wound to adsorb exudates. Care should be taken since they may shed fibres into the wound or adhere to the wound surface
- *Adhesive tapes:* used to keep dressing material in place. May be of the hypoallergenic type to decrease risk of skin irritation due to sensitivity to material.

> - Dressings used should not interfere with the process of healing

> - Surgical absorbents are preferred as secondary dressings to manage heavily exuding wounds where they are used on top of the primary dressing. In this way the risk of shedding fibres or adhering to the wound surface is eliminated.

Dressings

Characteristics of ideal dressing

- Maintain moist environment at the wound dressing interface
- Provide thermal insulation and mechanical protection
- Low or non-adherent
- Requires infrequent changing
- Free from particulate contaminants
- Safe, comfortable and mouldable
- Good absorption characteristics
- Impermeable to microorganisms
- Sterile.

Traditional dressings

The traditional dressings (e.g. cotton wool, gauze, lint) fail in a number of characteristics expected from a dressing, including that they require frequent changing, are not free from particulate contaminants and are not impermeable to microorganisms.

They are used on clean, dry wounds and as secondary dressings for absorbent and protective functions.

> There is no dressing that matches all the criteria required of an ideal dressing. Choice of dressing should be undertaken for each individual scenario to identify priority features required from the dressing.

Low adherent dressings

- Used for dry wounds or lightly exuding wounds
- May be used as the first layer in contact with the wound followed by other absorbent secondary dressings
- May have adhesive border or else require use of surgical tape to keep dressing in place
- Examples: Mepore (with adhesive border), Melolin.

Vapour-permeable films

- Allow vapour and oxygen to be interchanged across the dressing (water vapour permeable)
- Provide a moist healing environment and may provide a cooling of the wound surface
- Suitable for mildly exuding wounds, to protect minor skin damage in patients at risk and for prophylaxis of pressure sores. Also used as retention dressings for canulae and in stoma care
- Waterproof
- Advantage: very comfortable and convenient to use
- Disadvantage: excess exudate may accumulate as a bubble under the film and this may cause skin maceration; should be avoided in heavily exuding wounds
- Examples: Hydrofilm, Mepore Film, Opsite, Tegaderm.

Hydrogel dressings

- Consist of a large proportion of water (about 70–90% water)
- Promote moist healing
- Non-adherent and usually are amorphous materials that will take up the shape of the wound. A secondary dressing to cover the area is required
- Suitable for dry sloughy or necrotic wounds since they promote debridement. May be used in lightly exuding wounds since they absorb small amounts of exudates
- Examples: GranuGel, Hydrosorb, Intrasite gel.

Hydrocolloid dressings

- Contain methylcellulose, pectin and gelatin presented as a layer on a vapour-permeable film or foam
- Interactive dressings since they:
  - absorb fluid and form a gel which makes it easy to clear during wound dressing
  - promote formation of granulation tissue
  - provide pain relief
- Facilitate rehydration and autolytic debridement
- Suitable in acute and chronic wounds which are dry, sloughy or necrotic and light to moderately exuding wounds
- Advantage: do not require frequent wound dressing
- Waterproof
- Examples: CombiDerm, DuoDerm Extra Thin, Granuflex, Hydrocoll.

Foam dressings

- Consist of polyurethane foam
- Used for light–medium–highly exuding wounds depending on the type of product used
- Reduce hypergranulation tissue and so are indicated in patients with a tendency to develop keloids
- Advantage: do not require frequent wound dressing.

Alginate dressings

- Consist of alginates within the dressing
- The alginate component will gel when it comes in contact with exudates
- Used for moderately to heavily exuding wounds.

Other types

- Odour absorbing: contain charcoal that is used to adsorb odour.

Medicated tulle dressings

- Impregnated with an antiseptic (e.g. chlorhexidine) or an antibacterial (e.g. fusidic acid)

- Effectiveness over the application of the medication and a separate wound dressing is still not established.

Antiseptics

- The product should not interfere with the healing process
- Products that do not have an alcoholic base are preferred because there is a lower risk of irritation
- Physiological saline is an effective, safe and inexpensive product. Other products include chlorhexidine, povidone – iodine and cetrimide.

Practice summary

- It is important that the type of dressing used does not interfere with wound healing.
- Wound characteristics that influence choice of dressing include site of wound, whether wound is clean or infected and degree of exudate.
- Alginate dressings and foam dressings are preferred in medium–heavy exuding wounds. Hydrogel and hydrocolloid dressings are effective in medium exuding wounds.
- The use of irritant antiseptics and cleansers is not recommended; irrigation with physiological saline is the usual practice.
- *Note: in this chapter examples of dressings given reflect proprietary preparations.*

Questions

1. Compare hydrogel dressings and hydrocolloid dressings.
2. When are vapour-permeable adhesive film dressings recommended?
3. What are the advantages and disadvantages of povidone – iodine as an antiseptic?

Answers

1. *Hydrogels (e.g. Intrasite gel)*
   - Consist of 70–90% water
   - Promote moist healing
   - Cool surface of the wound
   - Suitable for dry or necrotic wounds, light exuding wounds.

   Hydrocolloids (e.g. Granuflex)
   - Contain methylcellulose, pectin, gelatin
   - Absorb fluid and lead to formation of a gel
   - Promote formation of granulation tissue and provide pain relief
   - Suitable in acute and chronic wounds, desloughing, exuding wounds.

2. Vapour-permeable adhesive films are suitable for relatively shallow wounds; can be used prophylactically to prevent pressure sores and as retention dressings.
3. Advantages: broad spectrum – active against most Gram-positive and -negative bacteria as well as most fungi, protozoa and viruses; indicated for skin disinfection, vaginal and oral infections; available in numerous dosage forms (e.g. solution, dry powder spray, mouthwash). Disadvantages: may stain skin and clothing; application of povidone–iodine to large wounds or severe burns may produce systemic adverse effects such as metabolic acidosis, hypernatraemia and impairment of renal function; regular use should be avoided in patients with thyroid disorders or those receiving lithium therapy.

Further reading

Morgan DA (1999). Wound management products in the Drug Tariff. *Pharm J* 263: 820–825.

Ohura T, Sanada H and Mino Y (2004). Clinical activity-based cost effectiveness of traditional versus modern wound management in patients with pressure ulcers. *Wounds* 16: 157–163.

Parnes A and Lagan KM (2007). Larval therapy in wound management: a review. *Int J Clin Pract* 61: 488–493.

Romanelli M, Dini V, Bertone M S and Brilli C (2007). Measuring wound outcomes. *Wounds* 19: 294–298.

49

Drug therapy in geriatric patients

Learning objectives:

- To identify problems in the use of medicines in the elderly
- To develop skills required in medicines management in older persons.

Background

Ageing is characterised by an inability to maintain homeostasis under conditions of physiological stress. This situation predisposes to health-related problems. Theories to describe the process of ageing describe a deterioration of the protein-synthesising mechanism.

Examples of conditions associated with age

- Osteoarthritis
- Osteoporosis
- Foot deformities
- Atherosclerosis
- Cerebral ischaemia
- Myocardial infarction
- Alzheimer's disease
- Parkinsonism.

Problems in the elderly that may interfere with drug therapy and disease progression

- Mental confusion
- Incontinence
- Postural instability
- Immobility
- Skin and muscle wasting.

Factors responsible for increased incidence of adverse drug reactions in the elderly

- Multiple disease states
- Increased use of medicines
- Over-prescribing
- Alterations in drug handling by the body
- Increased sensitivity to the effects of some drugs.

Pharmacist actions in geriatric patient care

- Participate in appropriate drug selection: consider other drugs being taken by patient, assess pharmacokinetic profile and impact of unwanted drug effects
- Ensure optimum use of medicines by patient: provide patient counselling, facilitate drug taking using medication reminder aids
- From time to time run medication reviews: examine all medications taken by patient to identify any duplication, conflicting therapy or drugs that may be withdrawn or doses that can be adjusted
- Identify drug-related problems: patient problems with drug or occurrence of side-effects

- Facilitate access to medications: provide domiciliary care.

Appropriate drug selection

When selecting drug therapy for the elderly, preference of one drug over another may be based on the pharmacokinetic profile of the drugs (e.g. lorazepam is preferred to diazepam because of its shorter half-life) or pharmacodynamic changes (e.g. calcium channel blockers preferred to beta-blockers in the management of hypertension in the elderly due to decreased responsiveness to beta-blockers).

Pharmacokinetic profile

Absorption

Age-related changes in upper gastrontestinal function include altered gastric pH, diminished blood flow and changes in motility. However, the significance of these changes on clinical outcomes is minimal.

Drug distribution

In older people, there is a decreased cardiac output which may lead to a decreased hepatic and renal blood flow. Changes in the body composition occur leading to a decrease in lean body mass and an increase in adipose tissues.

These changes will result in a decreased volume of distribution for drugs that are distributed primarily in water or lean body mass (e.g. digoxin – requires lower dose in geriatric patients). The volume of distribution of drugs that are primarily distributed in fat may be increased (e.g. diazepam – results in increased risk of accumulation with repeated use). There is also a decrease in serum albumin concentration which may affect degree of protein binding (e.g. phenytoin).

Drug metabolism

In older people, the total liver weight and the number of functioning liver cells are decreased. In addition, disease states and nutritional status may adversely affect liver function. This may result in a decrease in the elimination rate of drugs that are excreted in the liver (e.g. warfarin, long-acting benzodiazepines).

Renal elimination

Renal function decreases with age because there is a decline in glomerular filtration rate, tubular secretion, re-absorptive capacity and renal blood flow. Drugs that are eliminated by the kidney such as aminoglycosides, atenolol, digoxin, enalapril, fluconazole, fluoroquinolones, furosemide, lisinopril, methotrexate, spironolactone and thiazides may have reduced clearance in the elderly. Drugs where this factor may lead to side-effects and drug-related problems require dose adjustment (lower doses) in older people.

Pharmacodynamic changes

- Changes in receptor sensitivity (e.g. decreased responsiveness to agonists and antagonists at beta-adrenoceptors)
- Increased sensitivity to drug effects (e.g. anticoagulant effects of warfarin)
- Decline in some pathways: decreased cholinergic neurons in areas of the brain lead to a higher risk of drugs with anticholinergic properties (e.g. benzatropine, trihexyphenidyl, sedating antihistamines, tricyclic antidepressants, neuroleptics) inducing mental confusion
- Orthostatic hypotension: may be aggravated by alpha-adrenergic blocking drugs, diuretics, nitrates, phenothiazines, tricyclic antidepressants.

The use of drugs in the older patient is summarised in Table 49.1.

Use of medicines in the elderly

The occurrence of side-effects is higher in older patients. The reasons include:

- poly pharmacy
- doses used are sometimes too high in relation to reduced elimination
- doses used are sometimes too high in relation to decreased physiological responses (e.g. hypotensive drugs).

Adverse effects occurring in the elderly with antibacterial treatment are listed in Table 49.2.

Table 49.1 Use of drugs in the older patient

ACE inhibitors	Small initial doses to reduce risk of hypotension
Analgesics – opioids	Increased occurrence of side-effects: nausea, hypotension, central nervous system effects
Analgesics – NSAIDs	Avoid products with long half-life (e.g. piroxicam); increased risk of renal failure and gastrointestinal toxicity; may cause fluid retention
Beta-blockers	Increased risk of bradycardia and precipitation of heart failure
Benzodiazepines	Medicines with short half-life preferred to reduce risk of confusion and ataxia
Diuretics	Side-effects more common (hyponatraemia, postural hypotension, incontinence)
H_2-receptor antagonists	Excretion is reduced, increased risk of confusional states
Phenothiazines	Increased risk of tardive dyskinesia, anticholinergic symptoms
Warfarin	Smaller starting dose since anticoagulant effect is increased

ACE, angiotensin-converting enzyme; NSAIDs, non-steroidal anti-inflammatory drugs.

Ensuring optimum drug use by an elderly patient

- Rationalise therapy: minimise number of medicines to be administered
- Adopt simple dosage regimen: minimise frequency of drug administration
- Check that the patient understands how to take medication(s)
- Assess ability to comply:
  - for prescription medicines, access to prescription
  - access to pharmacy for getting medicines
  - ability to read label and instructions and handle container
  - ability to administer medication: use of self-injections, swallowing tablets or capsules, using an inhaler device
- Consider preparing medicines in a pill box where medicines are prepared according to the dosage regimen (assess product stability); use a memory aid to prompt patient to take medicines; use printed leaflets to explain dosage regimen.

Table 49.2 Adverse effects occurring in the elderly with antibacterial treatment

Drug	Adverse event
Aminoglycosides	Nephrotoxicity, ototoxicity
Broad-spectrum agents	Antibiotic-associated pseudomembranous colitis
Co-amoxiclav	Acute liver injury
Co-trimoxazole	Blood dyscrasias, hyperkalaemia
Tetracyclines	Oesophageal ulcers
Quinolones	Seizures

Factors to be considered when counselling on discharge medication/refill

- Identify literacy problems: ensure that patient knows clearly how to take medicines
- Number of prescribed and non-prescription medications administered: kept to a minimum
- Medication regimen: simple
- Identify administration problems: documentation necessary for patient to access medications on NHS where applicable, access to prescription

- Packaging and labelling: patient can access packaging and label is large, clear and can be read and understood by patient
- Occurrence of side-effects and identification of interactions: check occurrence of unwanted effects, even insignificant ones, that are bothering the patient and interactions
- Social functioning: patient requires social support and care at home to ensure adequate nutrition and independent living.

Medications review

- Identify indication for use of medicines
- Check suitability of dosage form and dose
- Assess outcomes of therapy
- Check for occurrence of side-effects
- Evaluate possibility of drug interacting with another drug or a medical condition.

Identifying drug-related problems

Discuss with patient medications used and health-related issues to identify any drug-related problems.

Problems with dispensed medication

- Illegible and unclear label
- Formulation
- Packaging
- Side-effects
- Use of non-prescription medicines.

Problems associated with formulation

- Swallowing tablets
- Measuring suspensions
- Using inhalers
- Instilling eye drops
- Using suppositories
- Applying creams.

Medicines management in older patients

- Medications Appropriateness Index: evaluates process of prescribing and administration of medicines
- Indicators of Preventable Drug Related Morbidity: evaluates outcome measurement, quality-of-life outcomes.

Falls in older people

- Common, devastating problem
- Associated with identifiable risk factors: weakness, gait, confusion, medications
- Fall prevention: assessment of fall risks by identifying risk factors and preparing a risk-reduction strategy which includes patient support and home help
- Fall management: in addition to looking into the physical damage, when falls in older people occur: pharmacist review of medications, physiotherapists to support patient in physical movements, social worker to assess patient needs at home.

Drugs and falls

- Drugs causing hypotension (e.g. antihypertensives)
- Drugs causing hypovolaemia (e.g. diuretics)
- Drugs causing incontinence (e.g. diuretics)
- Drugs causing undue sedation (e.g. benzodiazepines, antidepressants).

Practice summary

- When starting treatment, use a low dose and increase slowly, if necessary.
- Keep treatment as simple as possible using the minimum number of different drugs.
- Ensure that the patient or a responsible person clearly understands the treatment schedule.
- Avoid childproof containers for those who are unable to open them.

- Drugs may precipitate a health condition particularly in elderly patients. When patient presents with a condition and there is no obvious reason for that, consider each drug used and identify any correlation.

Questions

1. Why should diazepam be used with caution in elderly patients?
2. What precautions are necessary when NSAIDs are used in the elderly?

Answers

1. Diazepam has been shown to have an increased volume of distribution in the elderly due to the changes in the ratio of adipose tissue to lean tissue. Also, rate of metabolism is slower leading to increased risk of side-effects such as drowsiness and light-headedness the next day, confusion and ataxia.
2. Elderly patients have an increased risk of developing gastrointestinal side-effects and renal toxicity with NSAIDs. NSAIDs also cause fluid retention and should not be given to patients suffering from hypertension and/or heart failure. Therefore in elderly patients products with a short half-life should be adopted, use enteric-coated preparations and advise patient to take drug with or after food. NSAIDs should be used for the short term.

Further reading

Armour D and Cairns C (2001). *Medicines in the Elderly*. London: Pharmaceutical Press.

Fialova D, Topinkova E, Gambassi G, Finne-Soveri H, Jonsson P V, Carpenter I *et al.* (2005). Potentially inappropriate medication use among elderly home care patients in Europe. *JAMA* 293: 1348–1358.

Mansur N, Weiss A and Beloosesky Y (2009). Is there an association between inappropriate prescription drug use and adherence in discharged elderly patients? *Ann Pharmacother* 43: 177–184.

Zermansky A G, Alldred D P, Petty D R, Raynor D K, Freemantle N, Eastaugh J *et al.* (2006). Clinical medication review by a pharmacist of elderly people living in care homes – randomised controlled trial. *Age Ageing* 35: 586–591.

Zhang M, Holman C D J, Price S D, Sanfilippo F M, Preen D B and Bulsara M K (2009). Comorbidity and repeat admission to hospital for adverse drug reactions in older adults: retrospective cohort study. *BMJ* 338: a2752.

50

Drug therapy in paediatric patients

Learning objectives:

- To review management of common conditions associated with paediatrics
- To recognise differences in the handling of drugs by paediatric patients
- To grasp developments in the regulatory area with regards to development of medicines for use in paediatric patients.

Background

A large number of clients at the pharmacy are mothers of children who present common paediatric conditions. The pharmacist must be able to distinguish between minor ailments and potentially serious childhood conditions.

Weight

The average body weight at birth is 3.5 kg. A baby's body weight is monitored during the first year to assess child's growth. International agreement on age range and definition is shown in Table 50.1.

Vaccination programme

Table 50.2 shows a summary of the immunisation schedule.

Meningococcal group C conjugate vaccine

- Meningococcal disease in children is caused by *Neisseria meningitidis* serogroups B and C
- Immunisation provides long-term protection against infection by serogroup C of *Neisseria meningitidis*
- Indicated for children: doses given at 3 and 4 months; booster dose at 12 months
- Patients over 1 year up to 25 years: one dose.

Pneumococcal vaccine

- Directed against *Streptococcus pneumoniae* (pneumococcus)
- Recommended for childhood immunisation and in patients at increased risk: elderly patients, diabetic patients, patients with immune deficiency, chronic

Table 50.1 International agreement on age range and definition

Pre-term newborn infant	Born at less than 37 weeks' gestation
Term newborn infant	0–27 days
Infants and toddlers	28 days–23 months
Children	2–11 years
Adolescents	12–16/18[a] years

[a]Consensus not yet reached.

Table 50.2 Summary of immunisation schedule

Age	Vaccine
At 2 months	Diphtheria–tetanus–pertussis Polio *Haemophilus influenzae* type b Pneumococcal polysaccharide conjugate vaccine
At 3 months	Diphtheria–tetanus–pertussis Polio *Haemophilus influenzae* type b Meningococcal group C conjugate vaccine
At 4 months	Diphtheria–tetanus–pertussis Polio *Haemophilus influenzae* type b Pneumococcal polysaccharide conjugate vaccine Meningococcal group C conjugate vaccine
At 1 year	*Haemophilus influenzae* type b Meningococcal group C conjugate vaccine
During second year	Measles–mumps–rubella Pneumococcal polysaccharide conjugate vaccine
During fourth year	Diphtheria–tetanus Polio Measles–mumps–rubella
At 12–14 years	Tuberculosis (BCG vaccine) Human papillomavirus vaccine: 3 doses: second dose given 1–2 months after first dose and third dose given 6 months after first dose
At 16 years	Diphtheria–tetanus Polio

respiratory disease, cardiovascular disorders, renal and liver disease, asplenia, splenic dysfunction and cochlear implant

- Pneumococcal polysaccharide vaccine: polysaccharide from each of 23 capsular types of pneumococcus. Dose: single dose; recommended for children over 5 years and adults
- Pneumococcal polysaccharide conjugate vaccine: polysaccharide from each of seven capsular types of pneumococcus (conjugated to diphtheria toxoid) adsorbed onto aluminium phosphate. Dose: 2 months, 4 months and 13 months

Human papillomavirus vaccine

- Most effective if given before sexual activity starts
- There are two types of vaccine available: the bivalent vaccine and the quadrivalent vaccine. Since they are not interchangeable, repeated doses should be carried out with the same type of vaccine
- Prevents cervical cancer and other pre-cancerous lesions caused by the human papillomavirus (HPV) types 16 and 18
- The quadrivalent vaccine is also used for the prevention of genital warts and pre-cancerous lesions caused by HPV types 6, 11, 16 and 18
- The duration of protection from an entire course is still not known but at least 6 years' protection is given. If course is repeated same dosage regimen has to be followed

- Since vaccines do not protect against all strains, women should be advised that routine cervical screening should still be carried out.

Gastrointestinal problems in the neonate

- Colic
- Regurgitation and acute vomiting
- Constipation
- Diarrhoea.

Infantile colic

- Characterised by rhythmical bouts of screaming, each lasting a few minutes, in an otherwise thriving baby
- If baby is vomiting or crying persists for several hours: refer
- Change size of bottle teat. Incidence of colic is increased with the use of a teat with a large hole. Advise on use of infant formula milks specifically indicated to reduce colic
- Use simeticone with feeds.

Diarrhoea

- Oral rehydration salts (ORSs) are used
- Antidiarrhoeal preparations are contraindicated for use in children
- If baby is breast-fed, then breast milk can be given together with ORSs
- If baby is taking an infant formula milk, infant formula milk should be stopped and instead a soy-based formula introduced together with ORSs
- An oral vaccine against rotavirus which causes gastroenteritis in children is available for administration to infants over 6 weeks and before 16–24 weeks. Consists of two doses given with a 4-week interval.

Constipation

- Occurs due to inadequate food or fluid intake, withheld defecation and anal fissures
- Lifestyle changes: fluid intake and fibre, toilet training
- Stool softeners (lactulose) or bulk-forming laxatives (ispaghula) may be used, consider use of glycerin suppositories. Short-term use of stimulant laxative (senna) may be considered especially in patients with anal fissures
- Reduce laxatives slowly to prevent re-impaction.

Napkin dermatitis (nappy rash)

Prevention

- Frequent napkin change
- Avoid occlusive plastic pants
- Use barrier cream (see Chapter 47).

Management

- In many cases there is also occurrence of candidiasis. This is detected by the occurrence of white spots in the area. Antifungals, usually an imidazole cream, are required.
- Low-strength topical corticosteroids for a short time may be used to counteract inflammation.

> Use of corticosteroids in napkin dermatitis should be restricted as much as possible to hydrocortisone and the product should be used for only a few days. The occlusive effect of the nappy increases absorption of the steroid through the skin and increases risk of systemic side-effects.

Cradle cap

- Presents with scaling and crusting of scalp in infants
- Is a form of seborrhoeic dermatitis (see also Chapter 47)
- Usually appears within first 3 months and resolves spontaneously.

Management

- Rubbing olive oil/almond oil/baby oil into the scalp, leaving it overnight and then removing it by shampooing

- Proprietary products are available which have an emollient effect to counteract dryness associated with cradle cap.

Head lice (pediculosis capitis)

- Infestation spreads by head-to-head contact and is more common when children are in close contact (e.g. when children start school)
- Diagnosis is based on visual inspection and through the use of nit combs to detect active head lice and nits (eggs)
- Products used include carbaryl, dimeticone, malathion, the pyrethroids (permethrin and phenotrin)
- Resistance to anti-lice products develops and departments of public policy issue guidelines on effective products to use
- Malathion and permethrin are also used for scabies
- In addition to the use of medicated hair products the use of nit combs to remove nits should be emphasised.

Shampoo

- Advantages: pleasant to use, perfumed
- Administration: usual mode of application of a shampoo
- Disadvantage: requires repeated applications.

Lotion

- Advantages: effective (kills in one application), fast acting, treatment is complete with one application
- Disadvantages: may sting broken skin, strong smell.

Application of anti-lice lotions

- Rub into dry hair and scalp
- Allow to dry naturally
- Apply treatment at night
- Wash off after 12 hours
- Repeat procedure after 7 days
- Nit comb wet hair regularly until no more live lice appear on the comb
- Choose aqueous-based preparations in patients with atopic background, asthma and young children.

Drug dosing in children

Children dose may be calculated from adult doses using:

- age
- body weight
- body surface area
- combination of above.

Body surface area (BSA)

This is the most accurate way of calculating dose since many physical phenomena relate more closely to body surface area than to weight. The average BSA of a 70-kg human is 1.7 m^2.

$$\textit{Approximate dose for paediatric patient} = \frac{\textit{Surface area for patient } (m^2) \times \textit{adult dose}}{1.7}$$

- Young children may require a higher dose/kg than adults because of their higher metabolic rates
- Obese children would get a much higher dose than necessary when the dose is calculated on the body weight.

Pharmacokinetics

Absorption

- There are differences in gastrointestinal pH, blood flow, intestinal integrity and motility in neonates and children.

- Due to alkaline gastric pH in neonates, bioavailability of acidic drugs (e.g. phenytoin) may be decreased; bioavailability of weakly basic drugs or acid-labile drugs (e.g. penicillins, macrolides) is increased.

Drug distribution

- Plasma protein binding is decreased due to a lower concentration of binding proteins (during the first year of life). Decreased protein binding may occur with penicillins, diazepam, phenytoin and sulphonamides.
- Neonates are at increased risk of displacement of bilirubin from albumin-binding sites, resulting in kernicterus or bilirubin encephalopathy with administration of drugs that have a molar concentration which is much lower than that of albumin (e.g. ceftriaxone, sulphonamides).
- Increased permeability of drugs into neonatal tissues (e.g. distribution across the blood–brain barrier) may lead to increased volume of distribution and higher risk of unwanted central effects.

Metabolism

- Hepatic metabolism is lower than for adults due to decreased liver perfusion, hepatic enzyme capacity and biliary excretion.
- Reduced clearance of drugs such as chloramphenicol (decreased glucuronidation leads to the 'grey baby syndrome'), corticosteroids, diazepam, metronidazole, morphine, phenytoin and valproic acid.

Excretion

- In pre-term and neonates, glomerular filtration, tubular secretion and tubular re-absorption are decreased. These affect clearance of drugs such as gentamicin (decreased glomerular filtration), thiazides, morphine and penicillins (decreased tubular secretion).

Adverse drug reactions in children

Adverse drug reactions occurring most frequently in infants and children are listed in Table 50.3.

Reye's syndrome

This is an acute illness encountered exclusively in children and characterised by vomiting, central nervous system damage, hepatic injury and hypoglycaemia with a mortality rate of 50%. It is associated with aspirin intake in children. Aspirin is contraindicated in children.

Advice to parents regarding drug administration

- Avoid adding medicines to infant feeds
- Use oral syringes to calculate doses smaller than 5 mL.

Problems of use of medicines in paediatric patients

- Liquid formulation is preferred. However, some medicines, especially those that are not usually used in children, are not available in a suitable dosage form.

Table 50.3 Adverse drug reactions occurring most frequently in infants and children

Drug	Adverse drug reaction
Adrenocorticosteroids	Growth suppression
Chloramphenicol	Grey baby syndrome
Diazepam	Asthma
Phenothiazines	Extrapyramidal reactions
Tetracycline	Tooth staining, bulging fontanelle, growth inhibition
Rubella vaccine	Joint, muscular and neuritic reactions
Vitamin K	Kernicterus

- Taste may affect acceptability of medicine by the paediatric patient. Sometimes parents prefer a specific brand of a product due to the flavour.
- Problems with product availability in terms of presentation and formulation lead to extemporaneous preparation of medicines for children and to off-label use of medicines (e.g. beclometasone nasal spray in children under 6 years).
- Use of orphan drugs (drugs intended for diagnosis, prevention or treatment of diseases that affect only a small number of patients): many of these conditions are metabolic diseases occurring in paediatric patients (e.g. urea cycle disorders).

Licensing of medicines for paediatric use

- There is a lack of clinical trials providing evidence to support licensing applications for paediatric drug use due to technical problems in dosage form production and the expenses incurred.
- The European Medicines Agency (EMEA)[1] has issued new paediatric regulations:[2]
  As of 26 July 2008, for a valid application for a Marketing Authorisation, it is an obligation to submit results of studies conducted according to a paediatric investigation plan.
  As of 26 January 2009, for authorised, patented medicinal products there will be an obligation to submit results of studies for paediatric use when seeking a variation or an extension of the Marketing Authorisation for a new indication, new route of administration or new pharmaceutical formulation.

Practice summary

- Safe and effective therapeutic use of drugs in paediatrics is difficult due to limited evidence base and lack of appropriate dosage formulations.
- Risks of medication errors in paediatric patients are higher due to lack of appropriate dosing information, the requirement to prepare extemporaneous preparations for products that are not commercially available and miscalculation of doses.
- Pharmacokinetic changes in pre-term babies and paediatrics need to be considered when identifying medicines to be used in children.

Questions

1 Write briefly on (a) infantile colic and (b) napkin dermatitis.

2 Give reasons why the following preparations should be used with caution or are contraindicated in paediatric patients: (a) bisacodyl, (b) doxycycline, (c) prednisolone.

Answers

1 (a) Infantile colic is a common gastrointestinal problem in the neonate. It is characterised by rhythmic bouts of screaming, each lasting a few minutes, in an otherwise thriving baby. If baby is vomiting or crying persists for several hours referral is indicated. Non-pharmacotherapeutic measures could be suggested to decrease incidence of colic. Simeticone is used with feeds.

1 (b) Napkin dermatitis or nappy rash is a skin condition occurring in the nappy area presenting with soreness and redness. It may be aggravated with the occurrence of bacterial or candidal infections. Parents should be educated on measures to prevent napkin dermatitis: frequent napkin change, avoiding plastic occlusive pants and using a barrier cream. If condition occurs, treatment consists of using barrier and emollient creams if area is very dry. The use of imidazole creams should be considered when candidiasis is suspected.

2 (a) Bisacodyl is a stimulant laxative which should not be used in children due to the risk of causing electrolyte imbalance. Children are more prone to developing electrolyte imbalance.

2 (b) Doxycycline is a tetracycline that may cause tooth staining, bulging fontanelle and growth inhibition in children. Tetracyclines are contraindicated in children under 12 years.

2 (c) Corticosteroids cause growth suppression and are thus used with caution in children.

Further reading

Ghaleb M A, Barber N, Franklin B D, Yeung V W S, Khaki Z F and Wong I C K (2006). Systematic review of medication errors in paediatric patients. *Ann Pharmacother* 40: 1766–1776.

Jahnke C, Bauer E, Hengge U R and Feldmeier H (2009). Accuracy of diagnosis of pediculosis capitis. *Arch Dermatol* 145: 309–313.

Lowey A and Jackson M (2008). How to ensure the quality and safety of unlicensed oral medicines. *Pharm J* 281: 240.

Visscher M O (2009). Recent advances in diaper dermatitis: etiology and treatment. *Pediatr Health* 3: 81–99.

References

1 European Agency for the Evaluation of Medicinal Products. ICH Topic E 11. Note for guidance on clinical investigation of medicinal products in the paediatric population (CPMP/ICH/2711/99). London: EMEA, 2000.

2 Regulation (EC) No 1901/2006 and Amending Regulation (EC) No 1902/2006 of the European Parliament and of the Council.

51

Drugs used in pregnancy and during lactation

Learning objectives:

- To appreciate good practice of use of drugs in pregnancy and during lactation
- To identify lifestyle modifications to be recommended in pregnancy
- To develop skills to manage occurrence of minor symptoms in pregnancy and lactating mothers.

Background

During pregnancy, drugs used may adversely effect the developing fetus. Since the thalidomide tragedy in the 1960s, drug use during pregnancy takes into consideration the risk:benefit ratio due to passage of the drug across the placenta. In breast-feeding, a large number of drugs pass into breast milk and the clinical consequences depend on the amounts and type of drug used.

Teratogenicity

Since the thalidomide tragedy (see Chapter 1), medicines regulatory authorities have required that before becoming commercially available all medications are tested for teratogenicity on animals.

- *Teratogen:* a chemical entity that when present during critical periods of development is able to produce a congenital defect
- *Congenital defect*: minor or major malformations (anatomical or functional) in a baby which deviate from the norm (e.g. cleft palate associated with antiepileptic drugs).

Examples of drugs known or suspected to be teratogenic in humans

- Androgenic hormones
- Diethylstilbestrol
- Isotretinoin
- Lithium
- Phenytoin
- Tetracyclines
- Thalidomide
- Valproic acid.

Effects of teratogens

- Chromosomal abnormalities
- Impairment of implantation of the conceptus
- Resorption of early embryo and fetal death
- Structural malformations
- Intrauterine growth retardation
- Functional impairment (e.g. deafness)
- Behavioural abnormalities by the newborn
- Learning disability.

Factors affecting teratogenesis

- Time of exposure during pregnancy: greatest risk is associated with drugs administered between weeks 3 and 11 of pregnancy
- Dose administered
- Duration of treatment
- Mechanism by which drug affects development
- Rate at which drug crosses the placenta
- Genetic make-up.

Mechanism

Drugs cross the placenta by:

- ultrafiltration
- simple diffusion
- facilitated diffusion
- active transport
- pinocytosis
- passing through breaks in the placental villi.

Drug transfer across the placenta is governed by:

- concentration difference
- drug characteristics (lipid solubility, degree of ionisation, molecular weight).

> When using drugs in pregnancy, benefits should outweigh risks of treatment. Drugs should be avoided as much as possible, especially during the first trimester. Drugs that have been used and are backed up with clinical evidence and safety in pregnancy should be preferred over new or untried drugs and the lowest effective dose should be adopted.

Lifestyle modifications and pregnancy

Women planning a pregnancy and pregnant mothers should receive advice on lifestyle modifications to decrease risks to the fetus. They should consider alcohol and caffeine consumption, smoking and diet.

Alcohol and caffeine

Alcohol consumption, particularly regular intake, is associated with fetal alcohol syndrome. A safe level of alcohol consumption is not known. Pregnant women should be advised to refrain from alcohol consumption.

Intake of caffeine, which has stimulant effects, should be moderate and possibly limited to not more than three cups of coffee a day.

Smoking during pregnancy

Children whose mothers smoked during pregnancy were shown to lag behind non-exposed children in development and were associated with a decreased birth weight. The effects of smoking on the fetus include:

- fetal hypoxia caused by carbon monoxide
- intrauterine growth retardation caused by carbon monoxide and nicotine
- decreased fetal heart rate
- increased blood viscosity
- reduced fetal breathing movements
- reduced fetal movements.

Long-term effects of smoking in children:

- impaired physical growth
- impaired mental growth
- increased risk of childhood cancer
- increased frequency of bronchitis and pneumonia
- increased incidence of infant respiratory distress syndrome (dyspnoea and cyanosis).

> **Smoking cessation**
>
> During pregnancy, women should be motivated to quit smoking. Nicotine replacement therapy is not recommended during pregnancy because of lack of safety data. In patients who opt for nicotine replacement therapy, inhalators, gums and sprays at the lowest dose and frequency are the preferred dosage forms.

Diet and pregnancy

Pregnant women should be advised on a healthy balanced diet where calorie intake is increased during the pregnancy. Food intake should include foods rich in calcium and vitamin D (dairy products), iron (lean red meat) and folate (green vegetables). Vitamin supplementation, if used, should avoid excessive amounts of vitamin A.

Vitamin A

- Teratogenic in excessive amounts
- Avoid multivitamins containing vitamin A and fish liver oils
- Avoid food rich in vitamin A (e.g. liver).

Supplementation during pregnancy

Folic acid

- To reduce incidence of neural tube defects (e.g. spina bifida)
- Indicated as a supplement during pregnancy and in women planning a pregnancy.

Iron

- Foods rich in iron: red meat, green vegetables, nuts and beans
- Recommended supplementation, usually given in combination with folic acid
- Vitamin C supplementation (citrus fruit) improves absorption of iron.

Immunisation and pregnancy

- The use of immunising agents during pregnancy should be limited.
- Consider the use of tetanus toxoids (in case of accidents) and influenza vaccines according to the individual case.
- Rubella vaccination should be promoted to women planning a pregnancy.

Symptoms commonly presented in pregnancy

- Nausea and vomiting
- Gastrointestinal upset
- Constipation
- Haemorrhoids
- Common cold
- Headache and back pain
- Varicose veins, oedema and muscle cramps
- Vaginal thrush
- Pruritus.

Nausea and vomiting

- Occurs mostly during 14–16 weeks of pregnancy.

Aetiology

- Changes in endocrine system
- Hypersensitivity to proteins and fetal antigens
- Toxic and metabolic mechanisms.

Advice

- Eat small, frequent meals; avoid spicy meals
- Keep well hydrated, use oral rehydration salts if vomiting occurs.

Gastro-oesophageal reflux

Aetiology

- Increased pressure from uterus onto stomach
- Progesterone relaxes lower oesophageal tone
- Decreased gastrointestinal motility.

Advice

- Eat small frequent meals
- Avoid spicy and fried food
- Antacids that have a low sodium content may be recommended.

Constipation

Aetiology

- Increased pressure on colon
- Increased intestinal transit time
- Increased colonic absorption of water
- Use of iron supplements.

Advice

- Increase fibre intake
- Keep well hydrated
- Exercise
- Recommend use of bulk-forming laxatives as first-line treatment. An osmotic laxative may be considered. Stimulant laxatives should be used if a stimulant effect is necessary.

Haemorrhoids

- May develop or worsen during pregnancy.

Aetiology

- Increased pressure of uterus on the rectum
- Occurrence of constipation.

Advice

- Avoid straining at stool
- External products are preferred as opposed to suppositories. Astringents are preferred. Products containing topical anaesthetics and corticosteroids are to be used with caution.

Common cold

- Avoid use of drugs: they are not curative
- Avoid use of combination drugs
- Prefer topical rather than systemic administration of sympathomimetics (nasal decongestants). The use of saline nasal drops is recommended.

Headache and back pain

- Common complaints in pregnancy
- Headache occurs possibly due to intracranial vascular changes mediated by progesterone and oestrogen
- Analgesic of choice: paracetamol.

Varicose veins, oedema and muscle cramps

- Recommend use of support hosiery
- Advise patient to elevate legs
- Avoid high-heeled shoes.

Vaginal thrush (candidiasis)

- Patient should be referred.
- The use of imidazole intravaginal preparations should be recommended by a specialist after ensuring the safety of the application. Topical administration of imidazole preparations is preferred.
- Oral administration of itraconazole and fluconazole is not recommended due to reported toxicity in animal studies.

Pruritus

- Thought to be due to oestrogen-induced cholestatis
- Occurs as a generalised condition
- Recommend calamine lotion.

Chronic conditions

Epilepsy

Epilepsy in pregnancy is associated with an increased risk of congenital malformations including a higher risk of neural tube defects.

- Dose adjustments of antiepileptic agents (there may be increased dosage requirements during pregnancy) are required throughout pregnancy.
- Single antiepileptic therapy is preferred over multiple therapy.
- It is important that women taking antiepileptic drugs who are planning a pregnancy are counselled on the possible consequences and are given folic acid supplementation during the planning stage and continued during the pregnancy.
- After birth, the neonate is at risk of developing antiepileptic-associated neonatal haemorrhage. This is counteracted by the administration of vitamin K injection at birth.
- The benefits of treatment outweigh the risks.

Pregnancy and epilepsy

It has to be explained to the mother that compliance to antiepileptic drug therapy is essential for the well-being of fetus and mother.

Diabetes

Blood glucose control is essential during pregnancy and benefits of antidiabetic treatment overrule the risks of therapy.

- Insulin is the drug of choice during pregnancy.
- Sulphonylureas and metformin are relatively contraindicated during pregnancy (occurrence of neonatal hypoglycaemia reported).

Hyperpigmentation

This is caused by the deposition of melanin in the skin (melasma) during pregnancy. It may also occur in patients using oral contraceptives. Dark-brown patches occur on the face; these are accentuated by exposure to sun.

- Advise patient that darkening fades after childbirth.

Pharmacotherapy during pregnancy

Anti-infective agents

- Avoid use of co-trimoxazole, tetracyclines, griseofulvin, itraconazole and ketoconazole
- Recommended drugs: amoxicillin, erythromycin, co-amoxiclav.

Analgesics

- NSAIDs may cause delayed onset and increase duration of labour if taken during the third trimester.
- Recommended drug: paracetamol.

Drug use during pregnancy

- Avoid unnecessary medications including non-prescription medications
- Drugs licensed for infants generally do not pose a hazard
- Avoid long-acting preparations
- Monitor fetus during drug therapy
- Avoid new drugs.

Breast-feeding and use of medicines

Laxatives

- Agents that are not absorbed such as bulk-forming and osmotic agents are preferred.
- Short-term moderate use of stimulant laxatives may sometimes be prescribed in moderate doses.

NSAIDs

- Topical formulations are suitable
- COX-2 inhibitors: to be avoided, no clinical data
- COX-1 inhibitors: short-acting agents that do not have an active metabolite are preferred (e.g. diclofenac).

Antihistamines

- Preferably use a minimally sedating agent with a short half-life
- Newer antihistamines (e.g. cetirizine, desloratadine, loratadine): manufacturers advise avoidance.

Vitamins

- During lactation there is increased requirements for some vitamins and minerals (folate, vitamin B_2, B_6, B_{12}, C)
- Avoid use of megadose regimens.

Practice summary

- Use of drugs in pregnancy and lactating mothers should be avoided as much as possible.
- Benefits of drugs used in pregnancy and lactating mothers should outweigh risks to fetus and baby.
- Drugs used should be identified after careful evaluation of the symptoms, patient background and drug characteristics.

Questions

1 What advice should be given to a woman who is planning a pregnancy?
2 Give one example of an antihistamine which could be recommended to a lactating mother for systemic use.

Answers

1 To take folic acid supplementation 0.4 mg daily pre-conception until week 12 of pregnancy to reduce incidence of neural tube defects such as spina bifida. To take iron supplementation and eat foods rich in iron such as red meat, green vegetables, nuts and beans. Vitamin C enhances iron absorption. Woman should be advised to take up rubella vaccination prior to conception. If woman is a smoker, advise patient on importance of stopping smoking before pregnancy. Advice on the use of nicotine replacement therapy may be given for use before conception.
2 Older-type antihistamines are used, preferably a product with a short half-life such as diphenhydramine. Advise on risk of sedation.

Further reading

Every M and Hallam C (2003). Overview of pregnancy. *Pharm J* 270: 194–196

McElhatton P R (2003). General principles of drug use in pregnancy. *Pharm J* 270: 232–234.

McElhatton P R (2003). Drug use in pregnancy: part 1. *Pharm J* 270: 270–272.

McElhatton P R (2003). Drug use in pregnancy: part 2. *Pharm J* 270: 305–307.

Nathan A (2003). General care of pregnant women. *Pharm J* 270: 338–340.

52

Critical care therapeutics

Learning objectives:

- To appreciate use of parenteral preparations for fluid and electrolyte imbalance
- To develop skills required for using drugs and replacement fluids in critical care scenarios.

Factors that increase risk of death after intensive care

- Increasing age
- Greater severity of acute illness
- History of severe clinical conditions
- Requirement for emergency surgery
- Infections.

Principles of critical care therapeutics

- Critical care is associated with dysfunction in circulatory, respiratory, hepatic and renal systems.
- Routes of administration and doses of drugs should be based on physiological status of the individual patient.
- Critical care is more likely to be associated with the occurrence of adverse drug reactions due to number of medications used and type of medications used (narrow therapeutic index drugs).
- Monitor function of vital organs.
- Prevent occurrence of complications — infections, acute respiratory distress syndrome (ARDS).

Preservation of cardiovascular function

- Monitor fluid and electrolyte status
- Deterioration presents as arrhythmias, shock.

Preservation of respiratory function

- Monitor respiratory function
- Deterioration may be due to pulmonary oedema or pneumonia, and presents as respiratory failure.

Physiological markers used for health evaluation

- Body temperature
- Blood pressure
- Heart rate
- Respiratory rate
- Serum sodium
- Serum potassium
- Serum creatinine.

Prevention of occurrence of pulmonary embolism

Pulmonary embolism occurs due to prolonged immobility, tissue damage and activation of coagulation. In patients with prolonged bed rest, who have undergone recent surgery or have suffered a head trauma use heparin. Consider use of mattresses that avoid occurrence of pressure sores (see also Chapter 24).

> In critical care, patients may have interrelated pathologies. Try to summarise the information available and extract relevant issues.

Hypovolaemia

This condition is caused by loss of intravascular fluid as a result of trauma, vomiting, diarrhoea, haemorrhage, burns or dehydration. Symptoms include tachycardia and decreased urine output. Replacement solutions are used to correct hypovolaemia. These may be crystalloid solutions or colloid solutions.

Crystalloid solutions

These are isotonic solutions containing electrolytes:

- Sodium chloride 0.9%: may give rise to hypernatraemia presenting with oedema; use with caution in patients with impaired renal function, hypertension, cardiac failure, peripheral and pulmonary oedema.
- Lactated Ringer's solution (compound sodium lactate/Hartmann's solution/Ringer lactate solution): consists of sodium chloride 0.6%, sodium lactate 0.25%, potassium chloride 0.04%, calcium chloride 0.027%.
- Intravenous glucose: rarely used alone in hypovolaemia, usually used in combination with sodium chloride when there is a combined water and sodium depletion. Used alone when there is loss of water with no significant loss of electrolytes (e.g. hyperthyroidism, hypercalcaemia); also used to correct hypoglycaemia or for parenteral nutrition. When used as monotherapy, care should be taken since it may cause hyponatraemia and other electrolyte disturbances. Available as glucose 5%, 25%, 50% solutions or as solutions presenting a mixture of sodium chloride and glucose (e.g. 0.9% NaCl, 5% glucose and 0.45% NaCl, 5% glucose).

Colloid solutions

These are solutions containing plasma proteins or colloidal molecules. Since they contain large molecules, a smaller volume of fluid is required to produce the same volume expansion that would be obtained with crystalloid solutions.

Albumin

- Prepared from whole blood and contains soluble proteins and electrolytes
- Since it does not contain blood group antibodies, there is no need to match blood groups
- Contraindications: cardiac failure, severe anaemia
- Caution: history of cardiac or circulatory disease
- Patient monitoring: cardiovascular and respiratory function.

Plasma substitutes (dextrans: Dextran 40, Dextran 70; gelatin; etherified starch)

- Used to expand blood volume (e.g. in shock due to burns or septicaemia). They are also used short term until blood is available for transfusion after haemorrhage
- Caution: large volumes of some plasma substitutes may increase risk of bleeding, cardiac and liver disease, renal impairment
- Side-effects: hypersensitivity reactions, increase in bleeding time
- Patient monitoring: urine output.

Comparative prices of volume-expanding agents are shown in Table 52.1.

Hyperkalaemia

This condition is characterised by a potassium serum level >5 mmol/L.

Table 52.1 Comparative prices of volume-expanding agents

Product	Ratio for cost per 500 mL IV fluid
Albumin 5%	30
Albumin 25%	37
Dextran 40	7.5
Dextran 70	5
Ringer lactate	1
Physiological saline	1

- Aetiology: renal failure, acidosis, potassium-sparing diuretics
- Signs and symptoms: cardiac arrhythmias, muscle weakness.

Management

- Calcium gluconate or calcium chloride (intravenous): aim is to maintain cardiac function; prolonged use may cause hypercalcaemia
- Sodium bicarbonate (intravenous): lowers potassium levels; prolonged use may cause sodium overload
- Glucose solutions: given in regimen with calcium and bicarbonate and insulin in the emergency management of hyperkalaemia. Potassium moves across cell membranes with glucose in the presence of insulin. Glucose/insulin administration may be used for longer than the calcium and bicarbonate components. Dextrose 20% or Dextrose 50% may be used.

Hypokalaemia

This condition is characterised by a potassium serum level <3.5 mmol/L).

- Aetiology: diuretics, diarrhoea, alkalosis, vomiting, corticosteroids, renal tubular acidosis
- Signs and symptoms: cardiac abnormalities, muscle weakness, paralysis, weak pulse
- Caution: usually there is concomitant hyponatraemia; monitor serum sodium electrolyte levels.

Management

- Oral potassium solution is usually preferred unless patient is unable to swallow; gastrointestinal side-effects may occur.
- Intravenous administration of potassium: 20 mmol potassium in 1 mL mixed with sodium chloride 0.9%. Monitoring required includes ECG and serum potassium levels. Should not be administered rapidly since rapid infusion is toxic to the heart.

Practice summary

- Drug selection is based on: availability of dosage forms, drug suitability according to patient's characteristics (e.g. renal and cardiac function), drug interactions to be avoided
- Ensure documentation of drug administration
- Monitor use of parenteral solutions and assess route of administration
- Monitor for drug incompatibilities in solution and administration lines (e.g. drug–drug co-precipitation: gentamicin (positive charge) with cephalosporins/heparin (negative charge)
- Assess drug stability (e.g. intravenous co-amoxiclav has to be administered immediately after reconstitution)
- Follow up appropriate drug storage and labelling to avoid medication errors
- Patient monitoring: monitor hepatic, renal and cardiac function
- Identify and monitor occurrence of adverse drug reactions
- Assess risk of infection and adopt prophylactic therapy where appropriate: monitor anti-infective drug use and check that dose given is sufficient to ensure efficacy.

Question

1 When is potassium supplementation administered parenterally?

Answer

1 When hypokalaemia occurs, patient is at risk of developing arrhythmias and muscle cramps. Potassium supplementation is administered in patients receiving diuretics or those with hypokalaemia. Parenteral administration is considered for acute management of hypokalaemia when the risks of cardiac arrhythmias are high, such as in patients with very low serum potassium levels and cardiovascular disease and patients in whom administration of oral formulations is not possible.

Further reading

Anon (2009). Safe administration of intravenous potassium for treating hypokalaemia in hospital. *Clin Pharm* 1: 40.

Hess M (2007). *Integrating Critical Care Skills into Your Practice: A case workbook*. Bethesda, MA: American Society of Health-System Pharmacists.

Sexton J and Rahman M H (2008). Parenteral replacement of fluids and electrolytes: the basics. *Pharm J* 281: 571–574.

Acknowledgements

Bernard Coleiro, Consultant Physician, Department of Medicine, Mater Dei Hospital, Malta.

53

Recent advances in pharmacotherapy

Learning objectives:

- To appreciate developments in the availability of pharmaceutical drugs
- To highlight requirement to keep abreast of new developments in pharmacy and the use of medicines.

Background

A large number of drugs that are used today have been developed over the past 30 years (see also Chapter 1). Drugs that were developed over the past few years include:

- angiotensin II receptor antagonists (e.g. losartan)
- leukotriene receptor antagonists (e.g. zafirlukast)
- atypical antipsychotics (e.g. risperidone)
- antidepressants (e.g. venlafaxine)
- anti-obesity drugs acting on the gastrointestinal tract (e.g. orlistat)
- drugs for diabetes (e.g. repaglinide)
- bisphosphonates for the prevention of fractures in postmenopausal patients (e.g. alendronic acid)
- alpha-blockers to relax smooth muscle in benign prostatic hyperplasia (e.g. alfuzosin).

Recent developments in drugs acting on the cardiovascular system

Aliskiren

- Direct renin inhibitor
- Licensed for the management of hypertension.

Dabigatran etexilate and rivaroxaban

- Two oral anticoagulants indicated for the prevention of venous thromboembolism following hip or knee replacement surgery.
- Dabigatran etexilate acts as a direct thrombin inhibitor and rivaroxaban acts as a factor Xa inhibitor.
- Advantages: no need for coagulation monitoring.

Ivabradine

- Potassium channel antagonist that inhibits cardiac pacemaker current
- Indicated for the treatment of chronic stable angina pectoris in patients who have contraindication or intolerance to beta-blockers
- Lowers heart rate by its action on the sinus node
- Contraindications: severe bradycardia (less than 60 beats/min), recent myocardial infarction, recent cerebrovascular accident, unstable angina.

Rilmenidine

- Oxazoline compound with antihypertensive properties acting on medullary and peripheral vasomotor structures
- Selective for imidazoline receptors.

Recent developments in drugs acting on the central nervous system

Aripiprazole

- Atypical antipsychotic
- Causes little or no elevation of prolactin concentration.

Atomoxetine

- Indicated for attention deficit hyperactivity disorder
- Is a selective noradrenergic re-uptake inhibitor.

Bupropion

- Atypical antidepressant licensed for use as an aid to smoking cessation programmes.

Rufinamide

- An anticonvulsant agent that is a triazole derivative making it structurally different to other antiepileptic agents
- Marketed for patients with Lennox–Gastaut syndrome, a severe and difficult-to-treat form of epilepsy that usually begins in childhood.

Sibutramine

- Centrally acting anti-obesity agent that inhibits serotonin and noradrenaline re-uptake resulting in decreased food intake.

Varenicline

- Indicated for smoking cessation
- Partial nicotinic receptor antagonist designed to block the 'rewards' from smoking and to reduce the craving
- In 2007 – warning of possibility of occurrence of depression issued.

Recent developments in infectious disease management

HIV treatment – protease inhibitors

- Atazanavir, fosamprenavir
- Protease inhibitors are metabolised by cytochrome P450 enzyme systems and therefore have a significant potential for drug interactions
- Used with caution in hepatic impairment, diabetes (associated with hyperglycaemia) and haemophilia (increased risk of bleeding).

HIV treatment – integrase inhibitors

- Raltegravir prevents the covalent insertion or integration of the HIV genome into the host cell genome
- Indicated for use in HIV-infected patients showing HIV replication despite antiretroviral therapy
- To be used in combination therapy with other antiretroviral agents.

Micafungin

- An antifungal agent available for intravenous administration
- It acts by interfering with fungal cell wall
- Used for the systemic treatment of candidiasis and for the prophylaxis of candidiasis in patients undergoing haematopoietic stem cell transplantation.

Retapamulin

- Available as an ointment
- It is a pleuromutilin derivative that has bacteriostatic effects, particularly against *Staphylococcus aureus* and *Streptococcus pyogenes*.

Recent developments in diabetes management

Incretin mimetics/enhancers

Exenatide

- Available as injection for subcutaneous administration
- Increases insulin secretion, suppresses glucagon secretion and slows gastric emptying.

Sitagliptin

- Available as tablets for once-daily administration
- Increases incretin levels leading to increased insulin secretion and lower glucagon secretion.

Use of thiazolidinediones – rosiglitazone and pioglitazone

- To be used with care in patients with ischaemic heart disease due to increased risk of heart attack; risk of bone fracture increased.

Recent developments in drugs used in carcinoma

Fulvestrant

- An oestrogen receptor antagonist without the agonist effects seen with tamoxifen
- Licensed for oestrogen receptor-positive metastatic breast cancer in postmenopausal women
- Administered by deep intramuscular injection every 4 weeks.

Imatinib

- In chronic myeloid leukaemia, there is a chromosomal abnormality known as Philadelphia chromosome leading to abnormal tyrosine kinase activity.
- Imatinib is an oral signal transduction inhibitor that specifically inhibits the abnormal kinase activity associated with the Philadelphia chromosome.
- It is compared with conventional treatment: busulfan, interferon.

Lapatinib

- Oral protein kinase indicated for breast cancer with overexpression of HER2
- It is compared with trastuzumab which is available only for intravenous infusion.

Panitumumab

- Monoclonal antibody that is indicated in epidermal growth factor receptor (EGFR)-expressing metastatic colorectal cancer
- Used as monotherapy. Increased risk of toxicity when used in combination chemotherapy.

Temsirolimus

- A kinase inhibitor indicated for first-line treatment in advanced renal cell carcinoma
- Hyperglycaemia or hyperlipidaemia may occur as unwanted effects
- Monitoring required: full blood count, glucose and lipid profiles, renal function, symptoms of bowel perforation.

> New therapies, particularly in the area of malignancy, rely on pharmacogenetic expression of the disease. These treatment modalities represent personalised medication and apply particularly to patients who otherwise may experience treatment failure.

Extensions of existing therapies

- Sildenafil: acquired a licence for pulmonary arterial hypertension

- Clopidogrel: can be used in combination with aspirin in patients eligible for thrombolytic therapy, for the prevention of atherothrombotic events in ST-segment elevation acute myocardial infarction
- Pramipexole and ropinirole (antiparkinsonian drugs): licensed for restless legs syndrome.

New drugs and drug budgets

- Considerations of pharmacoeconomic evaluation
- Updating of guidelines and protocols on prescribing policies
- Drug use evaluation programmes
- Clinical expertise on new treatment modalities
- Require review by drug and therapeutic committees.

Drug patent

The originator company would like to retain market share from a product as much as possible once generic formulations become available soon after patent expiry. Strategies that can be adopted are to add value to the current patented product and therefore achieve an extension of the patent or post-patent expiry to compete with the competing manufacturer.

- Patent extension: adding value to product
  - new formulation
  - approved new indication
- Competing post-patent expiry
  - lobbying for P to POM switch
  - originator company marketing branded generic.

Practice summary

- New medications should be considered and drug information sought.
- Look out for updated information on drug profile for the first few years after release.
- Ensure patient safety and patient information when switching to a newer drug.

Question

1 What are the characteristics of the following drugs: (a) aliskiren, (b) varenicline?

Answer

1 (a) *Aliskiren* interferes with the production of angiotensin II which is a vasoconstrictor by inhibiting renin. Its efficacy is similar to ACE inhibitors and angiotensin II receptor blockers (ARBs).

(b) *Varenicline* acts by binding to nicotine receptors in the brain and causing a reduction of the craving sensation for nicotine and a reduced satisfaction when smoking. The drug is started 1 week before intended smoking cessation. Suicidal thoughts and behaviour have been reported. Patients should be advised to report immediately signs of these side-effects. The product should be used with caution in patients with a history of psychiatric illness, in renal impairment and during breast-feeding.

Further reading

Adcock H (2007). Clinical developments in 2006. *Pharm J* 278: 21–24.

Adcock H (2008). Clinical developments in 2007. *Pharm J* 280: 27–30.

Adcock H (2009). Clinical developments in 2008. *Pharm J* 282: 25–28.

PART 3

Responding to Symptoms in Community Pharmacy

54

Colds and influenza

Learning objectives:

- To understand common cold and drugs used in the management of symptoms
- To recognise influenza and methods of prophylaxis.

Background

The common cold and influenza are two conditions affecting the respiratory tract that are caused by a viral infection. Both are generally self-limiting. However, in some scenarios complications that have serious implications may occur. Transmission is by droplet inhalation.

The common cold

Also referred to as acute coryza or infectious rhinitis, this is a viral infection of the upper respiratory tract.

- Symptoms occur 18–48 hours after exposure. Onset is gradual
- Symptoms: sore or tickly throat (pharyngitis), sneezing, rhinorrhoea. Fever may occur in children
- Duration: 3–7 days
- Complications: secondary bacterial infection, otitis media particularly in children, sinusitis and laryngitis.

Factors that predispose to the common cold

- The 'iceberg concept': a number of viral respiratory tract infections do not cause any symptoms
- Factors that influence the body's immune response to the exposure to the virus include: nutrition, stress, smoking, emotional disturbances.

Why more colds in the cold?

- People spend time indoors in poorly ventilated homes
- Air is colder and this may allow the virus to replicate at a higher rate.

Influenza

During the viral infection, sloughing of epithelial cells in the respiratory system, submucosal inflammation and fluid extravasation occur.

- Incubation period: 1–4 days, average 2 days. Onset is rapid

- Symptoms: fever, headache, myalgia, severe malaise, non-productive cough, sore throat, rhinitis.

Influenza: high-risk patients

- Age >50 years
- Chronic medical conditions:
  - pulmonary disease
  - metabolic disease (e.g. diabetes)
  - renal dysfunction
  - immunosuppression
  - heart disease
  - liver disease
  - HIV
  - neurological disease
- Patients receiving immunosuppressants
- Residents of nursing homes or long-term care facilities
- People in close or frequent contact with anyone in the high-risk group.

Complications of influenza

- Croup in children
- Pneumonia, secondary bacterial infections
- Myositis
- Cardiac complications especially in patients with a history of cardiovascular disease
- Encephalopathy.

Inflammatory mediators associated with colds and influenza

- Prostaglandins
- Leukotrienes
- Bradykinin
- Thromboxane.

Assessing occurrence of symptoms

- Sore throat
- Rhinorrhoea
- Cough
- Aches and pain
- Temperature
- Earache.

When to refer

- Paediatric and geriatric patients
- Pre-existing heart or lung disease
- Sore throat lasting a week or more
- Hoarseness of more than 3 weeks
- Dysphagia
- Cough lasting 2 weeks or more
- Croup
- Sputum: yellow, green, blood stained
- Chest pain, shortness of breath, wheezing
- Facial pain and frontal headache
- Persistent fever
- Otitis media.

Croup (laryngotracheobronchitis) occurs mainly in paediatric patients and presents as a barking cough. Referral is recommended since sometimes condition may become life threatening.

Nasal decongestants

Nasal decongestants are sympathomimetic agents that act primarily on the alpha-adrenergic receptors causing peripheral vasoconstriction. They offer symptomatic relief from rhinorrhoea and nasal congestion. The products may be administered either topically (nasal administration) or orally (for a systemic effect).

Topical administration

- Dosage forms: drops, spray
- Disadvantage: rhinitis medicamentosa when product is applied for a prolonged period of time
- Examples: xylometazoline (0.05%, 0.1%) and oxymetazoline (0.025%, 0.05%)

- Advise patient to use topical nasal decongestants for a few days, usually not exceeding 7 days, to avoid occurrence of rhinitis medicamentosa.

Systemic administration

- Examples: pseudoephedrine, phenylephrine
- Side-effects: tachycardia, anxiety, insomnia, restlessness
- Caution: cardiac disease, hypertension, diabetes, hyperthyroidism, glaucoma, benign prostatic hypertrophy
- May be found in combination with antihistamines and cough preparations.

Other topical products

- Sodium chloride: 0.9%, safe product which can be used in paediatric patients and during pregnancy. Patient is advised to apply product as required to provide relief from congestion.
- Steam inhalations: intended to provide relief from nasal congestion. Volatile oils such as camphor and menthol may be added to the solution. Patient should be advised to be careful when using hot or boiling water to avoid injuries.

Antihistamines

- Examples: triprolidine, promethazine, chlorphenamine
- Decrease in sneezing and nasal secretions
- Side-effects: sedation, dry mouth, blurred vision, constipation, difficulty in urination
- The side-effect of sedation may be a required effect to induce sleep. Occurrence of sedation counteracts the side-effect of insomnia that is associated with systemic administration of nasal decongestants
- See also Chapter 25.

Cough suppressants

- To be used only for dry non-productive cough. Cough suppressants are contraindicated when there is a chesty cough
- They act by inhibiting medullary cough centre
- Products can be either opioids or sedating antihistamines
- Opioids: e.g. codeine, pholcodine, dextromethorphan (less potent, milder side-effect profile)
- Side-effects: drowsiness, constipation, nausea, vomiting
- Caution: asthma, hepatic and renal impairment, children, avoid under 1 year of age
- Antihistamines: e.g. diphenhydramine, promethazine.

Expectorants

- Examples: guaifenesin, ammonium chloride, ipecacuanha, squill
- Facilitate removal of mucus
- Evidence to support benefit from using expectorants very weak.

Mucolytics

- Examples: carbocisteine, bromhexine
- Facilitate expectoration by reducing sputum viscosity
- Used in patients with excessive mucus production.

Treatment controversies

Combined vs single therapy: combined preparations may contain products that are not relevant to a particular individual. Using different single products may be preferred to select active ingredients that are required to counteract symptoms in a particular individual. However, this approach is more expensive than a combination product and increases medicine handling requirements by patient.

Irrational combinations

- Cough suppressants + expectorants
- Antihistamines + expectorants.

Formulations that can be used with confidence in adults are shown in Table 54.1.

Table 54.1 Formulations that can be used with confidence in adults

Symptoms presented	Components of combination products
Fever, nasal congestion	Analgesic + sympathomimetic
Non-productive cough, congestion	Opioid antitussive + sympathomimetic
Productive cough, congestion	Guaifenesin + sympathomimetic
Sore throat	Demulcent pastilles or lozenges (see Chapter 56)

Patient advice

- Not to use topical nasal decongestants for longer than 5–7 days
- Not to use paracetamol with combination cold preparations that already contain paracetamol
- Drowsiness may occur with products containing sedating antihistamines or opioid antitussives.

Vitamin C supplementation

Vitamin C (ascorbic acid) is an antioxidant that neutralises the oxidising compounds released by neutrophils during a viral infection. Doses of 1–4 g/day decrease duration and severity of cold symptoms by 10–30%.

- Care: at high doses it interferes with diabetes urine tests and increases risk of production of urinary oxalate leading to renal stones.

Other products used for prophylaxis

- Garlic
- Echinacea
- Zinc
- Ginseng.

- According to the MHRA (UK), there is a lack of evidence of benefits and reports of side-effects from the use of sedating antihistamines, antitussives, expectorants and nasal decongestants in children under 6 years.[1]
- In children under 6 years the use of the following products is recommended:
  - paracetamol or ibuprofen: antipyretics
  - saline drops: to relieve nasal congestion
  - vapour rub: for children over 3 months to relieve nasal congestion
  - cough mixtures containing honey and lemon to relieve cough.

Influenza vaccine

- Inactivated vaccine containing different strains that are identified every year as the predicted predominant strains
- Administered in October–November
- Route of administration: intramuscular injection. A new formulation of the influenza vaccine has been granted a marketing authorisation by EMEA in 2008 for administration via the intradermal route. It is suggested that the route of administration allows for the antigen to be deposited in the dermal layer of the skin which is rich in dendritic cells that are associated with stimulating an immune response
- Aim of administration is to prevent secondary complications
- Target groups: high-risk patients
- Contraindication: hypersensitivity to eggs.

Antivirals

- Reduce replication of influenza viruses by inhibiting viral neuraminidase
- When used within 48 hours of onset of symptoms, reduce duration of symptoms
- Used for post-exposure prophylaxis of influenza. They may be used to prevent influenza in an epidemic.

Oseltamivir

- Available as capsules and suspension
- Cautions: renal impairment, pregnancy, breast-feeding
- Side-effects: gastrointestinal, headache, fatigue, insomnia, dizziness.

Zanamivir

- Available as a powder for inhalation
- Cautions: asthma and chronic pulmonary disease (avoid in severe disease), uncontrolled chronic illness
- Side-effects are rare and include bronchospasm and respiratory impairment
- Patient advice: if used in patients with asthma and chronic pulmonary disease, other inhaled drugs should be administered before zanamivir if concurrent administration is requires and a short-acting bronchodilator should be available to be used if bronchospasms occur.

The occurrence of fever warrants antipyretic treatment. In children paracetamol and ibuprofen are the drugs of choice; aspirin should be avoided. Patients should be kept well hydrated and in airy rooms. Avoid smoking. Using multiple pillows to elevate the head at night reduces the occurrence of post-nasal drip.

Practice summary

- Management of the common cold is based on counteracting symptoms presented.
- Topical nasal decongestants should not be used for a prolonged period. Sodium chloride 0.9% drops are preferred in very young children.
- Antitussive preparations should be used only when there is dry cough and should be avoided in patients with chronic respiratory disease and children under 1 year of age.
- The influenza vaccine should be administered yearly to patients at high risk of developing complications of influenza.

Questions

1. What is a disadvantage of topical nasal decongestants and what advice should be given to the patient to minimise occurrence of this unwanted effect?
2. Describe the nasal decongestant effect of phenylephrine. Name two side-effects that could occur with the systemic administration of phenylephrine. Name four conditions when phenylephrine should be used with caution.

Answers

1. Topical administration of nasal decongestants is intended only for short-term use (not more than 7 consecutive days) as prolonged use can result in rebound congestion (rhinitis medicamentosa). Patients should be advised to use the product for not more than 7 days.
2. Phenylephrine is a nasal decongestant that acts as a sympathetic nervous system agonist predominantly at the alpha receptors. It causes vasoconstriction of the nasopharyngeal and sinus passages, leading to relief from the symptoms of rhinorrhoea and nasal congestion. Side-effects include tachycardia and anxiety. Phenylephrine should be used with caution in

cardiac disease and hypertension, diabetes, hyperthyroidism and glaucoma.

Further reading

Barrett B, Harahan B, Brown D, Zhang Z and Brown R (2007). Sufficiently important difference for common cold: severity reduction. *Ann Fam Med* 5: 216–233.

Fleming D (2007). Assessing the accuracy of influenza diagnosis by community pharmacists. *Pharm J* 279: 441–444.

National Institute for Health and Clinical Evidence (2009). Amantadine, oseltamivir and zanamivir for the treatment of influenza: Review of NICE technology appraisal guidance 58. http://www.nice.org. uk/TA168.

Perrie Y (2006). Influenza: treatment and prevention. *Pharm J* 277: 399–402.

Reference

1 Anon. Cough and cold remedies no longer recommended for children under six years. *Pharm J* 2009; 282: 237.

55

The eyes

Learning objectives:

- To summarise use of topical agents in eye conditions
- To review presentation of common eye disorders
- To address management of glaucoma
- To appreciate principles of contact lens use and care.

Background

Preparations for the eye should be sterile. Eye drops in multiple-application containers used in domiciliary care should not be used for more than 4 weeks after first opening.

- *Eye drops:* drugs penetrate the globe, probably through the cornea; systemic effects may arise from absorption of drugs into the general circulation
- *Eye ointment:* applied to lid margins
- *Eye lotions:* solutions for irrigation.

Ocular symptoms most likely to be encountered in the pharmacy are red eyes, styes, swollen, painful eyelids and sore, gritty eyes. Responding to these symptoms requires special care to differentiate between minor disorders and potentially serious conditions that could have significant consequences.

Eyelid disorders

Stye (hordeolum)

- Local pyogenic infection involving the follicle or sebaceous gland of an eyelash
- Occurs on the outer surface of the eyelid as a palpable, tender nodule
- Presents with painful swelling and inflammation of the edge of the eyelid
- Management: hot compresses and application of local antibacterial eye preparations.

Chalazion

- Inflammatory granulomatous swelling on the eyelid or its margin
- Occurs due to blockage of one of the meibomian glands which lubricate the eyelid
- More common in adults than in children
- Management: surgical removal may be required, local antibacterial preparations may be considered if infection is suspected.

Blepharitis

- Inflammation of the margins of the eyelids
- Presentation: inflammation, scaling, pruritus, oedema, yellow crusts form on the eyelashes
- Causes: unknown, due to allergy, occurs with seborrheic dermatitis
- Management: cleanse the eye with saline solution and apply of local antibacterial preparations.

Contact dermatitis

- Presentation: swelling, scaling or redness of the eyelid, itching
- Could be due to make-up, soap
- Management: cold compresses, oral antihistamines.

Entropion and ectropion

- *Entropion:* turning inward of the eyelid
- *Ectropion:* eversion of the eyelid.

Entropion and ectropion are conditions that occur in old age and lead to eye discomfort and dryness.

Ocular surface disorders

Foreign substance contact

- Remove foreign particles with care.
- Refer in cases where metallic foreign bodies, chemical exposure or thermal damage has occurred.

Conjunctivitis

This is inflammation of the membrane that lines the eyelids (conjunctiva). It presents with erythema and swelling of the lids and can be acute or chronic. It may be due to:

- allergy: occurring in both eyes; watery discharge, itchiness and rhinitis may be concomitant symptoms.
- viral infection: occurring in both eyes; watery discharge, gritty feeling and usually patient also presents with respiratory viral infection (cold)
- bacterial infection: initially presents in one eye but may spread to both eyes; purulent discharge, gritty feeling and not usually associated with other symptoms.

Management

- Allergic: ocular decongestants, topical or systemic antihistamines
- Viral: artificial tears, ocular decongestants
- Bacterial: topical antibacterial preparations.

Dry eye

- Presentation of mildly red eye, gritty feeling or sensation of foreign body, excess tears
- Management: artificial tears which can be applied as often as required.

Subconjunctival haemorrhage

- May develop at any age following minor trauma, sneezing, coughing
- Alarming, but extravasation absorbed gradually within 2 weeks.

Accompanying symptoms indicative of referral

- Eyelid irritation: with history of trauma or with swelling and failed nodule treatment
- Red eye: with pain, blurred vision, photophobia, history of trauma, contact lens wear, foreign body sensation and possible contamination or vomiting.

Ophthalmic preparations

Topical antibacterial preparations

- Broad spectrum: chloramphenicol, ciprofloxacin, ofloxacin, gentamicin, framycetin
- Anti-staphylococcal activity: fusidic acid
- Available as monotherapy or in combination with corticosteroids

- Dosing schedule normally requires administration three to four times a day
- It is recommended to advise patient to continue treatment 48 hours after healing, about careful hand washing and to be careful when administering the drops or ointment in the lower conjunctival sac to avoid contamination of dropper.

When the application of eye ointments is relevant, it may be recommended to use the eye ointment at night and then complement therapy with the eye drops. Application of eye ointments is associated with blurring of vision and this may impact negatively on patient compliance if three to four times daily administration is requested.

Anti-inflammatory preparations

- Corticosteroids: e.g. betamethasone, dexamethasone
- Use: allergy, herpes simplex keratitis (+ aciclovir), post surgery
- Cautions: undiagnosed red eye since the use of the steroid may clear the symptoms while the underlying condition is not treated; precipitation of steroid glaucoma, steroid cataract and increased susceptibility to microbial infections.

Other anti-inflammatory agents

- Used for allergic conjunctivitis
- Antihistamines: e.g. antazoline, azelastine, emedastine, levocabastine
- Sodium cromoglicate and nedocromil sodium.

Decongestants

- Examples: phenylephrine, naphazoline
- Cause vasoconstriction and are useful in inflammation
- Chronic use may lead to rebound conjunctival congestion (conjunctivitis medicamentosa)
- Care: may mask diagnostic signs since redness and inflammation may be removed while underlying condition is not treated.

Others

- Aciclovir eye ointment used in herpes infections
- Tear deficiency products (e.g. hypromellose used in dry eyes)
- Diclofenac sodium available as eye drops used postoperatively
- Astringents: distilled witch hazel used in eye lotions for irrigation.

Products used in subfoveal choroidal neovascularisation

Verteporfin injection

- Indicated for age-related macular degeneration
- Administration by intravenous infusion over 10 minutes and then light activated using non-thermal laser
- Restricts growth of lesions.

Pegaptanib

- Vascular endothelial growth factor inhibitor
- Used in wet age-related macular degeneration
- Administration by intravitreal injection

Pharmacoeconomics in age-related macular degeneration

- Expensive therapy (starting from £520)
- The expense of drug therapy should be compared with the cost of loss of productivity and quality of life due to loss of peripheral vision.

Glaucoma

Glaucoma describes a range of ocular conditions where the intraocular pressure is too high for the eye to withstand without damage to the structure or impairment of function. The upper limit of normal pressure is 21 mmHg. The condition is classified into acute glaucoma (closed angle) and chronic glaucoma (open angle).

Acute glaucoma (closed angle):

- sudden onset of pain
- blurred vision
- dilated pupil
- if untreated can lead to blindness

- pain in and around eye
- nausea and vomiting.

Chronic glaucoma (open angle):

- more common
- insidious onset with loss of peripheral vision
- blurring
- halos around lights
- headaches
- feeling of fullness around eyes.

Drugs used in the treatment of glaucoma

Miotics

- Examples: pilocarpine, carbachol
- Parasympathomimetic agents
- Act on ciliary muscle leading to opening up of drainage channels in trabecular meshwork, resulting in increased aqueous flow
- Effective
- Disadvantages: small pupil, near vision.

Sympathomimetics

- Examples: adrenaline (epinephrine), dipivefrine (Figure 55.1)
- Increase in outflow and reduction of aqueous humour production
- Cause mydriasis
- Side-effects: red eye, conjunctival pigmentation
- Contraindicated in closed-angle glaucoma due to onset of mydriasis.

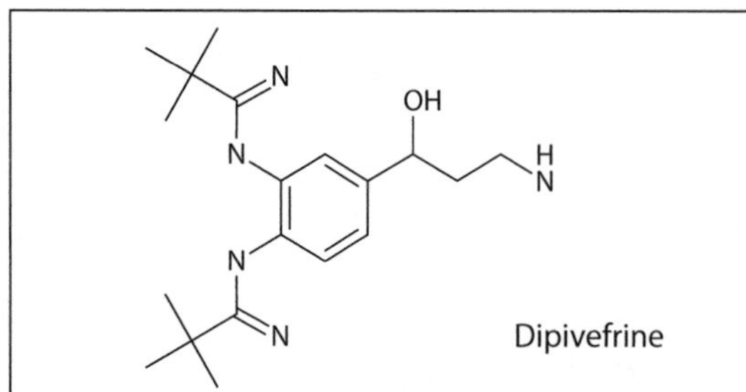

Figure 55.1 Chemical structure of dipivefrine. Prodrug of adrenaline (epinephrine).

Beta-blockers

- Examples: timolol (Figure 55.2), betaxolol (Figure 55.3)
- Reduce aqueous humour production
- Betaxolol has cardioselective properties whereas timolol is non-cardioselective
- Note: use in patients with asthma and obstructive airway disease should be avoided due to risk of bronchospasm if there is some degree of systemic absorption
- Contraindications: bradycardia, heart block, uncontrolled heart failure.

Carbonic anhydrase inhibitors

These decrease aqueous humour production.

Acetazolamide:

- available for oral administration
- side-effects: malaise, fatigue, muscle weakness
- long-term side-effects: electrolyte imbalances.

Brinzolamide and dorzolamide:

- available as eye drops
- used as monotherapy or in combination with beta-blockers

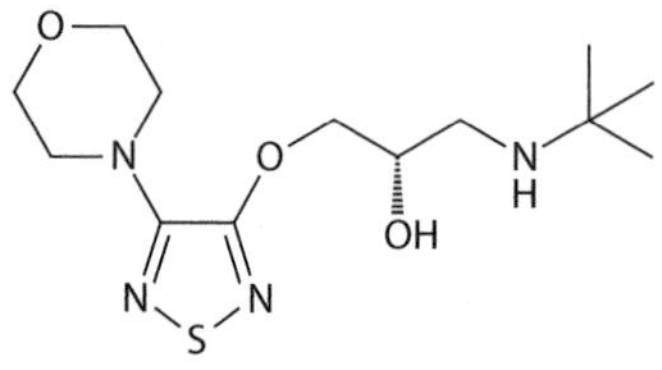

Timolol

Figure 55.2 Chemical structure of timolol (water solubility 2740 mg/L).

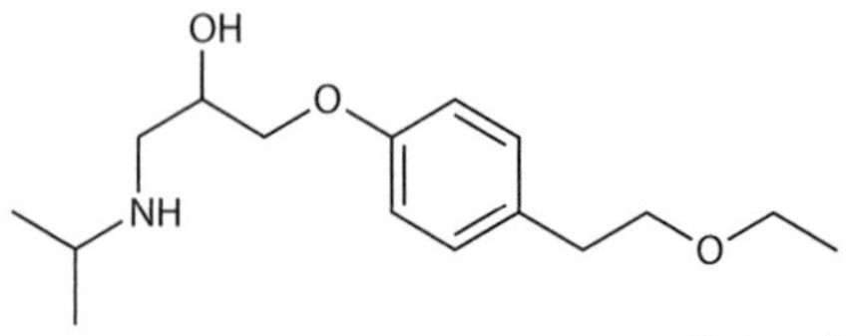

Betaxolol

Figure 55.3 Chemical structure of betaxolol (water solubility 451 mg/L).

- side-effects: bitter taste, burning and stinging of eyes common; other side-effects associated with systemic activity may occur including paraesthesia, flushing, headache, dizziness, fatigue, irritability, thirst, polyuria
- contraindications: renal impairment, hyperchloraemic acidosis, breast-feeding.

Prostaglandin analogues

- Examples: bimatoprost, latanoprost, travoprost
- Increase uveoscleral outflow and result in a decreased intraocular pressure in open-angle glaucoma
- May cause increase in brown pigmentation of iris
- Application once daily, preferably in the evening
- Available in combination products with timolol.

Glaucoma requires constant monitoring of the outcomes of therapy by evaluating intraocular pressure. When monotherapy is not effective, rather than increasing dosing frequency, combination therapy should be adopted.

Contact lenses

Contact lenses were first designed more than 100 years ago:

- 1940: hard lenses made of Perspex
- 1960: soft hydrogel lenses
- 1990s: disposable lenses.

Advantages

- Preferred to spectacles for cosmetic reasons
- Better peripheral vision
- Help to correct myopia, astigmatism.

Disadvantages

- Not suitable for people with allergies
- Manual dexterity required
- Tolerance may be reduced during pregnancy
- Diabetic patients and immunocompromised patients are at greater risk of developing eye infections.

- Soft contact lenses are the most popular type
- Extended-wear disposable: discarded after 4 weeks, intended to avoid complications associated with the accumulation of deposits.

Cleaning solutions

- Used for daily cleaning to remove fresh deposits of lipids, proteins and other contaminants
- Applied to both surfaces of the lens and digital pressure is used in a rotating manner in the palm of the hand.

Rinsing and disinfection solutions

- Rinsing: sterile saline solution
- Disinfectants: contain hydrogen peroxide. Lenses should be rinsed before insertion into the eye.

Multi-purpose solutions present the steps of rinsing, disinfection and storing in one product. These solutions are preferred since they are less time-consuming to use, only one type of product needs to be purchased and steps for maintenance and storage of the lenses are easy to follow. Care should be taken to use the solution that is appropriate for the type of lenses used (hard or soft lenses).

Comfort solutions

These are intended for instillation directly into the eye with the lenses on. They provide fluid to maintain adequate lens hydration and improve comfort.

Protein removal

These are used periodically after cleaning and before disinfection. They consist of proteolytic enzymes (e.g. papain) as tablets that are dissolved in saline. The lenses are soaked in this solution before being cleaned and rinsed. Protein removal tablets are suitable for soft and hard lenses.

The use of extended-wear disposable products eliminates the need for this step since at this stage the lenses are discarded.

Complications related to contact lens wear

Most complications are self-limiting if the lens is removed at the first sign of trouble. Complications could be as a result of:

- poor lens care
- inadequate hygiene
- overwear
- poor fitting.

Problems occur more in hot, dry environments.

Chronic conjunctivitis

- Red eye, itchy, mucus discharge
- Stop contact lens wear
- Disinfect and clean or change lenses for disposable lenses.

Ulcerative keratitis

- Rare but serious complication
- Precipitating factors include overnight wear and long intervals between cleaning.

Effects of systemic medications on contact lens use

- Reduced tolerance due to oral contraceptives: oestrogen component causes eyelid oedema, allergic conjunctivitis
- Anxiolytics, hypnotics, antihistamines: reduce blink rate
- Atropine, antimuscarinics, beta-blockers, TCAs: decrease tear volume
- Aspirin: appears in tears and may be absorbed by soft lenses resulting in ocular irritation and redness.

Effects of topical medications on contact lens use

- May damage contact lens and increase contact time of the drug
- Eye drops should be administered 30 minutes before inserting lens.

Practice summary

- Preparations administered in the eye should be sterile. Eye drops in multi-dose containers for domiciliary use should be discarded within 4 weeks of opening and those used in institutions should be discarded within 1 week of opening.
- Patients should be advised on the correct administration of eye drops and eye ointments.
- When using anti-infective preparations, care should be taken not to contaminate dropper.
- Administration of corticosteroids should be undertaken with care due to risk of misdiagnosis and risk of side-effects.
- In glaucoma more than one type of drug may be used to control intraocular pressure.
- Use of contact lenses requires strict adherence to recommendations for storage and lens use to avoid conditions related to contact lens wear.

Questions

1. Differentiate between chalazion and blepharitis.
2. What are the unwanted effects that could result from topical ocular administration of corticosteroids?
3. Giving examples, describe what is a miotic agent and comment on its use in glaucoma.

Answers

1. *Chalazion:* inflammatory granulomatous swelling on the eyelid or its margin. Occurs due to blockage of one of the meibomian glands

which lubricate the eyelid. More common in adults than in children. Management involves surgical removal and anti-infective agents. *Blepharitis:* inflammation of the eyelid margins characterised by inflammation, scaling, pruritus, oedema, formation of yellow crusts on the eyelashes. Causes may be unknown but may be associated with seborrhoeic dermatitis and allergy. Management involves cleansing the eye with saline solution and the use of topical antibacterial preparations.

2 Undiagnosed red eye, steroid glaucoma, steroid cataract, increased susceptibility to microbial infections.

3 Miotics (pilocarpine, carbachol) are parasympathomimetic drugs used in glaucoma. They act on ciliary muscle leading to opening up of drainage channels in trabecular meshwork, resulting in increased aqueous flow and a reduction in the intraocular pressure. A disadvantage is the short duration of action and products need to be applied four times daily. Ocular side-effects include burning and itching, blurred vision, conjunctival vascular congestion, myopia, vitreous haemorrhage and pupillary block.

Further reading

Elton M (2007). Ocular conditions from A to Z (i). *Pharm J* 278: 195–198.

Elton M (2007). Ocular conditions from A to Z (ii). *Pharm J* 278: 255–258.

Haque K (2007). Macular degeneration: symptoms and diagnosis. *Hosp Pharm* 14: 151–154.

Haylor V and Jones J (2007). Use of preserved eye preparations: is the Society's guidance still relevant? *Pharm J* 278: 186.

Titcomb L C (2000). Topical ocular antibiotics: part 1. *Pharm J* 264: 298–301.

Titcomb L C (2000). Topical ocular antibiotics: part 2. *Pharm J* 264: 441–445.

Titcomb L C (2000). Over-the-counter ophthalmic preparations. *Pharm J* 264: 212–218.

Titcomb L C (1999). Treatment of glaucoma: part 1. *Pharm J* 263: 324–329.

Titcomb L C (1999). Treatment of glaucoma: part 2. *Pharm J*. 263: 526–530.

56

Oral and dental problems

Learning objectives:

- To present symptoms of dental conditions
- To identify management of dental conditions
- To discuss oral hygiene and denture care
- To evaluate impact of drugs on dental conditions.

Background

Pharmacists are involved in responding to common dental problems such as tooth decay and gum disease. Oral and dental problems may present discomfort, interfere with food intake and pose social problems. The relevance of good oral health is an essential feature that needs to be emphasised.

Mouth ulcers

- Recurrent small ulcers that may repeatedly affect healthy people
- Present as round, single or clusters of greyish-white or yellow craters surrounded with raised red rim causing pain particularly on eating and drinking
- Occurrence is related to stress, trauma, infection, vitamin B and iron deficiency, and hormonal changes
- More common in the 20- to 40-year age group.

Questions to ask patient

- How old are you?
- How many ulcers are there?
- Where are they?
- What is their size and shape?
- Is there associated pain?

Referral indicated

- Large size: diameter >1 cm
- Ulcer that persists for more than 14 days
- Uneven coloration
- No associated pain or discomfort
- Patient is diabetic or in children under 10 years of age
- Signs of systemic illness (e.g. fever).

Treatment

- Corticosteroids (e.g. hydrocortisone, triamcinolone: available as an oral paste) reduce inflammation.
- Benzydamine, available as an oral rinse or buccal spray, reduces pain and discomfort.
- Choline salicylate, available as an oral gel, produces an analgesic effect.
- Local anaesthetics (e.g. benzocaine) available as lozenges and sprays.
- Chlorhexidine used as a mouth rinse to disinfect the oral cavity.

Teething

This is a condition occurring in paediatric patients that causes distress and discomfort.

- Anaesthetic topical preparations (e.g. benzocaine) can be applied every 20 minutes and are intended to provide relief
- Paracetamol may be used as an analgesic and for the associated pyrexia that may occur
- Non-pharmacotherapy: use teething accessories; some products can be placed in the freezer beforehand so as to provide a cooling effect when the child handles them and bites on them.

Dental pain

This may occur after extraction or after a new filling or due to an abscess. It may be triggered or worsened by heat or cold. For an abscess, the patient may also present with fever and facial swelling.

Referral should be considered if an abscess is suspected since anti-infective agents are required.

Treatment

- Systemic analgesics: paracetamol or NSAIDs unless contraindicated (see Chapter 31)
- Topical toothache tinctures.

Anti-infective agents used in dental conditions

- Co-amoxiclav
- Doxycycline
- Metronidazole.

Oral candidal infections

- Oral candidal infections cause oral thrush, denture-induced stomatitis and angular cheilitis
- Present with soreness, discomfort on eating and bad taste
- High-risk patient groups: paediatrics, patients who are administered systemic broad-spectrum antibacterial agents, patients with ill-fitting dentures, immunocompromised patients, use of inhaled corticosteroids.

Questions to ask patient

- Location of lesion?
- Size and shape of lesion?
- Associated pain?
- Use of medications?

Referral indicated

- Diabetics
- Duration more than 3 weeks
- Immunocompromised patients
- Painless lesions.

Treatment

Miconazole

- Inhibits biosynthesis of ergosterol which is a constituent of the fungal cell membrane
- Has some activity against Gram-positive bacteria
- Can be applied to children from birth
- Gel has to be retained in mouth for as long as possible
- Treatment to be continued for up to 2 days after symptoms subside
- Absorption from oral mucosa may occur: miconazole potentiates activity of warfarin, should be used with caution in pregnancy and breast-feeding, and is contraindicated in hepatic impairment.

Fluconazole

- Used in unresponsive infections and in chronic hyperplastic candidiasis (leukoplakia).

Miconazole may be used in combination with fusidic acid and hydrocortisone when concomitant bacterial infection is also suspected (e.g. angular cheilitis).

Cold sores

This is a condition caused by herpes simplex type 1 virus. It occurs on areas around the lips, is recurrent and is precipitated by stress, sun and the common cold.

- Contagious and painful condition
- Presents with a prodromal phase: burning, tingling and numbness occur before the occurrence of the cold sore.

Treatment

- Antiviral agents (e.g. aciclovir, penciclovir) used topically
- Should be used as soon as prodromal symptoms occur
- They reduce the duration of the condition. Higher effectiveness if treatment is started early.

Prophylaxis

Since exposure to the sun can precipitate the occurrence of cold sores, it is advisable to recommend the use of UV-blocking lip-salve as a preventive measure.

Patients should be advised that the condition is recurring and that they should recognise the prodromal symptoms so as to commence topical application of antiviral agent.

Halitosis

- Offensive unpleasant breath odour
- Source of social embarrassment
- Symptom of periodontal disease, diabetes, liver or kidney failure
- Treatment is to improve oral hygiene.

Xerostomia (dry mouth)

- Decreased salivary flow caused by salivary gland disease, drugs, irradiation of head and neck
- May be monitored by measuring saliva secretion
- Advise patients to use sugar-free lozenges, salivary substitutes and to avoid alcoholic mouthwashes
- Pilocarpine tablets are used in patients with dry mouth following irradiation of head and neck cancer or in Sjögren's syndrome.

Drugs that may cause dry mouth

- Antihistamines and anticholinergics
- Benzodiazepines
- Antidepressants (e.g. tricyclic antidepressant drugs)
- Antidiarrhoeals (e.g. loperamide)
- NSAIDs
- Antiparkinsonian drugs (e.g. levodopa, orphenadrine)
- Diuretics
- Proton pump inhibitors.

Gingivitis and periodontal disease

These are caused by an excess formation of plaque and plaque is visible, along with swelling and reddening of gums. Bleeding of gums also occurs after toothbrushing.

- Periodontal disease: spontaneous bleeding, taste disturbance and visible pockets
- Plaque: a film of soft material that forms on teeth which is composed of microorganisms and food. It calcifies by precipitating calcium salt from saliva and forms calculus.

Risk factors

- Smoking
- Poor nutrition
- Stress
- Medications
- Pregnancy
- Genetic predisposition
- Immunocompromised individuals.

Referral

- Spontaneous gum bleeding
- Bleeding caused by medications

- Unexplained bleeding
- Signs of systemic illness.

Proper oral hygiene is of great significance in the management of gingivitis and periodontal disease.

Oral hygiene

Toothbrush

- Small head size to be able to approach all areas of the mouth
- Multifaceted and dense for effective bristle action
- Medium texture
- Lifespan: should be changed regularly (every 3 months or earlier if bristles are visible from the sides when looking at the dorsal side of the brush) to achieve effective toothbrushing technique.

Electric models of toothbrushes

- Remove plaque more quickly
- Easier to handle for patients with reduced manual dexterity (e.g. people with rheumatoid arthritis).

Dental floss

- Used to clean inaccessible areas
- Unwaxed or waxed floss: choice depends on patient's preference
- Good technique should be ensured to avoid damage to buccal area.

Toothpaste

- Of little benefit in stain removal
- Serves to polish the surface of the tooth
- Use low abrasive dentifrices. Highly abrasive agents should be used with caution since these may damage dental enamel
- Fluoride-enhanced toothpastes present an anticaries activity.

Mouthwashes

- Assist in the removal of debris, mucus and purulent secretions
- May have an antiplaque activity (loosen plaque)
- Chlorhexidine: cationic antibacterial agent, proven activity against bacteria in dental plaque. However, it stains teeth yellow–black colour and therefore patients should be advised to rinse mouth with water after use to minimise teeth staining
- Other examples include: sodium chloride, hydrogen peroxide, hexetidine and povidone–iodine.

Lozenges and pastilles

Table 56.1 shows uses of lozenges and pastilles.

Denture care

- Dentures should be cleaned out of the mouth once or twice daily
- At night stored in water
- Special products to be used:
  - cleaning: denture toothpastes, denture cleaning tablets or powders
  - fixatives: pastes and cushions.

Oral adverse effects

Drugs that affect taste

- Cancer chemotherapy (e.g. tamoxifen, fluorouracil)
- Cardiovascular (e.g. amiodarone, enalapril)
- Antipsychotics (e.g. lithium, risperidone)
- Antidepressants (e.g. TCAs, SSRIs)
- Inhalation therapy (e.g. salbutamol, ipratropium, budesonide)
- Levodopa.

Table 56.1 Uses of lozenges and pastilles

Sore throat	Cough and catarrh	Oral thrush
Antiseptic	Menthol	Amphotericin
± local anaesthetics	Eucalyptus	Nystatin

Oral adverse effects associated with antiepileptics are listed in Table 56.2.

Other conditions

- Squamous cell carcinoma: a rare condition that may affect buccal mucosa which requires immediate referral
- Erythema multiforme (Stevens–Johnson syndrome): widespread ulceration of oral cavity
- Leukoplakia: precancerous state presenting as a white patch
- Lichen planus: erosive, ulcerated lesions on gingival tissues and buccal mucosa; requires administration of topical or systemic corticosteroids.

Practice summary

- Mouth ulcers tend to be recurrent but their repeated occurrence requires elimination of underlying factors which may require referral.
- Teething in children may warrant use of systemic analgesics in addition to topical anaesthetics and may present with extra-buccal symptoms.
- In dental pain, occurrence of an infection should be assessed.

Table 56.2 Oral adverse effects with antiepileptics

Drug	Adverse effect
Phenytoin	Gingival hyperplasia Erythema multiforme
Carbamazepine	Dry mouth Erythema multiforme Dyskinesias
Sodium valproate	Tendency to bleed

- Occurrence of oral candidiasis may be related to other drugs and to denture use.
- Cold sores are contagious and they are recurrent since the herpes virus remains dormant in the body.
- In oral hygiene, toothbrush used and proper toothbrushing technique are key factors to ensure maintenance of dental care.

Questions

1. What advice should be given to a patient who is complaining of dry mouth?
2. When should patients with gingivitis be referred?

Answers

1. Patients with a persistently dry mouth should be advised on the importance of good oral hygiene. Saliva lubricates the oral cavity and a dry mouth is associated with a higher risk of dental problems. Patients should be advised to adopt regular daily toothbrushing (using an anti-caries toothpaste, a medium textured small head toothbrush, proper brushing technique). An alcohol-free mouthwash helps to improve oral hygiene and provides a refreshing sensation. The use of sugar-free lozenges may help to increase salivation.
2. Patients with gingivitis should be referred when there is spontaneous gum bleeding to exclude bleeding caused by medications, unexplained bleeding and systemic illness.

Further reading

Garwood D (2003). Dental procedures. *Pharm J* 270: 551–553.

Garwood D (2003). Oral problems. *Pharm J* 270: 574–576.

Garwood D (2003). Oral hygiene. *Pharm J* 270: 619–621.

57

The feet

Learning objectives:

- To present symptoms of foot problems
- To develop skills for differential diagnosis of foot problems
- To identify management of foot problems.

Background

Untreated foot conditions such as corns and calluses, verrucae, athlete's foot and onchomycosis can have a negative impact on an individual's lifestyle. The use of support products to alleviate foot problems should be encouraged. Care needs to be exercised in the prevention and management of foot problems in diabetics and patients with compromised peripheral circulation.

Corns and calluses and verrucae

Corns and calluses

- Corn: a small, raised, sharply demarcated hyperkeratotic lesion with a central core; may be soft (occurring mostly between toes) or hard (occurring mostly on top of the toes)
- Callus: similar to a corn; ranges from a few millimetres to several centimetres in diameter. More common in adults
- Causes: pressure and friction; may be due to inappropriate footwear, bad posture during walking and activity.

Verrucae (warts)

- Contagious condition caused by human papillomavirus commonly affecting the feet as well as hands, anogenital region and face
- Appearance: scaly, rough papules, greyish with a black centre and a typical cauliflower-like appearance
- Causes: direct person-to-person contact, public showers, swimming pools
- Incubation period: 1–20 months, average 3–4 months.

Questions to ask patient

- Where is the sore located?
- Is the condition painful?
- Is it too uncomfortable to walk?
- During which activities do you notice pain?
- How long have you had the problem?
- Did it develop gradually?
- Is there any blistering, oozing or bleeding?
- Is the problem associated with a particular pair of shoes?

Questions to ask patient presenting with a foot problem

- Have you tried to treat the problem before?
- Have you suffered from the condition previously?
- Do you suffer from any medical problem?
- Are you taking any medications?

Factors that differentiate warts from corns and calluses are pain when pressure is applied to the area and the cauliflower raised appearance with reddish hue due to vascular damage in the area.

Referral indicated

- Diabetics
- Peripheral circulatory disorders
- Haemorrhage or oozing
- Corns and calluses are extensive and painful
- Extensive verrucae
- Proper self-medication was inadequate.

Immediate referral and counselling are required for patients presenting with:

- warts that grow and have changed colour
- warts that itch or bleed without provocation.

Treatment for corns, calluses and warts

- Salicylic acid in a plaster vehicle or salicylic acid as a liquid for topical application
- Treatment duration for corns and calluses is usually up to 14 days but for verrucae treatment duration is longer, even up to 12 weeks
- In verrucae, if treatment fails, referral is required for removal by cryotherapy.

Salicylic acid

- Has a keratolytic action
- Is contraindicated in diabetics due to the risk of irritation to the surrounding skin which may precipitate the development of a wound that may become infected
- Side-effects: local skin irritation
- Advice: adjunctive therapy; application of formulation containing salicylic acid should be specific to lesion to avoid skin irritation.

Adjunctive therapy

- Daily soaking in warm water
- Epidermabrasion: using a foot file, scrape away the excessive tissue
- Application of moisturising creams
- Use of adhesive pads to alleviate pain due to pressure
- In warts: patient should be advised on measures to prevent spread of infection to other members in the household and in common areas.

Irritation caused by the application of salicylic acid preparations may be avoided by applying petroleum jelly to the area surrounding the lesion to protect the skin from coming in contact with salicylic acid.

Bunion

A bunion is a deformity of the foot characterised by lateral deviation from the mid-line of the big toe.

- Causes: hereditary predisposition, footwear, manner in which person walks
- Protective pads may be used to reduce inflammation over the area that generally causes discomfort. Referral to a podiatrist may be necessary for surgical correction.

Athlete's foot (tinea pedis)

This is a fungal infection characterised by maceration, hyperkeratosis, pruritus, malodour, itching and stinging sensation. It commonly affects toe webs but may include sole, instep and toenails (onchomycosis). In onchomycosis, the toenail changes appearance to a yellowish colour. Systemic treatment is required in onchomycosis.

It is an infective condition that may be contracted from public places. Occlusive footwear precipitates the condition.

Questions to ask patient

- Where is the sore located?
- Is there toenail involvement?
- Is there redness, itching, scaling or bleeding?
- Did the problems begin with the use of new shoes, socks or soap?: to identify occurrence of contact dermatitis.
- Do your feet sweat a lot? (to eliminate hyperhidrosis)
- Do you notice an odour when you take off your shoes?
- Do you suffer from allergies?

The presentation of athelete's foot which has an infective component needs to be differentiated from hyperhidrosis and dermatitis. Characteristic signs of a fungal infection include itchiness and malodour.

Referral indicated

- Toenail involvement since systemic treatment is required
- Vesicular eruptions with purulent discharge due to probability of concomitant bacterial infection
- Condition disabling
- Diabetics
- Patients receiving immunosuppressive therapy.

Topical treatment of athlete's foot

- Imidazoles (e.g. clotrimazole, econazole, ketoconazole, miconazole) are effective. They may be used in combination with a steroid (hydrocortisone) for the first few days of treatment to reduce symptoms of inflammation.
- Tolnaftate: not as effective as imidazoles in the management of acute symptoms.
- Terbinafine (an allylamine): more effective than the imidazoles, but more expensive.

Dosage forms for topical administration of antifungals include creams, dusting powders and sprays. Dusting powders are more effective for application to footwear. Sprays may be easier to apply over a large area.

Systemic therapy for tinea pedis and onchomycosis

Systemic therapy may be required in toenail involvement or when the correct use of topical treatment failed.

- Tinea pedis: fluconazole (50 mg daily for 2–6 weeks) or itraconazole (100 mg daily for 30 days or 200 mg for 7 days) or terbinafine (250 mg for 2–6 weeks)
- Onychomycosis: itraconazole (200 mg daily for 7 days repeated after 21 days for two more courses) or terbinafine (250 mg daily for about 3 months).

Patient education and counselling

- In fungal infections, treatment is for a minimum of 2–4 weeks
- Proper foot hygiene: clean area regularly and dry properly, reduce risk of contamination to other members in the household
- Avoid occlusive footwear, change footwear regularly.

- Topical antifungal treatment in athlete's foot should be continued for a few days after symptoms have cleared to prevent re-infection
- Antifungal dusting powders containing tolnaftate may be used in footwear to prevent re-infection.

Ingrown toenails

These occur when a section of the nail presses into the soft tissue of the nail groove. The nail curves into the flesh of the toe corners and becomes embedded in the soft tissue of the toe, causing pain.

- Causes: incorrect trimming of nails, narrow or tight-fitting shoes
- Management: analgesia and refer for surgical correction. Anti-infective agents may be required if the area is infected.

Chilblains

- Itchy erythematous or purple swelling
- Predisposing factors:
  - low temperatures or extremes of temperatures
  - wet clothing
  - dehydration
  - smoking
  - circulatory disease.

Treatment

Rubefacients (e.g. salicylates, nicotinates, capsicum, camphor) provide symptomatic relief. They should not be applied if the skin is broken. In cases where there is broken skin, antiseptic creams are considered.

Hyperhidrosis

- Characterised by overactivity of the sweat glands, resulting in excessive perspiration
- Common in young adults
- Management: use of talc and zinc oxide dusting powders to adsorb excess sweat
- Advise patients to use non-occlusive footwear which reduces morbidity due to hyperhidrosis and decreases risk of athlete's foot.

Anhidrosis

- Abnormal absence of sweating
- Common in older people; presents with dry skin areas
- Management: use of moisturising creams.

Thromboses

- Arterial thrombosis: pain and loss of blood supply, cold and white in colour
- Venous thrombosis: swollen, blue/black in colour
- Atherosclerosis: pale and cold feet, local gangrene.

Practice summary

- Care should be taken when conditions occur in the feet in people with diabetes and in patients with compromised peripheral circulation.
- Avoid products containing salicylic acid in people with diabetes due to the risk of irritation that may lead to infection and skin lesions.
- Refer when patient is complaining of severe pain with sudden onset or if there is foot colour change or appearance is abnormal.
- Advise on proper footwear (comfortable, avoiding high heels and narrow pointed shoes) and to use alternate pairs of shoes so as to change footwear.

Questions

1. Explain what an ingrown toenail is and how its occurrence can be prevented.
2. When should referral be considered when a patient presents with a verruca?

Answers

1. An ingrown toenail occurs when a section of the nail presses into the soft tissue of the nail groove. The nail curves into the flesh of the toe corners and becomes embedded in the soft tissue of the toe, causing pain. An ingrown toenail can be prevented by correct trimming of the nails and avoidance of narrow tight-fitting shoes.
2. Immediate referral when patients present with verrucae that reportedly are changing in size

or colour and verrucae that itch or bleed without provocation. Referral is also necessary if patient has diabetes or peripheral circulatory disorders, if there is haemorrhage or oozing, if verruca is extensive and if proper self-medication has already proved inadequate.

Further reading

Keogh-Brown M R, Fordham R J, Thomas K S, Bachmann M O, Holland R C, Avery A J, *et al.* (2007) To freeze or not to freeze: A cost-effectiveness analysis of wart treatment. *Br J Dermatol* 156: 687–692.

Younes D A and Ahmad A T (2006). Diabetic foot disease. *Endocr Pract* 2006; 12: 583–592.

58

Ear problems

Learning objectives:

- To review characteristics of ear problems
- To discuss management of ear problems
- To develop skills to reduce risk of ototoxicity.

Background

The ear consists of three sections: the outer ear, the middle ear and the inner ear. Besides being an organ used to capture sounds, the ear (inner ear) is also a sensory organ involved with balance. Ear disorders may affect hearing or balance.

Disorders of the auricle

The auricle is a highly vascularized area. Its function is to direct sound waves into the ear. Conditions related to the auricle relate to skin disorders and include trauma, boils (furuncles) which are more common in young adults, dermatitis of the ear that may be due to contact with jewellery or cosmetics and itching or pruritus (see Chapter 47).

Disorders of the external auditory canal

Otitis externa

This is an inflammatory reaction that may be associated with infection due to bacteria (e.g. *Pseudomonas aeruginosa*) and fungi (e.g. *Aspergillus* spp., *Candida albicans*). It presents as a very painful condition in which chewing and manipulation of the pinna may exacerbate the pain. Oedema may occur and this may interfere with hearing.

- Moisture increases infection and the condition is associated with exposure to water (e.g. swimming: swimmer's ear).

Treatment

Topical administration of antibacterial agents (e.g. chloramphenicol, framycetin, gentamicin, neomycin and ofloxacin) is required. The use of aminoglycosides in patients with a ruptured tympanic membrane should be avoided. Since the infection may also be due to a fungal component and there is a risk of promoting a fungal infection with the use of topical antibacterial agents, a topical antifungal product such as clotrimazole or clioquinol (not to be used in perforated tympanic membrane) may be considered either as monotherapy or in combination with antibacterials.

- Topical corticosteroids: e.g. hydrocortisone, betamethasone, dexamethasone, flumetasone, prednisolone and triamcinolone. Corticosteroids are used in combination with anti-infective agents where inflammation and oedema are prominent.

- Sodium chloride 0.9% wash: used to clean ear from debris and as a soothing preparation.
- Aluminium acetate which has an astringent effect and acetic acid drops which have antifungal and antibacterial properties may be considered.

> - Exclude occurrence of underlying chronic otitis media before treating otitis externa
> - In otitis externa, systemic analgesics may be recommended in addition to topical treatment to counteract the pain.

Impacted cerumen (ear wax)

- Ear wax normally provides mechanical protection of the tympanic membrane
- Occurrence of impacted cerumen may be due to overactive ceruminous glands (some people are more prone to develop this condition), congenital anomalies (abnormally narrow ear canal), learning disability and changes in the consistency (drier) of the cerumen produced
- Presenting symptoms: ear discomfort and slight hearing loss, sensation of fullness in the ear. Symptoms may be precipitated by exposure to water since the wax will adsorb water and inflate
- Patients should be advised to avoid getting water in the ears (may use ear plugs during swimming or showering) and not to use cotton buds to remove impacted cerumen. The use of cotton buds may cause damage to the tympanic membrane since the impacted cerumen may be pushed further inside into the middle ear.

Application of topical products

- Drops warmed in the hands before use
- Patient is instructed to incline head and instil drops and remain in this position for a few minutes
- Repeat as necessary according to product used.

Products used to remove excess cerumen

- Fixed oils (olive oil and almond oil): to soften the wax
- Sodium bicarbonate: to break up the wax
- Sodium chloride: used as a rinse to soften wax
- Cerumenolytics: very safe products, but may cause irritation (e.g. docusate, paradichlorobenzene in chlorbutol, urea–hydrogen peroxide).

> Advise patient that use of cerumenolytics may not lead to an immediate effect and that repeated administrations for a few days may be required until cerumen is removed.

Disorders of the middle ear

Otitis media

- *Serous:* sensation of fullness in ear and hearing loss. Patient complains of popping and cracking noise when swallowing or yawning. Commonly occurs after a respiratory tract infection particularly in children and usually resolves spontaneously. It is due to the presence of fluid in the middle ear which does not drain completely. There are instances where the condition develops into a chronic serous otitis media (glue ear) where patient needs to be referred and assessed for the need of surgical draining. In children, occurrence of the chronic serous condition may affect hearing to an extent that it impinges on speech development. In chronic serous otitis media pain is absent.
- *Suppurative (purulent):* acute otitis media. Has an inflammatory and an infective component. Patient presents with pain, hearing loss, high fever and feeling ill. More common in children. Condition requires referral since systemic anti-infective agents are required.

Management

- Oral administration of antibacterials; considered drugs are usually amoxicillin or macrolides in penicillin-allergic individuals.
- Analgesics: oral administration of paracetamol or ibuprofen unless contraindicated.

Barotrauma

This occurs as a result of quick descent from a high altitude during air travel or travel to high altitudes. It results because the eustachian tube fails to ventilate, resulting in negative pressure in the middle ear. This causes suction and retraction of the tympanic membrane, leading to pain.

- Management: use of nasal decongestants (topical or systemic) to clear the condition. Products may be used prophylactically by patients who are at risk of developing barotrauma during travel
- Jaw movements such as chewing, swallowing and blowing may help alleviate the condition
- Occurrence of nasal congestion in patients with rhinitis (allergic or infective) predisposes to development of barotrauma.

Questions to ask patient presenting with earache

- Is there pain or discomfort?: assess degree of pain
- How long have you had it for? (Check onset)
- Is the pain constant or worsened by chewing or pulling at ears? (Pain that is associated with pulling at ears or touching auricle indicates an external ear problem)
- Do you have fever? (More likely to indicate otitis media)
- Have you attempted to remove ear wax during the last few days? (Ear wax removal with cotton buds or cerumenolytics may lead to irritation)
- Are your ear canals dry and flaky or wet and sticky? (Dry and flaky indicate an allergic reaction whereas wet and sticky indicate a purulent infection.)

Otosclerosis

This is immobilization of the stapes in the middle ear due to abnormal formation of new bone. It causes deafness.

- Occurs in women and is exacerbated by pregnancy
- Requires referral for surgical intervention.

Perforated tympanic membrane

- Causes: trauma, infection (otitis media)
- Outcome: usually heals spontaneously, sometimes surgery may be required.
  Degree of perforation affects degree of hearing loss
- Management: advise patient to restrict water entering ear and care should be adopted when using ear drops, particularly those containing aminoglycosides and clioquinol.

Questions to ask patient presenting with hearing loss

- When did you notice that your hearing is affected?
- Do you have a cold or influenza: nasal congestion? (May affect middle ear leading to temporary hearing loss)
- Have you been swimming during the past few days? (Increased risk of swimmer's ear)
- Are your eardrums damaged from a previous illness or injury? (To eliminate tympanic membrane damage)
- Have you been travelling recently? (To establish occurrence of barotrauma)
- Are you taking any medications? (Some medications may cause tinnitus and ototoxicity.)

Disorders of the inner ear

Labyrinthitis (otitis interna)

This is infection and inflammation of the inner ear. It can cause loss of hearing, vertigo, nausea and vomiting. The patient needs to be referred and antibacterial treatment is considered.

Vertigo

This is a sensation of instability, loss of equilibrium or rotation caused by a disturbance in the semicircular canal of the inner ear. It may be centrally induced or is due to peripheral system disorders (e.g. Ménière's disease (labyrinthitis) and vestibular neuronitis.

Management

Antihistamine products are used in nausea and vertigo (e.g. prochlorperazine, cinnarizine), as well as betahistine which is an analogue of histamine that is specifically indicated for vertigo, tinnitus and hearing loss associated with Ménière's disease (see also Chapter 18).

Questions to ask patient presenting with discharge

- Describe appearance and amount of discharge
- Was your ear itchy before discharge appeared? (To identify allergic component)
- Do you have any ear pain? (Ear pain that disappears with discharge indicates otitis media with ruptured tympanic membrane)
- Do you have diabetes? (Greater risk of developing infections)
- Are you taking any medications?

Ototoxicity

This is damage caused to structures within the inner ear which may lead to hearing or balance disorders.

- Cochlear damage: associated with tinnitus which may be constant or alternating. Tinnitus is described as a ringing or humming sensation
- Vestibular and stria vascularis damage: results in dysequilibrium and nausea
- Aminoglycosides: cause damage to the cochlea and stria vascularis, leading to deafness and vestibular disorders
- Loop diuretics: affect stria vascularis and the cochlea producing tinnitus and deafness
- Platinum compounds (antineoplastic agents): cause damage to the cochlea and stria vascularis leading to deafness. Risk is greater for cisplatin than for carboplatin and oxaliplatin
- Salicylates: in high doses cause damage to the cochlea, leading to tinnitus and hearing loss.

- As opposed to aminoglycosides, quinolones (e.g. ofloxacin) are not associated with ototoxicity. They may be preferred for topical administration in otitis externa where tympanic membrane damage cannot be excluded.
- Toxicity with loop diuretics is more likely with intravenous administration, particularly in patients with impaired renal function.
- The use of ototoxic products should be avoided in patients with a history of hearing loss and tinnitus.

Referral indicated

- Pain
- Deafness
- History of perforated eardrum
- Abnormal lesion on auricle
- Persistent vertigo
- Tinnitus
- Persistent wax.

Practice summary

- Analgesic ear drops should not be recommended for earache. The underlying condition should be identified.
- Cerumenolytic ear drops should not be recommended unless the presence of excess ear wax has been identified.
- Accompanying symptoms occurring with ear disorders that require immediate referral include nausea and vomiting (may be indicative of

internal otitis) and neck stiffness (may indicate meningitis).

Questions

1 What is barotrauma and how can it be mimimised?
2 Give one example of a product that could be used in the management of Ménière's disease. Describe the characteristics of Ménière's disease.
3 What advice should be given to a patient who is complaining of impacted cerumen?

Answers

1 Barotrauma results when there is a quick descent from high altitudes either during flying or when travelling in mountainous areas. The eustachian tube fails to ventilate, resulting in negative pressure in the middle ear, causing suction and retraction of the tympanic membrane triggering pain. Barotrauma can be minimised by using nasal decongestants either topically or systemically in high-risk patients or where nasal congestion is severe and by chewing, blowing or swallowing.
2 The symptoms of Ménière's disease are caused by increased pressure of the fluid in the labyrinth (consisting of the cochlea and vestibular system). The cause of the condition is not well understood. The patient suffers attacks of vertigo which may increase in severity and frequency. Patient presents with nausea and vomiting, tinnitus and a perceptive deafness. An example of a product that may be used is betahistine, which is a drug that is specifically indicated for Ménière's disease. Antihistamines and phenothiazines used in the management of nausea and vomiting may be considered.
3 To avoid using cotton buds and getting water in the ears since these may precipitate further the symptoms of impacted cerumen. Advice may be given on the use of cerumenolytic products.

Further reading

Allen S (2006). Outer and middle ear problems. *Pharm J* 276: 83–86.
Coco A S (2007). Cost-effectiveness analysis of treatment options for acute otitis media. *Ann Fam Med* 5: 28–29.

59

Musculoskeletal disorders

Learning objectives:

- To review characteristics of common musculoskeletal disorders
- To appreciate implementation of pharmacotherapeutic and non-pharmacotherapeutic approaches to musculoskeletal problems.

Background

Musculoskeletal disorders can affect bones, muscles or soft tissues (tendons, bursae). Pain is a characteristic symptom of musculoskeletal disorders. Evaluating onset and location of the pain helps to make a clinical decision as to the most appropriate line of action.

Questions to ask patient presenting with a musculoskeletal problem

- What is your age?
- Presenting symptom:
  - Is there pain, swelling?
  - Where is it?
  - How long have you had it?
- Patient history:
  - Do you have past or present injury?
  - Any medical conditions?

Description of injuries

Sprains and strains

- *Sprain:* overstretching of ligaments and/or joint capsule with tearing
- *Strain:* muscle fibres are damaged by overstretching and tearing
- In sprains and strains, mobilisation, strengthening and coordination exercises are recommended to decrease risk of scar tissue formation that may limit movement.

Whiplash

- Damage to the ligaments, vertebrae, spinal cord or nerve roots in the neck region, caused by sudden jerking back of the head and neck
- Typically associated with car accidents.

Coccygitis

- Injury to small spur of the vertebrae at the tip of the spine, the coccyx
- Generally onset is insidious and it is usually difficult for patient to recall injury.

Tennis elbow

- Excess force acting on the insertion of the tendons of the forearm muscles
- May be related to repeated activities including lifting heavy objects.

Description of overuse injuries

Muscle pain

- Stiff and painful muscles
- Common condition that occurs after patient carries out activities that are not normally undertaken (e.g. exercise by an individual used to a sedentary lifestyle).

Frozen shoulder

- Shoulder is stiff and painful
- Pain worse at night
- May relate to exposure to cold or exertion
- Referral is necessary for further assessment.

Arthralgia – painful joints

- May be due to arthritis
- Limitation of movement occurs
- Refer for further assessment.

Bursitis

- Inflammation of bursae
- Commonly occurs in the knees (housemaid's knee) in individuals who tend to kneel regularly and the elbows (student's elbow) in individuals who put pressure on their elbow while working at a desk.

Torticollis (wry neck)

- Painful condition where there is a spasm of one or more muscles in the neck due to straining of muscles
- May occur due to unaccustomed or repeated movement
- Neck mobilisation away from affected side is possible, but there is difficulty and pain in turning towards affected side
- Refer if patient has a history of arthritis or there is presentation of sharp pain.

Capsulitis

- Inflammation of the fibrous supporting tissue surrounding the shoulder joint
- Restriction of movement occurs
- May lead to development of frozen shoulder due to scarring or fibrosis of the muscles.

Back pain

- May occur after strenuous work (lumbago) or when patient undertakes activities that he or she is not used to doing (e.g. gardening).
- If severe and debilitating, causing difficulty with mobility or radiating from the back down to the legs, referral is required since symptoms indicate sciatica which requires further evaluation.
- If pain is just below ribcage in the middle part to side of back, or is associated with abnormality in passing urine, refer for assessment of occurrence of kidney problems.
- Chronic back pain (occurring for more than 3 months) indicates underlying pathologies rather than injury. Examples include osteoarthritis, inflammatory conditions (e.g. arthritis, ankylosing spondylitis).

Accompanying symptoms of back pain requiring referral

Occurrence of fever, bowel or bladder incontinence, numbness, worsening pain or referred pain to legs require referral.

When to refer musculoskeletal disorders

- Head injury
- Suspected fracture
- Deformity or severe swelling
- Possible adverse drug reaction
- Medication failure
- Arthritis
- Severe pain
- Back pain associated with urinary problems or numbness.

Management of painful conditions

- Non-pharmacological management
- Lifestyle modifications
- RICE regimen adopted in injuries (rest, ice, compression, elevation)
- Application of heat in chronic pain
- Pharmacological approach.

Non-pharmacological management of injuries

- Consider physiotherapy where relevant
- Advise patient on good posture and on exercise where indicated
- Consider use of support products (e.g. soft collars in whiplash, back supports in back pain, compression supports in sprains, foam supports in bursitis).

> **Non-pharmacological management of back pain**
>
> - Loss of excess weight
> - Lift things properly
> - Avoid sitting in same position for long periods of time
> - Good posture
> - Use of a firm mattress
> - Exercise: sit-ups, swimming, brisk walking.

RICE regimen

Rest

- Immobilisation is recommended for the first 24 hours.
- Prolonged rest for muscle injuries is usually discouraged because the collagen scar tissue formed is unable to contract and repair is associated with some loss of flexibility.

Ice

- Reduces the local blood flow
- Decreases the metabolic rate in peripheral cells
- Limits the extent of inflammation and degree of pain
- Administer cold pack for 30 minutes, repeating every 2 hours
- Care should be employed not to damage skin by application of cold compress. If ice is used, this should not be applied directly to the skin but first wrapped in cloth to avoid burning the skin.

Compression

- Application of pressure over the injured area
- Decreases bleeding and the flow of inflammatory exudates
- Use a compression bandage for at least 24 hours.

Elevation

- Raise injured area to aid drainage of fluid and reduce swelling.

Application of hot packs

Some patients find relief from pain, particularly due to chronic conditions, when heat is applied to the area.

Pharmacological approach

Analgesics

- Use of NSAIDs is usually warranted due to the requirement of an analgesic and an anti-inflammatory component. They may be used provided that patient is not asthmatic, is not suffering from or has a past history of peptic ulcer, and is not taking warfarin.
- NSAIDs may be administered topically, thus reducing risks with use of NSAIDs. Oral administration is considered when local administration is not providing the required pain relief.
- Paracetamol and compound preparations containing opioid analgesics may be considered in patients where NSAIDs cannot be recommended.
- See also Chapter 31.

Counter-irritants and rubefacients

- Cause vasodilatation inducing a feeling of warmth over the area
- The act of massage during the application of the product is known to relax muscles and it may disperse prostaglandins responsible for pain and inflammation
- Available in different formulations: sprays, lotions, creams
- Dosage regimen: four times daily
- Examples: methylsalicylate, nicotinates, menthol, camphor
- Disadvantage: strong smell associated with the active ingredients may be unacceptable to patients.

Muscle cramps

These are painful, sustained involuntary muscle contractions which are prolonged. They may be caused by dehydration, fatigue, imperfect posture, stress or potassium deficiency.

- Advise patient to drink water, exercise muscle to relax it
- Sometimes application of cold compress may offer relief and ibuprofen may be considered as an analgesic.

> Use of diuretics (not the potassium sparing ones) may lead to potassium deficiency if potassium supplementation is not adequate. This may present with muscle cramps.

Bruising (contusions)

This is an area of skin discoloration caused by the escape of blood from ruptured underlying blood vessels as a result of injury. Skin discoloration is initially red or pink, gradually becoming blue, green and yellow.

- Topical application of heparinoids which disperse oedematous fluid in swollen areas is considered.
- Heparinoids should not be applied on broken skin.

Practice summary

- A number of musculoskeletal problems occur as a result of an injury of which the patient may not be aware.
- Management of acute musculoskeletal problems requires recommendations related to use of support products and warrants referral to physiotherapists to control pain associated with the condition.
- Concomitant symptoms indicating organic illness or chronic conditions require referral for further assessment.

Questions

1. Write briefly on differential diagnosis of sciatica and its management.
2. Give one example of a non-steroidal anti-inflammatory drug that can be used topically as well as systemically.

Answers

1. Lumbago, sciatica and kidney problems may all present with back pain. Lumbago is back pain that occurs after strenuous work. If back pain is severe and debilitating, causing difficulty in mobility or radiating from the back down to the legs, then these factors are used to indicate the possibility of sciatica and the patient must be referred. If the back pain is just below the ribcage in the middle part to the side of the back or is associated with abnormality in passing urine, this suggests a kidney problem and the patient must be referred. Sciatica is managed using non-steroidal anti-inflammatory drugs such as

diclofenac as well as the B vitamins 1, 3 and 6 to strengthen the nervous system.

2 Diclofenac available as gel, gel patch, cutaneous solution, eye drops, tablets, dispersible tablets, capsules, suppositories and injection.

Further reading

Braund R (2006). Should NSAIDs be routinely used in the treatment of sprains and strains? *Pharm J* 276: 655–656.

Dickson J (2006). Promoting self care of joint pain. *Pharm J* 277: 285–288.

60

Abdominal pain, and perianal and perivulval pruritus

Learning objectives:

- To identify presentation of symptoms related to abdominal pain, perianal and perivulval pruritus
- To develop skills required for the management of these symptoms
- To appreciate the use of non-prescription medicines.

Background

The occurrence of abdominal pain is a symptom relating to a multitude of diagnoses (e.g. gastro-intestinal and urinary tract disorders) which requires assessment to identify the system affected.

Questions to ask patient presenting with abdominal pain

- Where does it hurt?
- How widespread is it?
- How strong is the pain?
- What is the duration of the pain?
- When did it start?
- What is your age?
- Are there any associated symptoms?

Differential diagnosis of abdominal pain

Table 60.1 lists the causes of abdominal pain and diagnosis of upper and lower abdominal pain is summarised in Figure 60.1.

Diagnosis of upper abdominal pain

Highly likely
dyspepsia
peptic ulcer
cholecystitis, cholelithiasis, renal colic
splenic enlargement, hepatitis, myocardial infarction
Very unlikely

Diagnosis of lower abdominal pain

Highly likely
irritable bowel syndrome
diverticulitis
appendicitis, endometriosis, renal colic
ectopic pregnancy, salpingitis, intestinal obstruction
Very unlikely

Figure 60.1 Diagnosis of upper and lower abdominal pain.

Table 60.1 Causes of abdominal pain

Organ	Condition
Oesophagus	Reflux oesophagitis
Stomach	Gastritis, gastric ulceration
Duodenum	Duodenal ulcer
Appendix	Appendicitis
Biliary tract	Gallstones
Colorectum	Diveriticulitis, diarrhoea, constipation, faecal impaction, motility disturbances
Non-specific	Crohn's disease, ulcerative colitis
Kidney	Pyelonephritis
Bladder	Cystitis
Male genitalia	Prostate
Female genitalia	Dysmenorrhoea, endometriosis, pelvic inflammatory disease

Acute cholecystitis and cholelithiasis

- Cholecystitis: inflammation of the gallbladder
- Cholelithiasis: gallstones in the bile duct (biliary colic)
- Onset is sudden in many cases occurring a few hours after a meal; fatty foods aggravate the pain
- Requires referral.

Renal colic

- Occurrence of urinary calculi in the urinary tract
- Severe colicky pain, associated with nausea and vomiting
- Good fluid intake recommended
- Requires referral.

Accompanying conditions of abdominal pain that warrant referral

- Pain is unbearable
- Continuous severe pain for more than 1 hour
- Pain has been present episodically for more than 7 days
- Vomiting
- Constipation
- Chronic back pain and occasional fainting; history of myocardial infarction: may indicate cardiovascular disorders.

Heartburn

Heartburn is the reflux of gastric contents that are particularly acidic in pH into the oesophagus, which cause an irritation of the sensitive mucosal surface.

Aggravating factors of heartburn

- Smoking
- Alcohol
- Caffeine, chocolate, fatty foods
- Posture.

Management of heartburn

- Decrease weight
- Small, frequent meals

- Raise head of bed to decrease occurrence of heartburn at night
- Use of antacids, preferably products containing alginates.

Referral is indicated

- Failure to respond to antacids
- Pain is radiating into arms: could indicate cardiovascular disorders
- Difficulty in swallowing: could indicate oesophageal problems
- Long duration
- See also Chapter 16.

Occurrence of heartburn in patients older than 50 years who do not generally have a history of heartburn or in patients where symptom has a long-standing duration raises concern. In these scenarios, referral should be considered to investigate serious conditions (e.g. carcinoma).

Indigestion (dyspepsia)

This is poorly localised abdominal discomfort usually brought about by excess food and alcohol. Management includes maintenance of good hydration, use of antacids to alleviate discomfort and if gastric pain is present use of H_2-receptor antagonists (e.g. ranitidine).

Constipation

- Ideally simple or functional constipation should be corrected by increasing fibre and fluid intake.
- For long-term use, bulk-forming laxatives (e.g. ispaghula husk) are preferred.
- Short-term use of stimulant laxatives (e.g. bisacodyl, senna) is justified to re-establish a bowel habit if dietary measures and bulk-forming laxatives have failed.
- The use of laxatives in children is undesirable; consider glycerin suppositories or enemas.
- Refer if constipation is not resolved in a week.
- Consider use of antispasmodic drugs (e.g. hyoscine), especially in patients suffering from gastrointestinal colic.
- Long-term drug treatment for constipation is indicated for:
  - drug-induced/surgical intervention-induced constipation
  - where straining exacerbates a condition (e.g. angina, haemorrhoids).
- See also Chapter 15.

Accompanying conditions with constipation that warrant referral

- Unexplained weight loss
- Blood per rectum
- Variable bowel habit
- Loss of appetite.

Laxatives should not be recommended if intestinal obstruction is suspected.

Diarrhoea

- Patients with diarrhoea should be referred to a doctor if it persists for more than:
  - 24 hours in babies under 1 year
  - 2 days in children under 3 years and the elderly
  - 3 days in older children and adults.
- Always refer children under 3 months.
- Risk of dehydration is higher in children and older persons.
- Oral rehydration salts are the mainstay of treatment. They replace lost water and electrolytes thus preventing dehydration.
- Loperamide may be used in adults as an adjunct to oral rehydration salts to reduce discomfort due to symptoms.
- See also Chapter 15.

Patients presenting with a change in bowel habit, bloody diarrhoea and signs of dehydration should be referred for further investigation to assess for the occurrence of inflammatory bowel disease and carcinoma.

Perianal and perivulval pruritus

This may be due to:

- cystitis
- vulvovaginitis (vaginal thrush)
- haemorrhoids (piles)
- pruritus ani.

Cystitis

This is inflammation of the bladder and urethra characterised by frequent urge to pass urine with a burning or stinging sensation on urination. It is caused by a bacterial infection (common micro-organisms involved include *Escherichia coli*, staphylococci and enterococci).

- Commonly occurs in women; occurrence in males is usually associated with underlying pathology (e.g. benign prostatic hyperplasia). Presentation in male patients requires referral.
- Presentation: dysuria, urinary frequency and urgency, nocturia, haematuria.
- Condition has an acute onset.

Management

- Alkalinising agents: salts consisting of sodium bicarbonate, sodium citrate, potassium citrate
- Dosage: three times daily for 48 hours
- Advice: increase fluid intake
- Alkalinising agents are relatively safe and free from unwanted side-effects. If condition does not resolve, patient requires antibacterial treatment. Usually trimethoprim, nitrofurantoin, co-amoxiclav (unless patient is hypersensitive), cephalosporins or quinolones are used
- Care when using alkalinising agents in patients with uncontrolled hypertension or electrolyte imbalance.

Occurrence of cystitis may lead to development of pyelonephritis which presents with symptoms of systemic infection including fever, chills and pain. This scenario requires referral. In acute pyelonephritis, antibacterial therapy is required (e.g. quinolone).

Vaginal thrush (vaginal candidiasis)

This is an opportunistic infection caused by *Candida albicans* occurring in women between 16 and 60 years of age. Symptoms include itchiness, creamy-coloured discharge and dysuria.

Precipitating factors

- Pregnancy
- Diabetes
- Immunosuppressants (e.g. oral steroids)
- Antibacterial drugs, broad-spectrum products.

Management

- Single-dose intravaginal imidazole preparations (e.g. clotrimazole, econazole, miconazole). Applied at night. Patient is advised to avoid nylon underwear and to use unperfumed soap. Imidazole creams are applied topically.
- Alternative option: povidone–iodine applied twice daily for 14 days. Disadvantages of povidone–iodine: it stains and inconvenience of dosage regimen.
- Systemic treatment may be considered in severe cases, in recurrent infection or failure of treatment with imidazoles.

Topical imidazole preparations should be recommended to the partner to avoid re-infection.

Table 60.2 Systemic treatment of vaginal thrush

Drugs	Fluconazole	Itraconazole
Dosage regimen	150 mg stat	200 mg twice daily for 1 day
Caution	Liver disease, renal impairment, breast-feeding, pregnancy	Renal impairment, pregnancy, heart failure, breast feeding
Common side-effects	Nausea, vomiting, diarrhoea, abdominal pain	Nausea, vomiting, diarrhoea, abdominal pain
Interactions	Warfarin, phenytoin, sulphonylureas, theophylline	Warfarin, phenytoin, statins, digoxin, calcium channel blockers

Systemic treatment of vaginal thrush is summarised in Table 60.2.

Referral indicated

- Diabetics: thrush may indicate uncontrolled disease; suggest review of diabetes control
- Strong smelly discharge: indicates bacterial vaginosis or trichomoniasis (where metronidazole or clindamycin is recommended)
- Recurrent attacks: evaluate for any underlying condition
- Pregnant women: specialist assessment required
- Women under 16 or over 60 years: very rare condition in these age groups.

Haemorrhoids

- Swelling and dilatation of the veins that line the anal canal
- May be internal haemorrhoids or protruding externally
- Symptoms: pain, itching and burning sensation, bleeding
- Precipitating factors: long standing, constipation or straining at stool, pregnancy.

A clinical classification of haemorrhoids is shown in Table 60.3.

Table 60.3 Clinical classification of haemorrhoids

Grade	Description	Surgical intervention
I	With bleeding	No
II	Prolapse on defecation	No
III	Prolapse requires manual reduction	Yes
IV	Permanent prolapse	Yes

Accompanying conditions requiring referral

- Altered bowel habit
- Tenesmus (feeling of incomplete evacuation)
- Weight loss
- Tiredness.

Anal bleeding could be a sign of minor conditions such as anal fissure but may indicate gastrointestinal haemorrhage due to ulceration or carcinoma.

Management of haemorrhoids – topical agents

- Anaesthetics (e.g. benzocaine): provide temporary relief from pain and itching, may cause sensitisation
- Astringents (e.g. bismuth, zinc): produce a protective coat

- Anti-inflammatory (e.g. hydrocortisone): effective in reducing inflammation
- Sclerosing agent (e.g. lauromacrogol 400)
- Fibrinolytic agent (e.g. mucopolysaccharide)
- Other examples: shark liver oil, yeast cell extract: provide a protective coat.

- Preparations with local anaesthetic or astringents are preferred for routine use. They may be applied twice daily and after each bowel movement.
- Ointments are preferred to suppositories.
- Products containing hydrocortisone may be useful when there is severe pruritus and inflammation or when other products were not effective. They should be used short term.

Management of haemorrhoids – systemic treatment

- Oral phlebotropic drugs that protect the endothelium, improve lymphatic drainage and increase venous tone
- They may be recommended in acute attacks or for chronic treatment.

Pruritus ani

- Dermatological disorders (e.g. atopic dermatitis)
- Allergic reaction
- Superficial infections and parasites: threadworm
- Liver disease
- Hyperhidrosis.

Threadworm infections

- Females of the worm *Enterobius vermicularis* migrate to the caecum and the anus at night to lay their eggs in the perianal area. They attach to the skin with a sticky, highly irritant fluid.
- Diagnosis based on sighting whitish worms on stools.
- Treatment offered to whole household due to risk of cross-infection.

Drug therapy for threadworms

- For example, mebendazole
- Causes death of the organism within 3 days
- Poorly absorbed from the gastrointestinal tract and so associated with minimal side-effects. Exerts a topical action on the organism in the gastrointestinal tract
- Adults and children over 2 years: 100 mg mebendazole stat dose, repeat after 2 weeks to ensure eradication.

Practice summary

- Presentation of symptoms of abdominal pain should be evaluated for signs of underlying pathology.
- Repeated presentation of symptoms of abdominal pain or perianal or perivulval pruritus require further assessment.
- Where laxatives are required for chronic use, bulk-forming laxatives or osmotic laxatives should be considered. In children and the elderly where faecal impaction is suspected, glycerin suppositories should be the drug of choice.
- In diarrhoea, oral rehydration salts are the mainstay of treatment and signs of dehydration should be identified.
- Management of haemorrhoids requires routine use of topical products or systemic phlebotropic agents.
- In cystitis a short course (2 days) of alkalinising agents is recommended together with advice to increase fluid intake. If condition deteriorates or symptoms do not subside, antibacterial therapy is recommended.
- In vaginal thrush treatment is based on single-dose intravaginal imidazole preparations with topical imidazole creams or single-dose oral fluconazole.

Questions

1 Explain the term anal fissure.
2 When is the use of a laxative not recommended for the management of a patient presenting with constipation?
3 Give one example of a topical agent and of a systemic product that could be recommended in vaginal thrush. For each example, state dosage regimen.

Answers

1 An anal fissure is a small split or tear in the anal mucosa that may cause painful bowel movements and bleeding. There may be blood on the outside of the stool or on the toilet tissue following a bowel movement. Anal fissures are extremely common in young infants but may occur at any age. Most fissures heal on their own and do not require treatment. The incidence of anal fissures decreases rapidly with age. Fissures are much less common among school-aged children than among infants.
In adults, fissures may be caused by constipation, the passing of large, hard stools or prolonged diarrhoea. They may occur after pregnancy and in Crohn's disease. Stool softeners and increased fibre in the diet are recommended.
2 No laxative should be recommended if intestinal obstruction is suspected.
3 Topical product: miconazole, dosage regimen: insert one ovule at night as a single dose. Systemic product: fluconazole, dosage regimen: stat dose 150 mg orally.

Further reading

Mashburn J (2006). Etiology, diagnosis, and management of vaginitis. *J Midwifery Womens Health* 51: 423–430.
Nickel J C (2005). Amoxicillin/clavulanate for the treatment of uncomplicated cystitis in women: a historical perspective. *Nat Clin Pract Urol* 2: 364–365.
Xu J, Schwartz K, Bartoces M, Monsur J, Severson R and Sobel J D (2008). Effect of antibiotics on vulvovaginal candidiasis: a metronet study. *J Am Board Fam Med* 21: 261–268.

61

Travel medicine

Learning objectives:

- To describe travel health risks
- To develop skills required in the recommendation of the preparation of medical first aid kits and the use of medicines in the management of travel-related disorders
- To appreciate pharmacist interventions that could be undertaken in travel medicine.

Background

Health risks associated with travel are due to:

- presence of disease at country visited
- hazards of travel (sickness, environmental, accidents).

Individuals need to receive information on prevention of travel health risks, preparing medical first aid kits and their use, and on the management of health-related problems during travel.

The support and information required depend on the destination (westernised countries or tropicals), duration of travel and type of travel (e.g. skiing holidays, back-packing, expedition).

Travel health hazards

- Infections (e.g. skin, respiratory tract, gastrointestinal)
- Accidents (e.g. traffic, sports associated)
- Travel sickness
- Dermatological (e.g. allergy, blisters, cuts and grazes)
- Acclimatisation
- Iatrogenic
- Chronic disease: deterioration or precipitation of chronic condition.

Medical kits for travel

When suggesting items for a medical kit, information on destination is required. In some countries (e.g. tropical or developing countries) it may be a problem to purchase basic medical first aid items, including bandages. Availability of medicines and quality of medicines that are accessible may vary in developing countries.

Products to be included in medical kits:

- chronic medication
- medications used occasionally (e.g. inhaled corticosteroids, oral NSAIDs)
- first aid products.

Considerations:

- Packaging: bulky packaging, liquid formulations are difficult to carry (e.g. alcohol swabs are preferred to surgical spirit)

- Controlled drugs: legal requirements between countries vary (e.g. amounts of narcotic products that can be carried may be restricted and need to be declared)
- Prescription-only medicines such as antibacterial agents (oral therapy, ear drops), prednisolone tablets for 'just-in-case' scenarios particularly if access to medicines may be limited in country and area visited.

First aid items for cuts and grazes

- Antiseptic (iodine based, surgical spirit)
- Plasters
- Crepe bandage
- Foot blister package
- Non-adherent dressing, hydrocolloid dressing (which is waterproof)
- Surgical tape.

Non-prescription medicines to include in medical first aid kits

- Analgesics, anti-inflammatory agents (e.g. paracetamol, ibuprofen)
- Antidiarrhoeals (loperamide) and rehydration therapy (oral rehydration salts)
- Antacids (e.g. aluminium–magnesium containing)
- Laxatives (e.g. senna)
- Motion sickness (e.g. promethazine)
- Oral antihistamines (e.g. loratidine)
- Cold preparations (throat lozenges, decongestants)
- Dermatological preparations: antifungal, hydrocortisone, antiseptic, soothing (e.g. calamine lotion) and moisturising cream.

Other products in medical pack that may need to be considered for specific regions include:

- insect repellents
- sunscreens
- water purification tablets.

Choice of antibacterial agents

- Broad spectrum
- Minimal risk of side-effects
- Hypersensitivity – if a medical first aid kit is being prepared for a group of individuals then one should consider possibility that some members may be hypersensitive. In such a scenario consider inclusion of macrolides
- Simple regimen
- Not expensive since product may not be used at all
- Antibacterial agents considered: co-amoxiclav and macrolides (respiratory and community-acquired pneumonia, urinary tract infections and wound damage), ciprofloxacin (bacterial travellers' diarrhoea and urinary tract infections), metronidazole (to be used in protozoa-induced travellers' diarrhoea).

> Accessibility to medications and to good-quality medicines may vary when travelling to foreign countries. Medical first aid kits should be adapted for particular travellers and specific type of travel.

Travel vaccinations

- Patients may be referred to the national immunisation centre for information on travel vaccinations.
- Live-attenuated vaccines (e.g. Bacillus Calmette–Guérin (BCG) vaccine, oral polio vaccine) offer immediate protection and tend to produce a more durable immunity than inactivated vaccines.
- Side-effects: discomfort at site of injection, mild fever and malaise. Some may produce a mild form of the disease.
- Contraindications: acute illness, anaphylaxis with a preceding dose of a vaccine, hypersensitivity to egg. Live-attenuated vaccines should be avoided in pregnant women.

Travel vaccinations are listed in Table 61.1.

> Risk of hepatitis A infection is increased when travelling to high-risk areas and frequent

Table 61.1 Travel vaccination

Name	Schedule	Lag time	Duration
BCG	One dose	2 months	N/A
Diphtheria/tetanus	Three doses at 1-month interval, booster one dose	After third dose immediate	10 years
Hepatitis A	One dose, booster after 6 months	4 weeks after first dose	6–12 months, 10 years
Hepatitis B	Three doses at 0, 1, 6 months	Effective after second dose but full effect after third dose, to be completed 10 days before	5 years
Polio (oral)	Dose at 0, 1, 3 months, booster one dose	After third dose immediate	10 years
Typhoid	One dose (parenteral)	10 days	3 years
Yellow fever	One dose	10 days	10 years

travellers should be advised to consider immunisation.

Problems related to air travel

- Motion sickness
- Jet lag
- Travel-related deep vein thrombosis
- Barotrauma
- Abdominal stretching.

Motion sickness

In motion sickness, the brain is responding inappropriately to certain types of 'unnatural' forms of motion. There is a physiological response to sensory mismatch.

- Predisposing factors: gender (females), age (3–12 years), mental state (anxiety), external factors (closed spaces)
- Symptoms: pallor, sweating, lightheadedness, nausea, vomiting, drowsiness.

For pharmacological treatment of motion sickness see Table 61.2.

Non-pharmacological treatment of motion sickness

- Sit in front seat when travelling in vehicles on the road, on the ship go on deck and follow horizon
- Avoid reading when vehicle is moving
- Follow movement direction
- Use of wrist bands, particularly useful in patients who cannot tolerate medications or when medications are contraindicated.

Motion sickness products are available in different dosage forms, namely transdermal patch, chewing gum and oral tablets. A disadvantage of motion sickness medications is the occurrence of sedation as a side-effect. Medication should be used to pre-empt occurrence of nausea and vomiting before there is onset of symptoms.

Jet lag

This occurs due to a disruption of the circadian rhythm, probably as a result of the effect of light on the retina which suppresses melatonin release from the pineal gland.

- Symptoms: daytime fatigue, sleeplessness at night
- Recovery after eastward flight is longer than that after westward travel.

Table 61.2 Pharmacological treatment of motion sickness

Drug	Minimum age (years)	Onset of action	Duration
Hyoscine	4	30 minutes	4–6 hours
Dimenhydrinate	2	30 minutes	3–6 hours
Promethazine	2	30 minutes	2–8 hours
Cinnarizine	5	2 hours	8 hours

Prevention and management of jet lag

- Sleep well for a few nights before departure
- Avoid critical tasks on arrival
- Adapt to local time and during flight adapt to destination time
- Avoid large meals, excessive caffeine and alcohol intake during flight
- Drink plenty of water
- Move about and exercise
- Melatonin supplements are licensed for this indication in some countries. Melatonin may be used to relieve jet lag and is taken before bedtime at the destination country.

When flying keep well hydrated, avoid alcohol and large meals, wear comfortable clothing and shoes, move around and perform leg–wrist–neck exercises.

Travel-related deep vein thrombosis

Risk of travel-related deep vein thrombosis increases in:

- previous or current DVT
- recent surgery or stroke
- paralysed lower limb
- myocardial angina
- unstable angina and uncontrolled heart failure.

The risks of travel-related deep vein thrombosis are shown in Table 61.3.

Prevention of travel-related deep vein thrombosis

- Maintain mobility and undertake ankle and foot movements during travel
- Avoid alcohol and caffeine
- Maintain good hydration
- Avoid crossing legs
- Wear support stockings during the flight
- Unless contraindicated, prophylactic aspirin 75 mg daily dose started a few days before travel and continued for a few days after reaching final destination.

Table 61.3 Risks of travel-related deep vein thrombosis (DVT)

Minor risk	Previous leg swelling Recent minor leg injury or minor surgery Extensive varicose veins Drugs: combined oral contraceptives, hormone replacement therapy
Moderate risk	Recent heart disease Pregnancy Recent major leg injury or surgery Family history of DVT

Recommendations to prevent travel-related deep vein thrombosis should be presented to all travellers. Emphasis should be given to those undertaking travel that is of a longer duration than 5 hours or those who have a minor or moderate risk.

Problems related to environmental hazards

- Sunburn
- Prickly heat
- Heat stroke

- Heat exhaustion
- Acute mountain sickness
- Decompression sickness
- Hypothermia
- Frostbite.

Sunburn

- Avoid sun between 11.00am and 3.00pm
- Wear light, loose-fitted clothes, hat, sunglasses
- Apply sunscreen with appropriate SPF:
  - apply 30 minutes before exposure, and repeat accordingly
  - should be water resistant
  - effectiveness may deteriorate on storage; check validity of product that has been opened for some time
  - protection against UVB and UVA (zinc oxide, titanium dioxide, camphor derivatives, benzophenones).

Prickly heat

This occurs due to blockage of sweat glands and leakage of sweat to surrounding epidermal tissue. It affects skin folds.

- Wear loose-fitting, light clothing
- Management: calamine lotion which can be applied repeatedly; hydrocortisone cream to be applied to small areas to remove inflammation; ascorbic acid supplementation for mucous membranes.

Heat stroke

This is a condition when sweat and thermoregulatory mechanisms fail. It is characterised by a rapid rise in body temperature.

- Symptoms: flushed, headache, confusion, delirium
- Factors that increase risk:
  - exertion
  - inappropriate clothing
  - drugs: diuretics, sympathomimetics
  - alcohol
  - sweating
  - dehydration
- Management: rehydrate, keep patient cool, use antipyretics.

Heat exhaustion

The primary factor in heat exhaustion is dehydration, resulting in insufficient sweat to cool the body.

- Symptoms: thirst, dry lips and mouth, decreased urine output, giddiness, neuropathy, slight rise in body temperature, rapid breathing, muscle cramps
- Management: rehydration.

Acute mountain sickness

This is reported to occur at altitudes of >2000 m and is probably related to a reduction in atmospheric pressure.

- Factors that increase risk: history of respiratory disorders, speed of ascent, physical exertion, cold
- Symptoms: headache, loss of appetite, nausea, vomiting, insomnia, dizziness, chest tightness
- May develop into high altitude pulmonary oedema, high altitude cerebral oedema
- Travellers should be advised on non-pharmacotherapeutic measures to prevent occurrence. They should be advised to seek referral if condition occurs.

When travelling to areas where there is the possibility of contaminated water:

- drink bottled water purchased in sealed containers
- avoid tap water even for toothbrushing
- avoid ice in drinks
- choose food that is freshly cooked and piping hot
- avoid salads, raw vegetables, fruit
- avoid ice creams
- avoid shellfish.

Practice summary

- Information on vaccination required for travel should be sought in advance of travelling since some vaccinations are associated with a time lag before immunity is achieved.
- Travellers should be advised to take the required amount of chronic medication for the duration of travel and also to take a supply of any medications that are required occasionally. It is advisable that chronic medications are carried in the carry-on luggage to avoid problems if checked-in luggage is mislaid or delayed.
- Good travelling practice should be adopted when flying to avoid dehydration, minimise impact of jet lag where applicable and decrease risk of deep vein thrombosis.
- When travelling to areas where there is a high risk of contaminated water, food and water hygiene are essential to minimise occurrence of disease (e.g. diarrhoea, hepatitis A).
- During travel the body is exposed to increased stress and individuals are at a higher risk of developing infections (e.g. common cold). The use of multivitamin preparations may be considered for individuals who are undertaking frequent travel, travelling to developing areas or at increased risk of developing infections.

Questions

1. List four factors that present a moderate risk of travel-related deep vein thrombosis (DVT). What prophylactic measures could be followed?
2. What considerations are necessary when recommending a product for prophylaxis of motion sickness?
3. What advice should be given to patients who present with prickly heat?

Answers

1. Recent heart disease, pregnancy, recent major leg injury or surgery, family history of DVT. Prophylaxis: consider use of support hosiery (stockings), prophylactic aspirin; advise on importance of proper hydration during travel and to maintain mobility and carry out ankle–foot exercises.
2. Age, duration required, onset of action, impact of side-effects.
3. Use loose-fitting, light clothing. Apply calamine lotion and prickly heat powders for symptomatic relief, consider use of hydrocortisone cream to reduce inflammation and take ascorbic acid (vitamin C) supplementation to prevent epidermal damage.

Further reading

Goodyer L I (2004). *Travel Medicine for Health Professionals*. London: Pharmaceutical Press.

PART 4

Pharmacy Information and Research

62

Pharmacy literature and medical information

Learning objectives:

- To appreciate use of pharmacy literature and medical information to support expertise on action and uses of drugs
- To familiarise oneself with use of formularies and pharmacopoeias
- To develop skills to use information presented on the internet.

Sources of information

Formularies

These are listings of drugs used in a particular setting. For example, the *British National Formulary* (BNF) is published jointly by the British Medical Association and the Royal Pharmaceutical Society of Great Britain in March and September every year.

> *The BNF includes key information on the selection, prescribing, dispensing and administration of medicines. Medicines generally prescribed in the UK are covered and those considered less suitable for prescribing are clearly identified. Little or no information is included on medicines promoted for purchase by the public.*[1]

Contents of BNF

- Drug monographs, e.g.
  - gastrointestinal system
  - cardiovascular system
  - respiratory system
  - central nervous system
  - endocrine system
- Notes on prescribing in palliative care, elderly people, dental practice
- Emergency treatment of poisoning
- Appendices:
  - interactions
  - liver disease
  - renal impairment
  - breast-feeding
  - intravenous additives
  - borderline substances
  - wound management products and elastic hosiery
  - cautionary and advisory labels for dispensed medicines

Drug monographs provide information on indications, cautions, contraindications, side-effects and dose. For preparations information on dosage forms is available; manufacturer, prescription-only status and price in sterling provided.

See also Chapter 68.

Pharmacopoeias

A pharmacopoeia is a compendium containing descriptions, standards and official assays for medical substances. The concept of pharmacopoeias has long been established. The publication in Nuremberg, Germany of the *Dispensatorium Pharmacorum Omnium* in 1546 is an early example and subsequently in 1561 in Basel such a publication was prepared which carried for the first time the term 'pharmacopoeia' in the title.

In 1618, the first *London Pharmacopoeia* was published. It included 1028 drugs and 932 compounds. With time, national pharmacopoeias replaced pharmacopoeias that were established for districts or cities. In the UK the Medical Act of 1858 established that the *British Pharmacopoeia* (BP) should be prepared as a single publication that encompasses information presented by those of London, Edinburgh and Dublin. More recently regional pharmacopoeias replaced the national document and today the *European Pharmacopoeia* (EP) is adopted within member states of the European Union. Attempts to harmonise the *US Pharmacopoeia*, the *Japanese Pharmacopoeia* and the *European Pharmacopoeia* are ongoing. In addition the World Health Organization issues the *International Pharmacopoeia*.

European Pharmacopoiea

- Published by the European Department for the Quality of Medicines within the Council of Europe.
- Establishes standard procedures for analysis and specifications of active substances, excipients, dosage forms and containers.
- Monographs are intended for regulatory authorities, quality control laboratories, manufacturers of active ingredients, excipients and medicinal products.

Other sources of drug information and therapeutics

- *Martindale: The Complete Drug Reference*
- *Monthly Index of Medical Specialities* (MIMS)
- Association of British Pharmaceutical Industry (ABPI)
- *Goodman & Gilman's Pharmacological Basis of Therapeutics*
- Medical dictionaries.

Martindale: The Complete Drug Reference

- Published by Pharmaceutical Press, London. *The aim of Martindale is to provide healthcare professionals with unbiased evaluated information on drugs and medicines used throughout the world. Martindale is based on published information and more than 37 500 selected references are included.*[2]

Journals

- *Pharmaceutical Journal* (*Pharm J*): published weekly by the Royal Pharmaceutical Society of Great Britain
- *American Journal of Health-System Pharmacy* (*AJHP*): published twice monthly by the American Society of Health-System Pharmacists
- *Journal of the American Pharmacists Association* (*JAPhA*): published twice monthly by the American Pharmacists Association
- *International Journal of Pharmacy Practice* (*IJPP*): published quarterly by Pharmaceutical Press and presents reviews and original studies in the areas of use of medicines and pharmacy practice
- *Clinical Pharmacist*: published by Pharmaceutical Press, United Kingdom and incorporates the journal *Hospital Pharmacist* which was published until 2008. It provides information on current practice that is of direct relevance to clinical pharmacy
- *Pharmacy World and Science* (*PWS*): presents articles that reflect studies which are practice oriented
- *British Medical Journal* (*BMJ*): published weekly by the British Medical Association
- *The Lancet*: published weekly and presents research studies in the medical and therapeutics field
- *Journal of the American Medical Association* (*JAMA*): published weekly by the American Medical Association.

The internet and pharmacy information

Traditional evaluation skills are necessary to assess information from the internet. These include:

- clear
- concise
- unbiased
- relevant
- referenced
- source identified.

Limitations to using internet sources for retrieval of drug information include that information may not be peer reviewed and it may reflect the views of the person or persons who posted the information. Therefore it is essential that internet sources are first evaluated prior to implementation.

Examples of useful websites

- Criteria for writing references: www.icmje.org
- *Pharmaceutical Journal*: www.pharmj.com
- *JAMA*: jama.ama-assn.org
- *The Lancet*: www.thelancet.com
- *BMJ*: group.bmj.com
- Pharmweb: www.pharmweb.net
- BNF: www.bnf.org
- *Merck Manual of Diagnosis and Therapeutics*: www.merck.com/pubs/mmanual.

Practice summary

- Sources of information used should be clear and reliable.
- Sources used should be updated to reflect current editions.
- Interpretation and evaluation of literature available should be carried out to support pharmaceutical care programmes, pharmacotherapeutic decisions and pharmacoeconomic evaluations.
- Drug information services are intended to provide adequate and timely drug information to health professionals.
- Medical and pharmacy literature is used in the preparation of educational programmes and written educational materials that are intended to be used by patients and their carers.

Questions

1. What is a pharmacopoeia?
2. Give examples of publications that could be used by a pharmacist when providing a drug information service.
3. What action should be taken to ensure quality service and reduce risks of errors in documenting drug information?

Answers

1. A pharmacopoeia is a compendium containing descriptions, standards and official assays for medical substances. Examples include the *British Pharmacopoeia* and the *European Pharmacopoeia.*
2. *British National Formulary, Martindale: The Complete Drug Reference, British National Formulary for Children, Stockley's Drug Interactions.*
3. Define the information requested. Use robust procedures in written format (e.g. use of check-lists). Ensure that information given is accurate, up to date and acquired from a reliable source. Verify data given (safe). Comply with legal and ethical requirements. Use resources of adequate quality and extent. Personnel sourcing and documenting drug information should be trained in this activity. Document all steps carried out, source of request, personnel pursuing the request.

Further reading

Baxter K, ed. (2007). *Stockley's Drug Interactions*. London: Pharmaceutical Press.

Dunlop D M and Denston T C (1958). The history and development of the British Pharmacopeia. *BMJ* **ii**: 1250–1252.

Kiley R (2003). *Medical Information on the Internet: A guide for health professionals*, 3rd edn. London: Churchill Livingstone.

Joint Formulary Committee (2008). *British National Formulary*, 58th edn. British Medical Association and Royal Pharmaceutical Society of Great Britain.

Paediatric Formulary Committee (2008). *British National Formulary for Children*. London: Pharmaceutical Press.

Sweetman S C, ed. (2007). *Martindale: The Complete Drug Reference*, 35th edn. London: Pharmaceutical Press.

References

1 Joint Formulary Committee *British National Formulary,* 57th edn. London: British Medical Association and Royal Pharmaceutical Society of Great Britain, 2009.

2 Sweetman S C, ed. *Martindale: The Complete Drug Reference*, 35th edn. London: Pharmaceutical Press, 2007.

63

Medical writing

Learning objectives:

- To describe the approach towards scientific writing of abstracts and reports
- To develop skills of scientific report writing.

Background

- *Review article:* critical evaluation of material that has already been published
- *Original paper:* an original study; usually presented in the format of: Introduction, Method, Results, Discussion.

Writing an abstract

An abstract is a summary describing the study and presenting salient points from the research. It should present:

- the issue and aims tackled
- method carried out
- salient observations
- inference of observations.

Preparing a report and papers for submission to journals

Scientific reports should be based on unbiased background information. Sound methodology needs to be presented. Data handling should be robust and reliable. Salient observations are emphasised and discussed.

- Set deadlines
- Write regularly
- Read when complete draft is ready
- Get reviews
- Check spelling and presentation.

Structure

- Table of contents: clear headings which indicate a consistent and systematic approach
- References: adopt style indicated and adhere to guidelines
- Opening page: check requirements for data that are essential.

> Report writing means rewriting. An attempt to draw a first draft may be difficult initially but once there is a draft it is easier to rearrange. Allocate enough time to be able to review drafts.

Introduction

- Discuss literature search
- Should not be an exhaustive historical review unless the report is looking at a review of works done. Background to the study should be presented.

Method

- Describe participants, apparatus and materials used
- Provide details on data handling and statistical analysis.

Results

- Use tables and figures to present data effectively
- Emphasise results that reflect salient observations.

Pie charts

- Used to express proportions
- Give a title and number
- Include label and figures (numbers or percentage) for each sector
- Do not include more than eight sectors
- Emphasise particular sector by separating sector from the rest.

Bar and line graphs

- Give each chart a title and number
- Label x and y axes
- Use bar chart to compare groups or show changes over time
- Normally use vertical positioning
- Adopt a horizontal positioning if using more than six compartments
- Use line charts to compare results over many points in time.

Tables

- Give title and number
- Give column headings
- Organise table systematically.

Discussion

- Describe whether results support or do not support original hypotheses
- Compare with other studies carried out previously or in other scenarios
- Comment on the implications of the study
- Review limitations of the study.

- For numbers smaller than 100, report in numbers
- For numbers greater than 100, report in percentage and numbers
- In tables and figures always include sample size
- Where statistical analysis is shown, indicate P value and specify significance
- Label columns, rows and graphs appropriately
- Do not repeat data presented in figures or tables in text or vice versa.

Referencing

- Compile list of references as you go along
- Check reference style that is required
- Textual references are easier to handle
- Avoid plagiarism: direct quotations vs paraphrasing. All quotations must be acknowledged as being quotes by using quote symbol and indicating source. For paraphrasing, reference should be indicated.

Reference lists and bibliography

- Document the write-up, report and paper with regard to sources used to provide the necessary background
- Provide the information necessary to identify and retrieve every source
- *Reference list:* cites works that specifically support the text
- *Bibliography:* cites work for background or for further reading.

Vancouver style of writing references

- Established in 1978 in Vancouver
- Maintained by the International Committee of Medical Journal Editors (ICMJE)

- Aims to maintain a standard approach to documenting sources used in a scientific report.

Articles in journals

- List the first six authors followed by *et al.*
- Title of journal abbreviated according to *Index Medicus* (see http://www.nlm.nih.gov).

Examples

Yeung V, Funnell R, Harrison R. Advice for pharmacists who need to comply with clinical trials regulations. *Pharm J* 2008; 281: 193–195.

Organisation as author

Royal Pharmaceutical Society of Great Britain. Protocols and staff training to be added to Code of Ethics. *Pharm J* 1996; 253: 124–127.

No author given

Anon. Creating a more professional image for a pharmacy. *Pharm J* 1991; 246: 304–305.

Books

Personal author

Waterfield J. *Community Pharmacy Handbook*. London: Pharmaceutical Press; 2008.

Chapter in a book

Kouimtzi M. Writing a research report. In: Stuart MC, ed. *The Complete Guide to Medical Writing*. London: Pharmaceutical Press; 2007, pp. 63–74.

Organisation as author and publisher

Health Education Authority (UK). *Helping People Change: Audit tool guidelines*. London: Health Education Authority; 1995.

Dictionary

Mosby's Medical, Nursing & Allied Health Dictionary, 5th edn. St Louis: Mosby; 1998. Bronchoscopy; pp. 231–232.

Electronic material

Lowey AR, Jackson MN. A survey of extemporaneous preparation in NHS trusts in Yorskshire, the North-East and London. Hospital Pharmacist [serial online] 2008; 15: 217–219 [cited 2008 September 9]. Available from: URL: http://www.pharmj.com/pdf/hp/200806/hp_200806_papers.pdf.

Referencing systems

- Vancouver system: numbered consecutively in the order in which they are first mentioned in the text; the references are listed consecutively by number at the end of the text:
  In 1968, Denzin and Mettlin described the pharmacy profession as an occupation 'which has taken some, but not all, of the characteristics commonly ascribed to the professions.'[1] *A study to test whether this practice affects service provided showed that pharmacists were similarly motivated irrespective of their area of practice.*[2]
- Harvard system: author–date citation, the references are listed in alphabetical order at the end of the text:
  In 1968, Denzin and Mettlin described the pharmacy profession as an occupation 'which has taken some, but not all, of the characteristics commonly ascribed to the professions.'

  A study to test whether this practice affects service provided showed that pharmacists were similarly motivated irrespective of their area of practice (Kronus, 1975).

  The total cost spent on health-care in major European countries has risen since the 1960s (Zayed and Manning, 1995).

  Participation of community pharmacists in practice-based research projects is a further contribution to professional developments (Ellerby et al, 1993).

Alphabetising the list of references for the Harvard system

- Letter by letter: nothing precedes something:
  King M J
  Kingsbury AL

- Order of several works by same first author:
  - by year: earliest first
  - one author and then two authors precede multiple author
  - same first, different co-authors; organise alphabetically according to co-authors
  - published in the same year, alphabetical order by title.

  Smith F. Referral of clients by community pharmacists in primary care consultations. *Int J Pharm Pract* 1993; 2: 86–89.

  Smith F, Salkind MR. Counselling areas: views of community pharmacists and clients. *Pharm J* 1988; 241(suppl): R7.

  Smith F, Salkind MR. Presentation of clinical symptoms to community pharmacists in London. *J Soc Admin Pharm* 1990; 7: 221–224.

  Smith F, Salkind MR, Jolly BC. Community pharmacy: a method of assessing quality of care. *Soc Sci Med* 1990; 31(5): 603–607.

Literature search

- Should be comprehensive
- Use key words
- Is an ongoing process throughout the study
- Identify common references.

Practice summary

- A literature search should be comprehensive and is an ongoing process throughout the entire study.
- Scientific writing should be based on statements that indicate facts and should avoid bias. Data presented should be robust, reliable and valid.

Question

1 Why is it important to reference medical writing properly?

Answer

1 To acknowledge the work of others and avoid plagiarism. To indicate when one is quoting other works, paraphrasing or summarising ideas put forward by others. To identify the reliability and the accuracy of the data, work quoted and sources used. To allow reader to locate sources used, read the original work and confirm data from cited works. To support the arguments made in the document. To identify which literature was consulted in drawing of conclusions. To follow harmonisation and academic robustness in medical writing.

Further reading

Stuart M C, ed. (2007). *The Complete Guide to Medical Writing*. London: Pharmaceutical Press.

64

Research methodology

Learning objectives:

- To appreciate aspects of research studies
- To identify processes involved in planning of a research study
- To develop skills required for oral communication and poster preparation during dissemination of a project.

Background

In a research study, principles of rigour need to be employed to ascertain a sound methodology and validity of results.

- Appropriate study design
- Reliability of data collection processes
- Validity of instruments
- Clear analytical procedures
- Interpretation of the findings in the light of the paradigms and methods employed.

Planning study design

- To contemplate advantages and disadvantages of different approaches and make choices:
  - balancing resources vs sample size
  - sampling procedures vs generalisability
  - number of mailings vs adequate response rate
- To undertake preliminary fieldwork and piloting studies.

See Figure 64.1 for processes involved in a research study.

> The planning stage of the research study is an important aspect since it may be very difficult to remedy steps that were not considered at this stage. For example, it would be impossible to interview patients before an intervention if the intervention has already commenced.

Research methods

- Quantitative methods.
  - survey research
  - focus groups
  - observation studies
- Qualitative methods
- Triangulation: more than one approach adopted.

Survey research

- Identification of suitable sampling frames
- Adoption of appropriate sampling procedures
- Achievement of good response rates
- Management of non-response

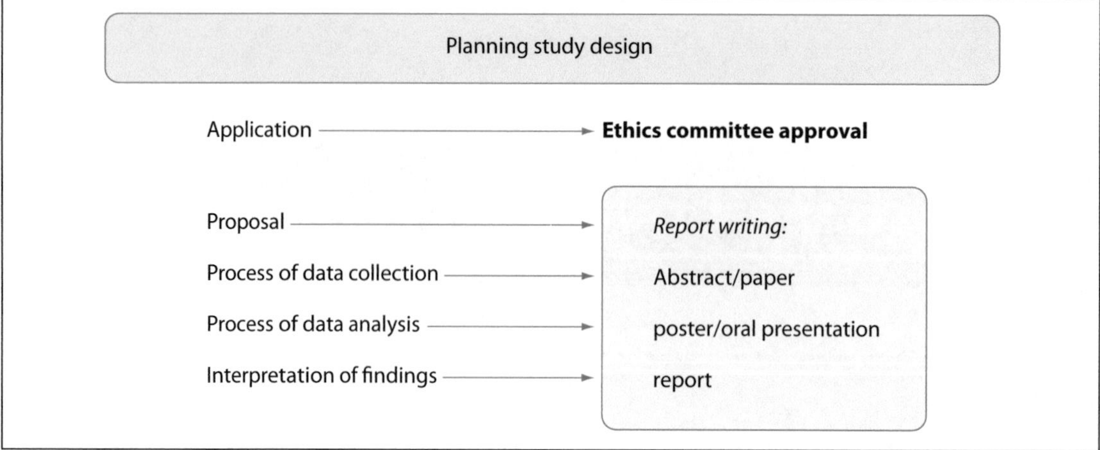

Figure 64.1 Processes involved in a research study.

- Development of survey instruments
- Ensuring validity, reliability and generalisability of data.

Focus groups

- A technique by which priorities of participants can be identified and insights gained into their reasoning and argument
- Interviewer needs to lead discussion and be able to discover as many issues relating to the area of study as possible
- The more concrete and detailed the account of each issue the better.

Observation studies

- Researcher has control over quality and completeness of data.
- Data relate to actual events and not to estimates or reports by participants.
- Major disadvantage is the 'Hawthorne effect' where participants being observed, knowingly or unknowingly, modify their behaviour.

Terms used in research investigations

- *Incidence:* the frequency of occurrence
- *Prevalence:* the number of individuals experiencing a condition
- *Risk:* the number of events that occur in a defined time period divided by the average population at risk
- *Standardised mortality rate (SMR):* the observed crude death rate divided by the expected crude death rate
- *Cost-effectiveness analysis (CEA):* the examination of the costs of two or more programmes that have the same clinical outcome as measured in physical units (e.g. lives saved, reduced morbidity)
- *Cost–utility analysis:* estimates patient preference for a particular intervention in terms of the patient's state of well-being. The product of utility and life-years gained provides the term quality-adjusted life-years (QALY).

Quality-adjusted life-years (QALY) is a technique used to determine the most efficient and effective treatment that should be made available to patients. QALY is meant to measure outcomes of healthcare (e.g. pain relief, anxiety reduction, morbidity improvement and life extension). The use of QALY in determining benefit of drug action has to be made in the light of ethical issues, social justice and moral legitimacy.

Longitudinal (cohort) study

- A clearly defined group of individuals studied in a period of time
- Enables collection of data on the course of events providing information on timing of events
- Limitations: time factor, follow-up and attrition, expenses required to run the study for a long period of time that is essential for follow-up.

Cross-sectional study

- Data related to one point in time.

Repeat cross-sectional studies

- Data collected at more than one point in time
- Not necessarily completed by same individuals.

Controlled study

- Experimental vs control group
- Double-blind: participants and researchers are not aware of how the groups are divided
- Single-blind: participants do not know in which group they are
- Matching between groups is required to eliminate bias due to external factors (equating experimental and control groups) (e.g. for age, gender, level of education).

Sampling vs generalisability

- Sampling frame: list of population eligible for study
- Sampling unit: single member of a sampling population
- All sampling units: sampling frame
- Random (probability) sampling is desirable as this allows the application of probability statistics and generalisation of the data to the population from which the sample is drawn (Figure 64.2).

Simple random sampling

- Every sampling unit has an equal chance of being selected
- Use of table of random numbers or throwing a dice to pick up sampling units that are selected
- Unbiased sample is obtained
- May not pick up all elements in a population.

Stratified random sampling

- Population is divided into subgroups or strata (e.g. districts, age).
- Subgroups are identified from expert opinion, literature review and should be related to outcome of study.
- The method employed in simple random sampling is undertaken for each subgroup.
- Advantage: better representation of elements in the population that may affect the study hypothesis.

Systematic random sampling

- Sampling is carried out in a repetitive manner
- Example: 200 patients are required from a sample frame of 1000 patients
- Therefore select 1 every 5 (1000/200)
- Still requires random identification of first unit.

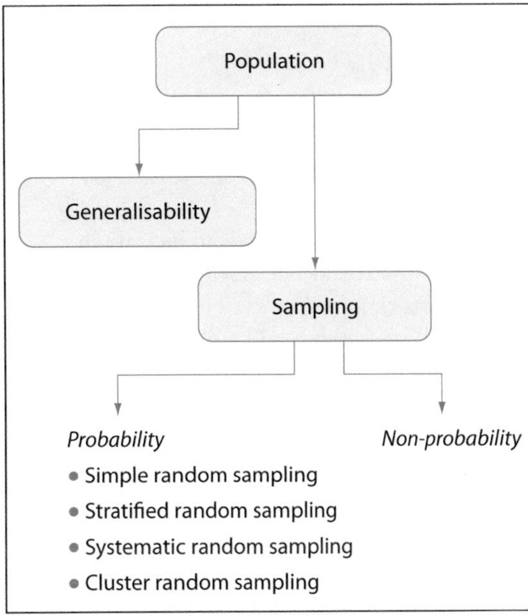

Figure 64.2 Sampling.

Cluster random sampling

- Random selection of clusters of units
- All members of cluster are included
- Example: cluster shopping areas and then include all units (pharmacies) in shopping areas identified
- Used in large surveys.

Non-probability sampling

This is adopted when participants or units are chosen based on judgement regarding characteristics of the population and objectives of the survey. For example:

- surveys of hard-to-identify groups (e.g. drug abusers)
- survey of specific groups (e.g. cancer patients)
- piloting stage.

Examples of non-probability sampling include:

- convenience sampling – participants available and ready to participate
- snowball sampling – relies on previously identified members
- focus groups – representatives of population.

Sample size

- Any subset of sampling units from a population
- Sample size represents a proportion (5%) of the population
- Increasing sample size leads to increase in precision of results but may require more costs and more time
- Sample size is estimated by deciding the level of accuracy expected (standard error)
- When planning the study and recruiting sampling units, it is essential to account for non-response error (uninterviewable, not found, refusals, not suitable for analysis). So a greater number of sampling units should be used to make up for the attrition that will occur during the study so as to achieve the required sample size by the end of the study.

Promoting response and minimising response bias

- Interview technique adopted as opposed to self-administration
- Identify larger number of eligible sampling units than needed (a balance is required since increasing the number increases the costs)
- Keep results anonymous and confidential
- Be realistic about the eligibility criteria and timeframes established.

Problems associated with sampling frames

- Always select a larger sample initially in order to compensate for omissions
- Incomplete frames – data on sampling units missing
- Clusters of elements – sampling units listed in clusters and identification of individual sampling units is impossible
- Blank elements – unlabelled sample for analysis, small volume of sample to enable analytical analysis, blank or incomplete questionnaire.

Designing questionnaires

- Clearly establish the objectives of the questionnaire: what information is needed? Refrain from asking questions that bring information that is not related to these objectives
- Types of questions used:
  - open-ended
  - close-ended: Likert scale, two-way, ranking
- Questions should be worded to avoid bias
- Adopt appearance and layout that make the document easy to complete
- During the pilot phase assess applicability, validity and reliability testing
- Use language that is appropriate for the audience.

When designing questionnaires bear in mind the method of administration and data analysis.

Administering questionnaires

- Questionnaires may be carried out as self-administered questionnaires
- Questionnaires may be carried out by interview: formal, semi-structured, unstructured. The interview method ensures response rate but more time is required from the research group
- Aim for a response rate >60%.

Observation studies

These capture what people actually do, compared with what people state that they do, which is reported in a questionnaire.

- Number of visits, duration, time of visit
- May be carried out as covert or overt
- Analysis of qualitative or quantitative data.

Data collection and analysis

Goals

- Accuracy and precision
- Minimal errors
- Elimination of inter- and intra-observer variability.

Statistical analysis

- Describe population parameters
- Sample data: gender, age (frequency distribution, mean, range)
- Quantitative data: frequency distribution, mean, standard deviation.

Software packages, e.g. SPSS (Statistical Package for the Social Sciences), BMDP (Biomedical Data Package) and Minitab Statistical Software may be used to calculate:

- Significance levels: Pearson's chi-squared or Mann–Whitney test on non-parametric data (nominal or ordinal data); Student's *t*-test or analysis of variance (ANOVA) on parametric data (interval and ratio data)
- Tests for correlation: Pearson's product moment correlation, regression analysis
- Reliability of scales (questionnaires): Cronbach's alpha.

Significant testing is based on the laws of probability which determine the probability that the differences would have occurred in any case (by chance). The probability level usually accepted is expressed as P values less than 0.05, implying that it is 95% certain that the difference is not due to chance.

Evaluation of research study

- Purpose of study: clear objectives stated and addressed
- Background research: exhaustive and provides an appropriate background
- Appropriate research design: methodology adopted is sound and robust to generate data that meet the specified objectives
- Research population: the study population is a correct representation of the sampling frame
- Validity and reliability of data: data collection is validated (method of analysis used or the questionnaire employed)
- Analysis of data: statistical handling of the data uses indicated parameters
- Correct interpretation of results: extrapolation of the inferences that can be drawn from the data obtained is sensible and statistically sound
- Valid conclusion: conclusion reached is based on the results obtained and links with the established objectives.

Dissemination

- Undertaken in the form of: oral presentations, posters, abstracts, journal articles, reports, workshops and seminars
- Present objectives, describe methodology and results
- Style, length, referencing system depends on type of dissemination activity undertaken.

Oral communication

Presentation skills

- Personal approach: enthusiastic
- Time: never go over the time allocated
- Amount of time spent on various aspects of the talk should be balanced, e.g. appropriate time dedicated to the introduction, methodology, results and discussion
- Practice: practise the presentation to identify areas that are not clear
- Appropriate to the audience: direct level of detail according to the audience background
- Enjoy it: being stressed and anxious makes it difficult to achieve a good delivery.

Audiovisual aids

- Use simple fonts such as Arial or Times New Roman at a 24 font size, double spacing, bold type
- Use a dark background and do not use more than four colours per slide
- Use upper- and lowercase letters rather than all uppercase
- Each slide should contain only one main idea, table or figure
- Do not write more than six to eight lines per slide and use the middle area of the slide
- Use phrases rather than complete sentences
- Round numbers to the nearest whole numbers
- Limit tables to five rows and six columns
- In graphs label x and y axes
- Provide headers for tables, figures, graphs
- Review slides for typographical errors, clarity and sequence.

Title slide

- Keep it brief and understandable
- Avoid inclusion in the title of phrases such as 'a report of', 'an analysis of', 'with reference to', 'with special emphasis', 'the use of'.

Structure

- Organise the presentation according to a systematic approach: Introduction, Aim(s), Method, Results, Conclusion
- Use the audiovisual aids to keep track of the stages within the structure of the presentation.

Method

- A brief overview of what was done
- Describe sampling
- Activity: analysis – give summary of procedure done, survey – details on content
- Use flowcharts to help audience follow the steps.

Results

- Report sample size
- Patient characteristics: mean age, age range, gender
- For numbers smaller than 100, report in numbers
- For numbers greater than 100, report in percentage and numbers.

Posters

- Use only a few words to present an issue
- Include point-form presentation, sketch figures, flowcharts
- Be consistent and adopt a systematic approach
- Use symbols (e.g. bullets)
- Use colours and pictures appropriately.

Journal articles

Papers should be submitted according to the instructions to author provided by the identified journal.

These would include word count, number of figures and tables, referencing system, structure of article (e.g. abstract, keywords, introduction, methodology, results and discussion) (see also Chapter 63).

Practice summary

- Planning and documentation of every step are required.
- The proposal outlines objectives of the study, methodology to be followed, expected results as well as budget and timeplans.
- Dissemination of the project could be undertaken through oral communication, posters and abstracts. Relevant results should be identified and emphasised.

Questions

1. Differentiate between simple random sampling and stratified random sampling.
2. Explain what is a focus group.
3. Explain what is a longitudinal study.

Answers

1. *Simple random sampling:*
   - Every sampling unit has an equal chance of being selected
   - May not pick up all elements in a population.

   Stratified random sampling:
   - Population is divided into subgroups or strata (e.g. districts, age)
   - Subgroups are identified from expert opinion, literature review and should be related to outcome of study.
2. A focus group is based on a technique in which priorities of participants can be identified and insights gained into their reasoning and argument. A discussion is undertaken and led by the lead investigator to discover as many issues relating to the area of study as possible. The more concrete and detailed the account of each issue, the better. Interventions by focus group members should be recorded.
3. A sample is followed up for a period of time. It enables collection of data on the course of events providing information on timing of events. Limitations: time factor, follow-up and attrition, expenses.

Further reading

Durham T A and Turner R J (2008). *Introduction to Statistics in Pharmaceutical Clinical Trials*. London: Pharmaceutical Press.

Edgar A, Salek S, Shickle D and Cohen D (1998). *The Ethical QALY: Ethical issues in healthcare resource allocations*. Surrey: Euromed Communications Ltd.

Smith F (2002). *Research Methods in Pharmacy Practice*. London: Pharmaceutical Press.

Smith F, Francis S A and Schafheutle E (2008). *International Research in Healthcare*. London: Pharmaceutical Press.

Stuart M C, ed. (2007). *The Complete Guide to Medical Writing*. London: Pharmaceutical Press.

PART 5

Pharmacy Systems

65

Primary care health services

Learning objectives:

- To appreciate the expectations of society from primary care health services
- To identify pharmacist actions at the primary care health services level.

Background

Healthcare delivery systems can be classified:

1. Primary care: physician, pharmacist, dentist
2. Secondary care: specialist treatment, hospital care
3. Tertiary care: highly specialised inpatient care.

There is also:

- Self-care: diagnosis, treatment and prevention of disease conditions by the individuals themselves.

Primary healthcare

Improves the nation's and the individual's health not only in the treatment of disease but also in the maintenance and promotion of health.

Objectives

- To provide a consumer-oriented service
- To raise standards of care
- To promote health and prevent illness
- To provide patients with the widest range of choice in obtaining high-quality primary care
- To decrease the demand for secondary care in the hospital setting.

Targets of primary care health services

- Prevention of disease
- Early diagnosis, treatment and/or referral
- Treatment of ailments not requiring admission to hospital or specialist treatment.

Features of primary care health services

- Accessible
- Available
- Relevant to the community
- Cost-effective.

Programmes within primary care services

- Sanitation
- Maternal and child health
- Immunisation
- Management of minor diseases
- Provision of essential drugs
- Management of injuries
- Prophylaxis and disease prevention.

Setting

- Government-funded health centres
- Private clinics
- Private community pharmacies.

Payment of service

- Government
- Patient
- Third party insurance company.

Factors influencing primary healthcare

- Developments in medical technology, pharmaceutical technology, diagnostics, surgery
- Rising costs
- Unlimited demand.

Pharmacy services

Community pharmacists act as coordinators and navigators of patient care within primary healthcare. They also:

- participate in formulary development in collaboration with prescribers in the area
- provide domiciliary services to housebound patients
- educate the community
- provide professional services to nursing and residential homes in the area.

Home care services

Delivery of home care medications, and monitoring of patients receiving therapy at home including patients receiving home intravenous therapy and home parenteral fluid treatment.

Ambulatory care

Primary care-based services and services provided from office-based specialists and hospital visits on an outpatient basis.

The pharmacist in primary healthcare collaborates with other healthcare professionals in the sector and across the other levels of service provision on a regular basis. The pharmacist in primary healthcare is also the link between different specialists participating in patient care (e.g. the diabetologist and the obstetrician and gynaecologist for pregnant patients with diabetes).

Pharmacy primary healthcare

Scenario in Europe

- Healthcare organisation: government
- Healthcare funding: government ± social security
- Healthcare expenditure: between 6% and 12% of GDP is spent on healthcare.

Scenario in the USA

Over the past few years the USA has decreased the rise in healthcare costs by encouraging the population to invest in managed care plans.

- Managed care: structured network of providers of healthcare formed to offer quality care, including preventive care at the lowest cost.

Supplementary and pharmacist prescribing

In the UK, supplementary prescribing role for the pharmacist was established in 2003 and pharmacist prescribing was established in 2005. Overview of process:

- Meeting patient and interviewing patient to establish patient's background
- Documentation: care management plan which is co-developed with a prescriber, identify clinical guidelines followed (e.g. practice hypertension protocol)

- Patient access to clinic: referred by health professionals or seek direct attention
- Patient monitoring: evaluate treatment outcomes
- Decision-making: prescribe or refer.

Practice summary

- Pharmacist actions at the primary healthcare level include education about disease prevention and healthy lifestyle, responding and managing minor symptoms, recommending referral where indicated and patient monitoring.
- By acting as navigators and coordinators of patient care, pharmacists in the primary care setting may contribute to increase collaboration within the primary care level and with other care levels. This will increase the provision of seamless care and decrease risk of drug-related problems due to the patient moving from one interface to another.

Question

1 What are the requirements for a screening programme to be provided from a community pharmacy as part of primary care health services?

Answer

1
- Condition addressed must have serious implications (e.g. produce significant morbidity or mortality).
- Condition is common.
- There is effective therapy or action that can be taken.
- Screening test must be reasonably quick, easy and inexpensive.
- Screening test must be safe and acceptable to individual being screened and to the pharmacist providing the service.
- Sensitivity, specificity and positive predictive values must be known and acceptable. Probability of occurrence of false positives and false negatives must be within reasonable, acceptable limits (see Chapter 11).
- Adequate and accessible information about the condition and the screening test must be provided.
- There must be adequate follow-up for individuals with a positive result. A pharmaceutical care plan needs to be drawn up beforehand (see Chapter 12).
- Treatment or preventive measures recommended should be acceptable to individuals.
- The setting where the service is provided should be adequate (see Chapter 5).
- Personnel providing the service and carrying out the screening test should be properly trained.
- Documentation including a referral system is established.

Examples of common screening programmes that may be provided from community pharmacies include hypertension, lipid profile, blood glucose.

Further reading

Jepson G M H (2001). How do primary health care systems compare across Western Europe? *Pharm J* 267: 269–273.

Lavender G (2005). Opportunities in primary care: diary of a pharmacist supplementary prescriber. *Pharm J* 274: 151–152.

Smalley L (2005). Supplementary prescribing in action – an example from primary care. *Pharm J* 274: 213–214.

66

Community pharmacy management

Learning objectives:

- To appreciate principles required in community pharmacy management
- To develop skills essential in the management of personnel, designing pharmacy layout and handling of stock.

Background

Perception of the community pharmacist

- Accessible health professional
- Provides advice to patients on health issues
- Professional charge is not clear: patrons believe that they can receive counselling without being charged
- Patients may feel more comfortable in a pharmacy setting rather than a clinic environment

Changes occurring in the community pharmacy setting

- Availability of new drugs
- Ageing population
- Alternative dispensing systems: automated dispensing, domiciliary services, mail order, internet services
- Change to non-prescription medicine status.

Challenges in the community pharmacy setting

- Financial viability
- Preservation of market share as opposed to competition from supermarkets, internet pharmacy and other sources to get drugs
- Cost containment
- Keeping up with ethical and legal considerations; the misconception that having a good business aspect is inconsistent with good clinical practice is very often discussed
- Use of computer technology to connect with prescribers and maintain patient's profile
- Time management to allow for new patient contact interventions required.

Business operations

- Accounting: keeping records
- Finance: monitoring cash
- Personnel management: managing people, training and development
- Production: time-and-motion studies
- Administration: payments, legal requirements, ordering.

Personnel management

- Appointing and dismissing of staff: issuing contracts and drawing up job descriptions
- Health, safety and welfare
- Training and development.

Good management improves the satisfaction of patients with professional pharmacy services and meets expectations regarding the quantity and quality of the care received.

Starting a pharmacy

- Plan the business
- Stategic planning and identifying legal form of business (proprietor, partnership, company)
- Capital needs: obtain financing
- Location and licences
- Set up records
- Insure the business
- Manage the business.

Plan the business

For businesses where the pharmacy already exists and is being taken over, this step is essential to evaluate costs incurred in acquiring a business.

- Review history: for already existing businesses, the sales and profit; for a new pharmacy look at potential for clients
- Assess condition of facilities and identify and cost any upgrades necessary
- Estimate maximum realistic profit that can be generated
- For already existing businesses, assess ability to transfer goodwill to new owner.

Strategic planning

- Identify targets according to timeframes where the business should be
- Assess the impact of changes on targets
- Develop and implement procedures and policies.

Capital needs

- Establish how to finance starting up business: enquire with banks regarding loans and repayments and work out how these conform with the expected profits
- Set-up capital:
  - buying or renting business and/or premises
  - insurance
  - fixtures
  - equipment
- Stock
- Start-up capital:
  - capital needed to get it started immediately prior to opening or during the first few weeks
  - decorative fixtures
  - office supplies
- Operating capital:
  - expansion
  - cash shortages.

Location

- Population: community demographic data
- Competition with other businesses
- Availability of physicians and primary care clinics, collaboration with prescribers in the area
- Retail shops close by may serve as a positive point in that the area is considered as a shopping centre
- Traffic direction may hinder access to the pharmacy or may have a positive influence on patron's choice, availability of parking space.

The accounting system for a pharmacy should be developed in a way that it is easily understandable and serves the needs of the pharmacy. Financial records are required both for internal and for external reasons.

Product lines

- Decision on what to stock:
  - not to delay dispensing a prescription
  - not recommended to keep a product just in case someone needs something because overstocking may lead to money tied in stock or to stock that will become shop soiled or past its expiry date

- Carry out study sales
- Identify prescribers in the area and define drugs that they prescribe.

Buying merchandise

- Right quality
- Right quantity
- Right supplier
- Right time.

Policies and procedures

Specific policies and procedures are needed for specific tasks to explain the procedure and who is authorised to:

- place orders and receive merchandise
- update legal records
- keep financial records
- check stock, update and maintain formulary.

Sources of supply

- Reliability
- Order-processing time
- Delivery
- Risk
- Credit extension.

Merchandise control

- Expiry date
- Shop-soiled items
- Slow moving merchandise
- Stock levels.

Services offered

- Methods of payment for clients: acceptance of credit cards
- Provision of domiciliary services and delivery to institutions and house-bound patients
- Dispensing services: emergency prescription dispensing, unit-dose dispensing, containers
- Patient profile cards
- Point-of-care testing: blood pressure monitoring, blood tests (see Chapter 11)
- Patient monitoring, medication review and patient counselling
- Controversial issues: advertising and slashing prices, discounts.

Personal selling skills

- Identifying prospective customers
- Approaching clients
- Attracting attention to the services provided
- Handling queries
- Follow-up of interaction with clients.

Design and layout

Physical environment

- Promote atmosphere that is pleasing, conducive to shopping and professional
- Psychological effect or feeling created by physical characteristics of the pharmacy.

Pharmacy layout

- Planning the internal arrangement of departments and allocating the amount of space for each department
- Designed to direct 'traffic' around the pharmacy
- Space allocated to specific departments depending on profitability
- Maximising exposure of products.

Product presentation

- Most saleable and profitable items in the most prominent locations
- Products arranged by pack size, colour, brand, price
- Eye-level positions rather than bottom or top shelves
- Prepare impulse purchase items on counter
- Identify fast moving products.

Shop-window display

- Pleasing
- Matches image projected by the pharmacy
- Simple
- Clean and neat.

A large number of purchases from the pharmacy with regard to non-prescription items and parapharmaceuticals occur as a result of impulse buying. Methods used to attract clients to the pharmacy and to display the stock, and the stock displayed, influence impulse buying.

Financial operating processes

Journals

- Purchases journal: to record credit purchases (supplier, amount, when payment is due)
- Sales journal: to record accounts receivable
- Cash disbursements journal: to record purchases paid.

Balance sheet

A balance sheet is a statement of the financial condition of the business at a given point in time. It reflects what is owned by the pharmacy, what it owes and what the owner has invested.

Assets

- Current assets: convertible into cash within a year (e.g. short-term stock)
- Fixed assets: not used within 1 year (e.g. computer, office equipment)
- Intangible assets: goodwill.

Liabilities

- Amounts owed to creditors.
- May be current liabilities (must be paid within 1 year) or long-term liabilities (e.g. bank loans).

Computers in pharmacy

- Used for stock control, purchases and supplies
- Used for professional services.

Computer use for professional services

- Electronic patient records
- Presenting point of access to patient information on the web
- Management of prescribed medicines
- Promotion of healthy lifestyles: development of compact discs
- Pharmacy webpage, on-line pharmacy services.

Computer audit

- Password to limit access to authorised personnel
- Back-up copies
- Keep up regular physical counts of stock and expiry dates.

In converting from a manual system to a computerised system or from one computer system to another it is advisable to keep a parallel version (the old system) for some time. This reduces the risk of errors. However, it is more expensive.

Advantages of computerisation

- Improved business information
- Increased work quality
- Better organisation of business
- Record keeping: patient profiles
- Stock status immediately available and controlled.

Disadvantages of computerisation

- Initially demanding on staff
- Conversion from manual to computerised system may be traumatic
- Generates a large amount of information which may be of little value to business but distracts attention from major issue
- Investment required: computer hardware and peripherals (e.g. printers), software, back-up and storage.

Steps in acquiring a computer

- Identify the activities that will be carried out with the computer system
- Select adequate hardware (including right memory) and software
- Select the vendor that provides the system according to specifications required and has after-sales services
- Install system and train the users.

Practice summary

- The financial aspect of a community pharmacy is important to make the business viable.
- A sound working relationship with clients, personnel and other health professionals improves the running and development of the business.
- Pharmacy layout, stock presentation and shop window dressing influence the professional image that is projected by the pharmacy.
- An understanding of the potential of computer-driven technology within the business is essential to identify activities that would be of benefit to the pharmacy.

Question

1 How can satisfaction with pharmacy services be improved?

Answer

1
- Establish targets and objectives
- Assess standards of professional pharmacy services (see Chapter 70).
- Measure patient satisfaction using reliable tools
- Identify areas for improvement.

Further reading

Desselle S P and Zgarrick D P (2005). *Pharmacy Management*. New York: McGraw-Hill.

Kayne S B (2005). *Pharmacy Business Management*. London: Pharmaceutical Press.

Tootelian D H and Gaedake R M (1993). *Essentials of Pharmacy Management*. St Louis: Mosby.

67

Hospital pharmacy services

Learning objectives:

- To become familiar with professional pharmacy services provided in hospitals
- To identify pharmacist actions within hospital pharmacy services.

Background

Hospital classification

- Ownership: public or private
- Type of care provided: primary, secondary or tertiary
- Teaching affiliation: provision of specialist training within the institution.

Organisational structure of the hospital

- Hospital director
- Financial officers
- Director of pharmaceutical services
- Director of nursing
- Human resources manager
- Medical resources
- Physiotherapy, occupational therapy department.

Organisation of pharmaceutical services

Director is in charge of:

- financial management
- purchasing drugs and equipment
- inter-departmental affairs
- quality assurance
- provision of professional services.

Purchasing of equipment

- Enteral and parenteral infusion pumps (e.g. patient-controlled analgesia pump, see Chapter 31)
- Computer systems
- Refrigerator and narcotic cupboards
- Counting systems, tablet counter, containers
- Laminar airflow hoods
- Gloves
- Balance.

Considerations when purchasing equipment

- Specifications, functionality
- Reliability of the equipment
- Personnel training
- Cost
- Maintenance
- User-friendliness
- Portability
- Lease vs purchase.

Professional hospital pharmacy services

- Medicines supply to inpatients and outpatients
- Clinical pharmacy
- Drug information service
- Drug and therapeutics committee
- Infection control committee
- Medical gases
- Cytotoxic dispensing
- Special units (e.g. total parenteral nutrition, extemporaneous preparation)
- Developing systems of seamless care: integrating community and hospital pharmaceutical services.

Medicines supply to inpatients

Pharmacist could be involved in:

- prescription sheet design to ensure an easy-to-follow documentation of medicines to be administered
- medicines storage and medicine stock levels at ward level.

Dispensing medicines for the wards

- List of ward stock items maintained updated
- Topping up of ward stock: maintain practical stock levels to ensure that wards have the required medicines in the appropriate amounts and avoid hoarding, stock wastage, pilferage
- Consider unit-dose dispensing: may lead to increased pharmacist time during dispensing of medicines to wards but it is an efficient system that reduces medication errors. Cost-effectiveness of the system employed needs to be assessed.

- Pharmacists must ensure that the quality of the medicines used in the hospital remains intact until they are administered to the patient. This is achieved by ensuring proper storage and handling of medicines even in the wards (e.g. rotation of stock, removal of damaged or expired products, stability and incompatibility of parenteral admixtures).
- The pharmacists' approach towards nurses should be based on a teamwork approach inviting nurses to ask questions when they require information and to cooperate to ensure appropriate management of drugs on the wards.

Definition of ward stock

- Medicines where at least five or six patients are receiving it at the same time
- Products should not be expensive
- Products should have a good shelf-life
- No major contraindications to their use and no requirements for specialist care and supervision
- Include commonly used items (e.g. paracetamol tablets)
- Label: name of drug, strength, instructions for use (e.g. dilution/reconstitution), storage requirements, no dosage instructions and patient names
- Items used without prescription (e.g. disinfectants, antiseptics).

Controlled drugs

- Stock record books are kept. Unused stock of these books should be kept in a secure place
- Medicines stored in a locked box on ward
- Signature upon receipt of stock and when administering drug doses.

Ward drug storage areas

- Controlled drugs cupboard
- Cupboard for medicines intended for internal use
- Cupboard for medicines intended for external use
- Area to store disinfectants
- Refrigerator to store drugs: temperature controlled with thermometer being used calibrated, clean and lockable
- Clean area for intravenous fluids.

Monitoring ward stocks

- Pharmacy staff should establish a working relationship with nurses and ward manager
- Ensure cleanliness and hygiene
- Advise on appropriate storage conditions
- Remind ward staff to carry out stock rotation when new stock is received
- Correct stock levels
- Ensure appropriate monitoring of refrigerators
- Check controlled drugs cupboard.

- Drugs to be stored in a refrigerator include total parenteral nutrition (TPN) solutions, reconstituted antibacterial suspensions and cytotoxic drugs, insulin, vaccines
- Items and drugs that are not to be stored in refrigerator include heparin, blood and urine specimens, food, inflammables
- A good procedure is to prepare a list on the door of the refrigerator of all the items that require storage in a refrigerator
- Check that all items in the refrigerator require to be stored in a refrigerator (usually between 2 and 8°C).

Specific pharmaceutical dosage forms: eye preparations

- Good practice is required to prevent cross-infections
- Eyes are at greater risk of developing an infection when an injury has occurred or a surgical intervention was carried out
- Use of single-dose preparations preferred but some preparations may not be available in this presentation and costings have to be considered
- For preparations presented as multiple dose, the product should not be used for more than 1 week; separate bottles are used for each eye, and new bottles used postoperatively
- See also Chapter 55.

Pharmacists' actions in the development of protocols to standardise practical nursing techniques on the wards

- Blood sugar monitoring technique
- Use of patients' own medicines
- Administration of injections
- Intravenous additives
- Medicines administration
- Nebuliser therapy
- Urine testing
- Ordering and storage of medicines.

Drug and therapeutics committee

Aims are:

- to maintain a hospital formulary (see Chapter 68)
- to develop and implement policies on drug use including, for example, generic substitution, therapeutic guidelines and cost-containment policies.

Infections control committee

Aims are:

- to review use of anti-infective agents
- to develop and implement policies and guidelines regarding the use of anti-infective agents
- to develop policies for wound management.

Drug information services

Aims are:

- to respond to queries from different departments and other care settings
- to evaluate drug usage
- to investigate drug activity and coordinate clinical trials activity (this activity may be shared with the quality assurance unit)
- to coordinate reporting programmes for adverse drug reactions and medication errors

- to provide poison information
- to produce publications
- to educate and provide professional development for professionals.

See also Chapter 62.

Wound management committee

Aims are:

- to design protocols for wound management
- to liaise with the infections control committee to identify antibacterial agents that are less likely to develop bacterial resistance
- to use proper wound treatment and appropriate dressings
- to keep wound treatment cost-effective
- to address factors precipitating wound development (e.g. uncontrolled diabetes).

Clinical pharmacy services

Pharmacists should use their professional knowledge to foster the safe and appropriate use of drugs by patients in a teamwork approach. They should also aim to solve medication errors, detect drug–drug interactions and identify drug-induced disease.

Services provided include:

- therapeutic drug monitoring
- pharmacokinetic dosing
- patient education
- medication counselling
- drug utilisation review
- participation in pharmacotherapy decision-making and in patient follow-up.

Pharmaceutical care should also:

- focus on patient outcomes
- identify potential and actual drug-related problems
- resolve actual drug-related problems
- prevent potential drug-related problems.

Documentation of pharmacist actions in pharmacy-held patient records should contain information on:

- age, weight and height
- medical history
- allergic or adverse drug reaction history
- renal function
- hepatic function.

See also Chapter 12.

Practice summary

- Pharmacy services are provided to support the rational and safe use of medicines and to ensure teamwork in the therapeutic process.
- Pharmacists can give advice on storage of medicines, stock levels for ward stock, information on methods of drug use and drug administration, participate in development of therapeutic protocols and in clinical trials, and participate in patient care and patient monitoring.
- Pharmacists practising in a hospital involved in the clinical pharmacy services are in a position to promote seamless care when the patient is transferred back to the primary care level.
- Pharmacists in the hospital setting should be involved in the wards and outpatient clinics to establish collaboration with the prescribers and nursing staff so as to liaise with them as a team when providing the pharmacy professional services.

Question

1 How can a hospital pharmacist monitor the proper storage of ward stocks?

Answer

1
- Discourage overcrowded storage areas
- Encourage cleanliness and hygiene
- Insist on proper insect control
- Check stock rotation

- Correct stock levels in consultation with the ward manager
- Ensure appropriate storage including the refrigerator used for medicinal products
- Check for proper labelling and identify sources of contamination or mixing up of drugs.

Further reading

Stephens M, ed. (2002). *Hospital Pharmacy*. London: Pharmaceutical Press.

68

Formulary systems

Learning objectives:

- To review processes required for the development and maintenance of formularies
- To identify benefits and controversies associated with formulary systems.

Background

> *A formulary is a continually updated list of medications and related information, representing the clinical judgement of physicians, pharmacists and other experts in the diagnosis, prophylaxis or treatment of disease and promotion of health. A formulary includes, but is not limited to, a list of medications and medication-associated products or devices, medication-use policies, important ancillary drug information, decision-support tools, and organizational guidelines.*[1]

Selection of drugs for inclusion in a formulary

Drugs are selected for inclusion on the basis of their:

- efficacy
- safety
- patient acceptability
- cost.

Historical perspective on the development of hospital formularies

1778	*Lititz Pharmacopoeia* developed for a specific military hospital
1954	*Hospital Formulary for Selected Drugs* for the University of Michigan Hospital
1959	American Society of Health-System Pharmacists (ASHP) issued the American Hospital Formulary Service in loose leaf format so as to retain the idea of selectivity for specific institutions.

Subsequently:

1975	World Health Organization List of Essential Drugs – a list of drugs necessary for the provision of basic healthcare
1978	ASHP produced guidelines on production and maintenance of a formulary system which were subsequently updated regularly.

See also Chapter 62.

Types of formularies

- National formularies (e.g. *British National Formulary* (BNF))
- Hospital formularies
- Local formularies
- Joint hospital–local formularies.
- *Open formulary system*: the formulary recommends drugs and non-formulary drugs are still routinely available
- *Closed formulary system:* restricted drug list: only medicines included in the formulary may be used.

Reasons to develop formulary system

- To ensure quality and appropriateness of drug use in a particular practice
- To teach appropriate drug therapy especially relevant for junior doctors
- To promote evidence-based and cost-effective drug therapy
- To cut down on the range of drugs in use
- To encourage the use of therapeutic protocols.

Benefits of a formulary

- Cost-effective prescribing
- Rational prescribing
- Use of a restricted range of drugs results in better knowledge of drug use
- Better stock management
- Improvement in communication between prescribers and pharmacists
- Promotes seamless care between hospital practitioners and primary care practitioners.

Number of drugs to be included in a formulary

- A formulary for general practice should include enough drugs to treat 80–90% of all common conditions met in the practice in addition to emergency drugs.
- Having too many drugs in a formulary defeats its purpose of cost-reduction, effective and rational selection.
- Having too few drugs in the formulary makes the formulary an ineffective and useless resource.

Objections to development of a formulary

- Deprives the prescribers of the freedom of prescription
- Allows for purchase of inferior quality drugs
- Does not always reduce the cost to the consumer.

Formulary development

- Team work approach is required
- Decision whether to adapt another formulary or develop a completely new formulary
- Instil a culture of willingness to accept change
- Should be flexible and adapt to ongoing needs of prescribers and patients.

Formulary system

- Inclusion and exclusion criteria
- Process to monitor drug use and establish policies on drug use
- Adverse drug reaction reporting activities
- Provision of reference material on drugs included in formulary.

Formulary management system

- Has to be flexible and dynamic
- Regular updates to reflect current practice (e.g. biannual or annual editions)
- Inclusion of new drugs released on the market: consider issue of safety, cost, indications, me-too drugs
- Withdrawing drugs: discontinued drugs, drugs no longer prescribed
- Procedure to meet non-formulary requests.

Key issues for a successful formulary system

- Communication with end-users
- User-friendly
- Professionally presented.

Content of a formulary

- Introduction
- Follow a basic drug information system (e.g. reference to *British National Formulary*)
- Use a classification system (e.g. pharmacological or symptomatic)
- Include drug costs and cost of treatment
- Notes on inclusion criteria and selection of drugs.

Formulary presentation

- Pocket sized
- Binding: loose-leaf allows for flexible adaptations but may present problems with long-term use
- Use colour to facilitate presentation of material
- Cover: durable and attractive design
- Font size to make appropriate reading
- Availability in electronic format.

Inclusion criteria

- Efficacy
- Side-effect profile and contraindications
- Interaction profile
- Pharmacokinetic profile
- Patient acceptability: taste, appearance, ease of administration
- Generic availability, cost.

Ethical implications of developing a formulary system

- Interfering with non-pharmacological basis for choice of product
- Formulary system may provide for generic substitution or therapeutic substitution
- Interactions with the pharmaceutical industry may influence the formulary system.

Non-pharmacological basis of therapeutics

At the macro level, prescribing trends that influence the individual prescriber include:

- cost
- availability of product
- traditions and education of society (e.g. may influence dosage form selection)
- health issues
- stability and power of pharmaceutical industry
- medical teaching.

At the micro level, the individual prescriber is influenced by:

- peer groups
- society
- control measures and regulations by health authorities
- pharmaceutical industry.

Generic substitution

This is the dispensing of a different brand or an unbranded drug product for the drug product prescribed.

Therapeutic substitution

This is the dispensing of a particular drug entity in place of a therapeutically similar but chemically different drug product.

Opposition to therapeutic substitution is based on three factors:

- lack of scientific and clinical evidence
- clinical studies suggesting that not all drugs of similar classes are equivalent
- holistic approach in drug therapy.

Practice summary

- A formulary provides information on the drugs and medical devices that are used in a particular institution.
- For successful implementation, the formulary requires regular updating, and participation of different members of the health professions in decisions relating to its development and maintenance.
- Presentation of the formulary should be easy to use and follow, and attractive. Electronic access to the formulary should be supported.

Question

1 List factors influencing inclusion of drugs in a formulary.

Answer

1
- Efficacy (e.g. demonstrated in clinical trials)
- Toxicity (e.g. for equally effective drugs, select the least toxic)
- Adverse effects (e.g. include drugs with same indication but different side-effect profiles)
- Contraindications (e.g. avoid drugs with serious teratogenic effects)
- Interactions (e.g. select drug with least clinically significant interactions)
- Pharmacokinetic profile (e.g. include drugs with short half-lives, include drugs minimally affected by hepatic or renal impairment)
- Formulations available (e.g. drugs available for both oral and parenteral administration allow for smooth transition from parenteral to oral therapy)
- Generic form available: usually cheaper
- Cost: encourage cost-effective prescribing
- Use (e.g. certain categories of drugs such as anaesthetics may not be relevant to the formulary setting)
- Type of formulary: specialised or generic
- Precautions (e.g. avoid drugs that require special storage requirements).

Further reading

Serracino Inglott A, Azzopardi L M, Zarb Adami M and Camilleri J (1999). Analysis of a formulary for a geriatric hospital. *Pharm J* 263: R43.

Winfield A J and Richards M E ed. (2002). *Pharmaceutical Practice*, 3rd edn. London: Churchill Livingstone.

Reference

1 American Society of Health-System Pharmacists (ASHP) Expert Panel on Formulary Management. ASHP Guidelines on the Pharmacy and Therapeutics Committee and the Formulary System. *Am J Health-Syst Pharm* 2008; 65: 1272–1283.

69

Medicines regulatory affairs

Learning objectives:

- To introduce principles of regulatory affairs for medicinal products
- To appreciate requirements of EU Good Manufacturing Practice, EU Good Distribution Practice and EU Good Clinical Practice
- To identify interventions of qualified persons.

Background

Within the pharmaceutical industry, regulatory considerations are implemented across all stages of the development of a medicinal product (from the investigational medicinal product stage to the distribution stage). The main principle underlying the regulatory framework is to ensure safety, quality and efficacy of the product.

European Medicines Agency (EMEA)

- Decentralised body of the European Union
- Forms part of a network of national agencies, is a service provider for the network and has a coordinating role within the network
- Mainly responsibile for the protection and promotion of public and animal health, through the evaluation and supervision of medicines for human and veterinary use
- Responsible for scientific evaluation of applications for a European marketing authorisation (centralised procedure) for medicinal products
- Coordinates the pharmacovigilance network for European countries.
- Coordinates good manufacturing practice, product- and process-related inspections at manufacturing sites run by national regulatory bodies (e.g. MHRA in the UK)
- Liaises with other international medicines regulatory bodies (e.g. in the USA, Canada and Japan)
- See also Chapter 1.

Authorisation of medicines

- Manufacturers of medicinal products must hold a marketing authorisation for each product manufactured and sold for human consumption
- Medicinal products are granted a marketing authorisation to ensure their efficacy, safety and quality
- Marketing authorisation could be granted:
  - either as a national procedure at the level of the national agency
  - or as a European procedure at the level of the EMEA – centralised procedure[1]

- In an attempt to harmonise the presentation of data for the application for registration of medicinal products for human use in the EU, the USA and Japan, the Common Technical Document (CTD) was developed. This document compiles the data required to be presented for an application for a marketing authorisation into five sections: administrative and prescribing information, summaries and overview, information on product quality, non-clinical study reports and clinical study reports.

Application for a marketing authorisation

Details required for marketing authorisation (MA) application include:

- formulation
- source of active pharmaceutical ingredients (APIs)
- process of manufacture
- site of manufacture, testing
- packaging and labelling.

Centralised procedure for application for a marketing authorisation

The centralised marketing authorisation application procedure was started in 1995.

- The pharmaceutical company files one application and if the application is successful receives marketing authorisation in all EU member states, Norway, Iceland and Lichtenstein.
- The Committee for Medicinal Products for Human Use (CHMP) is responsible for carrying out assessment of the applications and handling post-authorisation requests for variations or extensions to existing marketing authorisations.
- For medicinal products for human use, the centralised procedure is *obligatory* for products derived from high-technology or biotechnology, products used in rare diseases (orphan drugs), products used in AIDS, cancer, neurodegenerative disorders, diabetes, and autoimmune and viral disease.
- The procedure may be used for new active substances and products that bring therapeutic or scientific progress and for generic medicines once data exclusivity periods granted to originator products authorised through centralised procedure expire (10 years).

Counterfeit medicinal products are products that are deliberately and fraudulently mislabelled with respect to identity, amount or source of drug. This is an escalating global problem. All stakeholders involved with the manufacture, distribution and use of medicinal products are responsible for combatting medicines counterfeiting by reporting any incidents to the national medicines regulatory authorities.

EU Good Manufacturing Practice (EU GMP)

This ensures that medicinal products are consistently produced and controlled to the quality standards appropriate to their intended use and as required by the marketing authorisation.

- GMP is concerned with both production and quality control.
- Pharmaceutical manufacturers require a manufacturing licence (ML) which is renewable periodically and is issued by the regulatory authority.
- Inspections are carried out to verify EU GMP compliance.

Manufacturing licence

- Location of site
- Authorised activities and processes
- Authorised dosage forms
- Authorised personnel: production manager, quality control manager, qualified person(s).

Compliance with EU GMP

- Directive 2003/94/EC[2] outlines EU GMP requirements
- Facilities of site (premises, equipment, environment)
- Staff (key personnel, training)
- Quality system (standard operating procedures [SOPs], documentation, records, internal audits, batch release).

> A pharmaceutical manufacturer in the EU producing medicinal products and investigational medicinal products for human use cannot function without a manufacturing licence.

Qualified person (QP)

The primary legal responsibility of the QP is to release batches of medicinal product prior to use in a clinical trial (investigational medicinal product; IMP) or prior to release for sale.

The responsibilities of a QP are:

- to ensure that standards of good practice in manufacturing are complied with at all times
- to ensure that each batch of medicinal products has been manufactured and tested, and complies with EU directive and EU GMP
- to ensure that each batch of medicinal products has been manufactured in accordance with the requirements of the marketing authorisation.

> All personnel in the pharmaceutical industry should be aware that the medicinal product will be used by patients and that it is important to safeguard quality, safety and efficacy.

Investigational medicinal products (IMPs)

- Directive 2003/94/EC[2] also takes into consideration manufacture of investigational medicinal products.
- This ensures that trial participants are not placed at risk and that the results of clinical trials are not affected by inadequate safety, quality or efficacy arising from unsatisfactory manufacture.
- It ensures consistency between batches and that changes during the development of an IMP are adequately documented and justified.

> **Special features required for the production of an IMP**
>
> - Labelling: highlighting status as an IMP
> - Destruction of unused and returned IMPs after clinical trial.

Good clinical practice (GCP)

- Regulated by Directive 2001/20/EC[3] and Directive 2005/28/EC[4], which stipulate requirements related to clinical trials
- Compliance by pharmaceutical sponsor (paying for the trial), contract research organisation (handling the trial), investigational trial sites (where clinical tests are carried out) and clinical trial laboratories (where analysis is carried out).

EU Good Distribution Practice (EU GDP)

This ensures that medicinal products are consistently stored, transported and handled under suitable conditions as required by the MA or product specification.

- Wholesalers have to appoint a responsible person (RP) who is responsible for ensuring that EU GDP is implemented.

Compliance with EU GDP

- EC Directive 92/25/EEC[5] outlines EU GDP requirements.
- Personnel (training)
- Quality system (SOPs, documentation, records, internal audits)
- Premises and equipment
- Storage including during transportation
- Returns, recall procedure (tracing system).

All pharmaceutical distributors in the EU should hold a licence for wholesale dealing in medicinal products.[6]

Pharmacovigilance

- EU requirements described in Directive 2001/83/EC[6]
- Activity that describes collection, verification and presentation of adverse reaction reports
- Encourages exchange of information between EU member states
- The Marketing Authorisation holders must ensure that they have an appropriate system of pharmacovigilance in order to assume responsibility and liability for their products on the market and to ensure that appropriate action can be taken when necessary
- Marketing Authorisation holders should have at their disposal a person responsible for pharmacovigilance in the different states
- The national regulatory authority is the body coordinating pharmacovigilance.

Pharmacovigilance relies almost exclusively on the spontaneous reporting systems which allow healthcare professionals, including pharmacists, to report adverse drug reactions to a central agency. In the UK, suspected drug adverse reactions may be reported by completing the Yellow Card, copies of which are available with the British National Formulary.

Practice summary

- Pharmaceutical manufacturers and regulatory authorities have a duty to ensure that patients are properly protected and that medicinal products meet appropriate requirements for safety, quality and efficacy.
- Key personnel should have access and be familiar with European and national guidance documents and legislation relating to the manufacture, clinical trials and distribution of medicinal products for human use.

Questions

1. What is a marketing authorisation?
2. Summarise the requirements to comply with EU Good Distribution Practice.

Answers

1. Medicines are granted a marketing authorisation to ensure their efficacy, safety and quality. The national procedure to obtain a marketing authorisation is in agreement with the national agency while the European procedure is an EMEA-centralised procedure.
2. EU Good Distribution Practice ensures that the quality, efficacy and safety of the product is maintained during the distribution chain. A quality system is required to outline standard operating procedures (SOPs) for all processes

carried out in the wholesale activity. Personnel should receive training in the processes and the SOPs which has to be documented. Documentation of all processes (receipt, sale, recall of medicines) has to be kept and a tracing system for the products handled is required. Premises and equipment used for storage should be controlled, including cold storage in the store and during transportation. The wholesaler has to appoint a responsible person who is responsible for overseeing the implementation of EU GDP.

Further reading

Department of Essential Drugs and Other Medicines, World Health Organization (1999). *Counterfeit Drugs: Guidelines for the development of measures to combat counterfeit drugs*. Geneva: World Health Organization.

Franklin N (2007). Effective compliance with EU GMP Part II in active substance manufacture: How did these GMP requirements arise? *Indust Pharm* 14: 6–9.

Harman R J (2004). *Development and Control of Medicines and Medical Devices*. London: Pharmaceutical Press.

Medicines and Healthcare products Regulatory Agency (2007). *Rules and Guidance for Pharmaceutical Distributors*. London: Pharmaceutical Press.

Medicines and Healthcare products Regulatory Agency (2007). *Rules and Guidance for Pharmaceutical Manufacturers and Distributors*. London: Pharmaceutical Press.

Robson A S, Bawden D and Judd A, eds. (2001). *Pharmaceutical and Medicines Information Management: Information management*. London: Churchill Livingstone.

References

1 Regulation (EC) No. 726/2004 of the European Parliament and of the Council of 31 March 2004 laying down Community procedures for the authorisation and supervision of medicinal products for human and veterinary use and establishing a European Medicines Agency.

2 Directive 2003/94/EC of 8 October 2003 laying down the principles and guidelines of good manufacturing practice in respect of medicinal products for human use and investigational medicinal products for human use.

3 Directive 2001/20/EC of the European Parliament and of the Council of 4 April 2001 on the approximation of the laws, regulations and administrative provisions of the Member States relating to the implementation of good clinical practice in the conduct of clinical trials on medicinal products for human use.

4 Commission Directive 2005/28/EC of 8 April 2005 laying down principles and detailed guidelines for good clinical practice as regards investigational medicinal products for human use, as well as the requirements for authorisation of the manufacturing or importation of such products.

5 Directive 92/25/EEC of 31 March 1992 on the wholesale distribution of medicinal products for human use.

6 Directive 2001/83/EC of the European Parliament and of the Council of 6 November 2001 on the Community code relating to medicinal products for human use as amended by Directives 2002/98/EC, 2004/24/EC, 2004/27/EEC.

70

Quality standards in community pharmacy practice

Learning objectives:

- To appreciate the need for quality standards
- To identify structure and presentation of quality standards
- To review issues that are assessed in quality care standards.

Quality in community pharmacy

A number of questions are posed by healthcare regulators, financing agents and consumers regarding the assessment and evaluation of professional pharmacy services provided from community pharmacy. Two main issues are whether professional services provided from community pharmacies meet the required standards and then what the required standards are.

> In today's market-oriented, economics-driven society, all professions face the question: what do I do for my customers that makes my contribution unique? (Peter Kielgast, Past-President, International Pharmaceutical Federation)[1]

A basic critical analysis of community pharmacy identifies two strengths and three weaknesses:

Strengths:

1. A large number of pharmacists are practising in this sector
2. Accessibility to patients and other healthcare professionals is good

Weaknesses:

1. The apparent loss of the traditional role when compounding was replaced with industrial manufacturing
2. Deprofessionalisation due to practice offered from a business platform
3. Economic scenario that requires proof of value-added services to support professional fee.

Milestones

- Quality policy and assessment for professional services identified by professional bodies (e.g. International Pharmaceutical Federation)

- Establishment of pharmacy standards in different countries
- Inclusion of perception of consumers and other health professionals in the quality assessment for some standards.

International Pharmaceutical Federation (FIP) Good Pharmacy Practice Guidelines

1993	Adopted in Japan[2]
1997	In Vancouver presentation of revised version endorsed by the WHO Expert Committee on Specifications for Pharmaceutical Preparations[1]
1998	In The Hague adoption of the guidelines on Good Pharmacy Practice in Developing Countries[3]
2003	In Sydney presentation of results from the Working Group on Quality Care Standards.[4]

Quality and professional services

Within the scenario where the community pharmacist is participating in all aspects of drug therapy, from evaluating a prescription to monitoring the effectiveness of a patient's treatment and to piloting changes in pharmacotherapy, standards of care are required to ensure that this is a valid contribution.

Quality care standards look at administration and infrastructure of the pharmacy and at professional services such as pharmacist interaction with patients, recommendation of non-prescription medicines, dispensing of prescription medicines, diagnosis and pharmacotherapy monitoring, and planning.

Quality care standards and pharmacist actions when dispensing prescription medicines are shown in Figure 70.1.

Quality care standards

The description of quality care standards can be based on whether they are adopting an area-specific approach where particular professional services are addressed or whether a generic approach is adopted. For a generic approach standards are intended to address more than one type of service.

Quality care standards and pharmacist actions when responding to symptoms are shown in Figure 70.2.

Examples of area-specific standards

- Drug information and counselling developed by the Nordic Pharmacy Association[5]
- Provision of pharmacist-recommended medicines developed by the Pharmaceutical Society, Australia[6]
- Prevention of errors in drug dispensing developed by the Japan Pharmaceutical Association.[7]

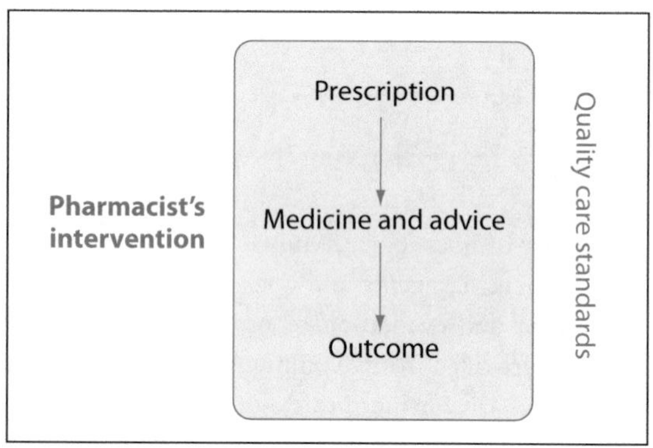

Figure 70.1 Quality care standards and pharmacist actions when dispensing prescription medicines.

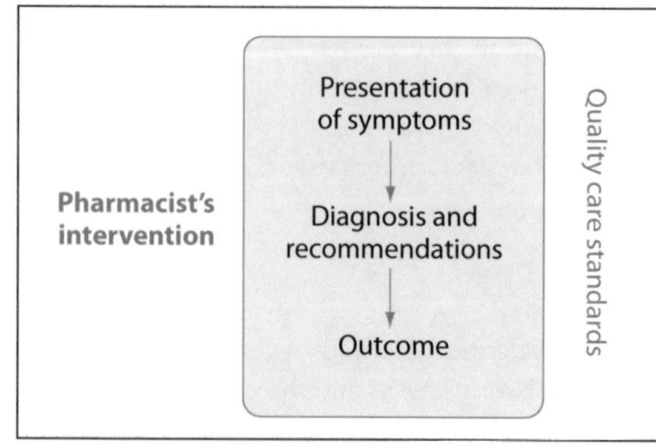

Figure 70.2 Quality care standards and pharmacist actions when responding to symptoms.

Presentation

The presentation of standards can be described as guidelines or as an audit tool.

Guidelines

Guidelines are presented to create a quality environment, to promote responsibility for quality, to present aims and objectives of service provided and to present standard procedures.

Examples

Extract from Dutch Pharmacy Standard by the Royal Dutch Association for the Advancement of Pharmacy (KNMP):[8]

> *Informing and advising the patient*
>
> *The pharmacist's first concern is the welfare of the client. He will respect the client's own responsibility.*
>
> *The pharmacist supports the client to make well considered decisions regarding the use of medicines and health care products.*

Extract from the standard by the American Pharmaceutical Association (APhA):[9]

> *Information Evaluation*
>
> *The pharmacist evaluates the subjective and objective information collected from the patient and other sources then forms conclusions regarding: (1) opportunities to improve and/or assure the safety, effectiveness, and/or economy of current or planned drug therapy; (2) opportunities to minimize current or potential future drug or health-related problems; and (3) the timing of any necessary future pharmacist consultation.*

Audit

Standards that are presented as audits outline procedures to be followed and adopt a quantitative approach. After using the standards as an audit tool a score is obtained providing tangible results.

Example

Extract from the standard Validation of Community Pharmacy Method developed by the Department of Pharmacy, University of Malta:[1]

Greeting the patient	*Score*
I. The pharmacist gives immediate attention to the patient in an orderly way	*3*
II. The pharmacist greets the patient with a friendly message	*2*
III. The pharmacist addresses the patient by name	*2*
IV. The pharmacist is recognised by the patient or introduces himself to the patient	*3*

Areas included in generic standards

The FIP report by the Working Group on Quality Care Standards[4] analysed 18 generic standards submitted by international pharmacy organisations and identified the areas included in the generic standards as listed in Table 70.1.

Extracts from quality care standards from different countries

Extemporaneous preparations

Example from the standards developed by the Indian Pharmaceutical Association:[10]

> *Written standard operating procedures as well as standard formulations should be maintained for commonly made extemporaneous preparations.*
>
> *Batch numbers of each medicine used for compounding should be recorded.*

Handling of stock

Example from the standards developed by the National Association of Pharmacy Regulatory Authorities in Canada (NAPRA):[11]

> *Pharmacists manage drug distribution by performing or supervising the functions of*

Table 70.1 Areas included in generic standards by international pharmacy organisations

No. of pharmaceutical organisations	(n = 18)
Extemporaneous preparations	15 (83%)
Handling of stock	14 (78%)
Interaction with patients	13 (72%)
Non-prescription medicines	13 (72%)
Setting of the pharmacy	13 (72%)
Documentation systems	12 (67%)
Dispensing prescription medicines	11 (61%)
Equipment	10 (56%)
Health promotion	10 (56%)
Research and professional development	9 (50%)
Audit	7 (39%)
Diagnostics	7 (39%)
Pharmacotherapy monitor/plan	7 (39%)
Domiciliary services	4 (22%)
On-line services	4 (22%)
Pre-registration training	4 (22%)
Parapharmaceuticals	3 (17%)
Customer perceptions	2 (11%)

acquisition, preparation, and distribution of drugs to ensure the safety, accuracy and quality of supplied products.

Example from the standards developed by the Royal Pharmaceutical Society of Great Britain, UK:[12]

[Pharmacists] must ensure that pharmaceutical stock is stored under suitable conditions, taking into consideration the stability of the drug.

Interaction with patients

Example from the standards developed by the Indian Pharmaceutical Association:[10]

The pharmacist must work out strategies to make time to provide professional counselling with regard to use of medicines and related products, so as to improve the quality of the patient's life.

Non-prescription medicines

Example from Validation of Community Pharmacy Method, Department of Pharmacy, University of Malta:[1]

Management of the condition – diarrhoea	*Score*
i. The pharmacist recommends electrolyte replacement salts with or without medications to reduce diarrhoea	*10*
ii. The pharmacist recommends regular fluid intake	*5*
iii. The pharmacist recommends medications to reduce diarrhoea	*4*

Non-prescription medicines

Example from the standards developed by the Royal Pharmaceutical Society of Great Britain, UK:[12]

[Pharmacists must ensure that] when a patient or their carer requests advice on treatment, sufficient information is obtained to enable an assessment to be made of whether self-care is appropriate, and to enable a suitable product(s) to be recommended.

Setting of the pharmacy

Example from standards developed by the Pharmaceutical Association of Israel:[13]

The pharmacy externally should have a professional appearance, in such a way that it can be easily distinguished as being a pharmacy.

A predominant sign should indicate it is a pharmacy in at least two of the major ethnic languages used in the location.

Dispensing prescription medicines

Example from standards developed by the Pharmaceutical Society of Uganda:[14]

A pharmacist or his/her designee must see every prescription for a medicine and make a judgement as to what action is necessary.

For each prescription, the date of issue, the quantity of drug supplied, the balance due and the signature of who dispenses the prescription must be indicated in red ink.

Health promotion

Example from standards developed by the Association of Finnish Pharmacies:[15]

Health promotion is an important aspect of the activity of a community pharmacy. Prevention of diseases and health promotion are among the central objectives of Finnish health policy.

Parapharmaceuticals

Example from standards developed by the Association of Finnish Pharmacies:[15]

Part of the herbal drugs and homeopathic products are sold exclusively from pharmacies. Therefore, the staff shall also get acquainted with the use of these products.

On-line services

Example from the standards developed by the Royal Pharmaceutical Society of Great Britain, UK:[12]

Patients must be readily able to identify who is operating an internet site from a registered pharmacy premises.

Initiating quality assurance of professional services in a community pharmacy

- Prepare standard operating procedures for specific areas such as preparation of extemporaneous preparations
- Carry out a self-assessment audit on a specific process (e.g. steps carried out during dispensing a prescription).

Further considerations

- Who should run the method: the profession or an outside body?
- Cost of quality system: costings of the system, how are these going to be shared?
- Voluntary or mandatory: it is recommended to start off on a voluntary basis with a lot of incentives, otherwise success rate may be low.
- Reward for improving quality: to support pharmacies to undertake required upgrading.

Practice summary

- Community pharmacists contribute to patient care in multiple processes by identifying, resolving and preventing medicine-related problems and facilitating access to safe and effective pharmacotherapy. Such interventions can be provided by the pharmacist as distinct from those by other skilled people because of the scientific approach given to pharmacists during their pharmacy education.
- Quality care standards are processes carried out to confirm the effectiveness of the pharmacist in a community setting.

Questions

1 List four salient points that may be evaluated in the process of greeting the patient at a pharmacy.
2 List five essential steps to be evaluated in quality assessment of the process of dispensing a prescription in a community pharmacy setting.

Answers

1 Patient is given immediate attention; patient is greeted in a friendly message; if patient is known to pharmacist, he or she is addressed by name; pharmacist is wearing professional attire and can be identified by the patient.

2 Prescription is evaluated, checked for validity (date of issue, prescriber), drug required identified, quantity to be dispensed prepared and patient advised on use of medication according to instructions on prescription.

Further reading

Azzopardi L M, Salek S, Serracino Inglott A and Zarb Adami M (1998). Development of external validation tools for community pharmacy. *Pharm J* 261: R20.

Azzopardi L M, Salek S, Serracino Inglott A and Zarb Adami M (1999). An innovative auditing system: validation of community pharmacy. *Pharm J* 263: R64.

Azzopardi L M, Salek S, Serracino Inglott A, Zarb Adami M and Buhagiar A (2001). Validating tools for the monitoring of community pharmacy services. *Pharm J* 267: 303–305.

Azzopardi L M, Serracino Inglott A, Zarb Adami M and Salek S (2003). Development of external methods to evaluate the quality of pharmacy services offered by community pharmacists. *Qual Assur J* 7: 248–257.

References

1 Azzopardi L. *Validation Instruments for Community Pharmacy: Pharmaceutical care for the third millennium*. New York: Pharmaceutical Products Press, 2000.

2 International Pharmaceutical Federation. Standards for quality of pharmacy services, 1997. http://www.fip.nl/files/fip/Statements/latest/Dossier%20004%20total.pdf.

3 Working group on GPP in Developing Countries. Good Pharmacy Practice in developing countries: Recommendations for stepwise implementation, 1998. http://www.fip.nl/files/www2/pdf/gpp/GPP_CPS_Report.pdf.

4 Working Group on Quality Care Standards. Report presented at International Pharmaceutical Federation Annual Congress, 2003.

5 Nordic Pharmacy Association. Guidelines for drug information and counselling for pharmacies in the Nordic countries, 2003. http://www.apotekerforeningen.dk/pdf/international/NA_guidelines.pdf.

6 Pharmaceutical Society of Australia. Standards for the provision of *pharmacist only* and *pharmacy* medicines in community pharmacy, 1999. http://www.psa.org.au.

7 Japan Pharmaceutical Association. Emergency measures to be taken by JPA member pharmacies to prevent errors in drug dispensing, 2002.

8 Dutch Pharmacy Standard by the Royal Dutch Association for the Advancement of Pharmacy (KNMP). Dutch pharmacy standard, 1996.http://www.knmp.nl.

9 American Pharmaceutical Association. Principles of practice for pharmaceutical care, 1995. http://www.caremark.com/portal/asset/Principles_of_Practice_for_Pharmaceutical_Care.pdf.

10 Indian Pharmaceutical Association. Good pharmacy practice guidelines, 2002. http://www.ipapharma.org

11 National Association of Pharmacy Regulatory Authorities. Model standards of practice for Canadian pharmacists, 2003. http://www.nbpharmacists.ca/LinkClick.aspx?fileticket=mj6rtHn%2FGpI%3D&tabid=261&mid=695.

12 Royal Pharmaceutical Society of Great Britian. Code of ethics for pharmacists and pharmacy technicians, July 2008. http://www.rpsgb.org/protectingthepublic/ethics.

13 Pharmaceutical Association of Israel. Standards of practice in community pharmacy.

14 Pharmaceutical Society of Uganda. Standards for pharmacy practice in Uganda, 2001.

15 Association of Finnish Pharmacies. Guidelines for a professional community pharmacy in Finland, 1997.

Bibliography

American Society of Health-System Pharmacists (2006–2007). *Best Practices for Hospital and Health-system Pharmacy: Position and guidance documents of ASHP*. Bethesda, MA: American Society of Health-System Pharmacists.

Azzopardi L M (2000). *Validation Instruments for Community Pharmacy: Pharmaceutical care for the third millennium*. Binghampton, NY: Pharmaceutical Products Press.

Brunton L L, Lazo S J and Parker K L, eds (2006). *Goodman & Gilman's Pharmacological Basis of Therapeutics*, 11th edn. New York: McGraw-Hill.

Edwards C and Stillman P (2006). *Minor Illness or Major Disease? The clinical pharmacist in the community*, 4th edn. London: Pharmaceutical Press.

Gard P, ed. (2000). *A Behavioural Approach to Pharmacy Practice*. London: Blackwell Science.

Greene R J and Harris N D (2008). *Pathology and Therapeutics for Pharmacists*, 3rd edn. London: Pharmaceutical Press.

Joint Formulary Committee (2009). *British National Formulary*, 58th edn. London: British Medical Association and Royal Pharmaceutical Society of Great Britain.

Koda-Kimble M A, Young L Y, Kradjan W A, Guglielmo B J, Alldredge B K and Corelli R L, eds (2005). *Applied Therapeutics: The clinical use of drugs*, 8th edn. Maryland: Lippincott Williams & Wilkins.

Lee M, ed. (2004). *Basic Skills in Interpreting Laboratory Data*, 3rd edn. Bethesda, MA: American Society of Health-System Pharmacists.

Murdaugh L B (2005). *Competence Assessment Tools*, 3rd edn. Bethesda, MA: American Society of Health-System Pharmacists.

Nathan A (2006). *Non-prescription Medicines*, 3rd edn. London: Pharmaceutical Press.

Nathan A (2008). *FASTtrack Managing Symptoms in the Pharmacy*. London: Pharmaceutical Press.

Randall M D and Neil K E (2009). *Disease Management: A guide to clinical pharmacology*, 2nd edn. London: Pharmaceutical Press.

Reid J L, Rubin P C and Walters M R (2006). *Clinical Pharmacology and Therapeutics*, 7th edn. Oxford: Blackwell Publishing Ltd.

Richards D and Aronson J (2006). *Oxford Handbook of Practical Drug Therapy*. Oxford: Oxford University Press.

Rutter P (2004). *Community Pharmacy: Symptoms, diagnosis and treatment*. Edinburgh: Churchill Livingstone.

Sweetman SC, ed. (2007). *Martindale: The complete drug reference*, 35th edn. London: Pharmaceutical Press.

Walker R and Edwards C (2003). *Clinical Pharmacy and Therapeutics*, 3rd edn. Edinburgh: Churchill Livingstone.

Waterfield J (2008). *Community Pharmacy Handbook*. London: Pharmaceutical Press.

Whalley B J, Fletcher K E, Weston S E, Howard R L and Rawlinson C F (2008). *Foundation in Pharmacy Practice*. London: Pharmaceutical Press.

Wiffen P, Mitchell M, Snelling M and Stoner N (2007). *Oxford Handbook of Clinical Pharmacy*. Oxford: Oxford University Press.

Williams D A and Lemke T L (2002). *Foye's Principles of Medicinal Chemistry*. Baltimore, MD: Lippincott Williams & Wilkins.

Wright J, Gray A H and Goodey V (2006). *Clinical Pharmacy*. London: Pharmaceutical Press.

Index